Recent Understanding of Colorectal Cancer Treatment

Edited by Keun-Yeong Jeong

Published in London, United Kingdom

Recent Understanding of Colorectal Cancer Treatment
http://dx.doi.org/10.5772/intechopen.100844
Edited by Keun-Yeong Jeong

Contributors
Sean Ramcharan, Cortland Linder, Vanessa Cubas, Tom Evans, Julia Merchant, Rakesh Sinha, Daniel Sur, Alecsandra Gorzo, Claudia Burz, Keun-Yeong Jeong, Marisa D. Santos, Pedro Nuno Brandão, Lucia Lacerda, Igor Monsellato, Francesca De Stefano, Gianfrancesco Intini, Carlo Gennaro, Ali Chahrour, Ryan Holman, Orane Lorton, Pauline C. Guillemin, Alexis Ricoeur, Andrea Peloso, Rares Salomir, Samaa Abdullah, Byron Baron, Isaac Micallef, Cinzia Tesauro, Josephine Geertsen Keller, Birgitta R. Knudsen, Kamilla Vandsø Petersen, Olusola Bolaji Adewale

First published in London, United Kingdom, 2022 by IntechOpen
IntechOpen is the global imprint of INTECHOPEN LIMITED, registered in England and Wales, registration number: 11086078, 5 Princes Gate Court, London, SW7 2QJ, United Kingdom

British Library Cataloguing-in-Publication Data
A catalogue record for this book is available from the British Library

Additional hard and PDF copies can be obtained from orders@intechopen.com

Recent Understanding of Colorectal Cancer Treatment
Edited by Keun-Yeong Jeong
p. cm.
Print ISBN 978-1-80356-131-8
Online ISBN 978-1-80356-132-5
eBook (PDF) ISBN 978-1-80356-133-2

For EU product safety concerns:
IN TECH d.o.o., Prolaz Marije Krucifikse Kozulić 3, 51000 Rijeka, Croatia,
info@intechopen.com or visit our website at intechopen.com.

Meet the editor

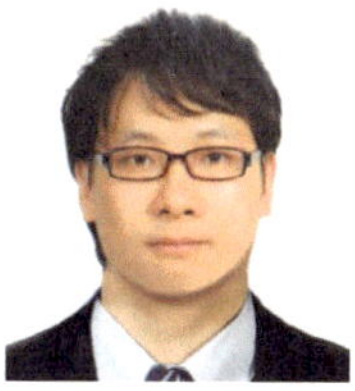

Keun-Yeong Jeong serves as the chief executive officer and chief technology officer of PearlsinMires. He received his Ph.D. in Medicine from Korea University and a BS in Biochemistry from Chungbuk National University, South Korea. He completed his postdoctoral fellowship at Yonsei University College of Medicine, South Korea. Prior to founding PearlsinMires, Dr. Jeong focused on investigating the treatment of cancer and general diseases. He has noticeable scientific achievements to his credit, including many peer-reviewed publications and patents. Dr. Jeong developed promotion methods for the treatment of solid cancers utilizing stem cells, radiation, and peptides. He is the founder of PearlsinMires and a primary contributor to a core technology related to the company's anticancer drug platform.

Contents

Preface IX

Section 1
Introduction 1

Chapter 1 3
Introductory Chapter: Efforts to Conquer Colorectal Cancer from the Past to the Present
by Keun-Yeong Jeong

Section 2
Diagnostics, Basic to Clinical 7

Chapter 2 9
Utilising Proteomics and Organoid Cultures for Predicting Treatment Response in Colorectal Cancer
by Isaac Micallef and Byron Baron

Chapter 3 37
Simple and Fast DNA-Based Tool to Investigate Topoisomerase 1 Activity, a Biomarker for Drug Susceptibility in Colorectal Cancer
by Josephine Geertsen Keller, Kamilla Vandsø Petersen, Birgitta R. Knudsen and Cinzia Tesauro

Chapter 4 53
Colorectal Cancer Stages, Progress, Genetic Predisposition, and Immune Surveillance
by Samaa Abdullah

Section 3
Surgical Care by Robotics 65

Chapter 5 67
Robotic Rectal Resection for Rectal Cancer: State of the Art
by Francesca De Stefano, Gianfrancesco Intini, Giulia Costantini, Carlo Gennaro, Ali Chahrour and Igor Monsellato

Section 4
Radiology Based Care 87

Chapter 6 89
Magnetic Resonance-Guided Focused Ultrasound in the Treatment of Colorectal Cancer Liver Metastases
by Ryan Holman, Orane Lorton, Pauline C. Guillemin, Andrea Peloso, Alexis Ricoeur and Rares Salomir

Section 5
Considering Advanced Therapeutics 121

Chapter 7 123
Multidisciplinary Management of Early Rectal Cancer
by Sean Ramcharan, Vanessa Cubas, Cortland Linder, Thomas Evans, Julia Merchant and Rakesh Sinha

Chapter 8 143
Immunotherapy for Colorectal Cancer in the Era of Precision Medicine
by Daniel Sur, Alecsandra Gorzo and Claudia Burz

Section 6
Supportive Care 169

Chapter 9 171
Nutrition: A Natural and Promising Option in Colorectal Cancer Intervention
by Olusola Bolaji Adewale

Chapter 10 187
Understanding Sphingolipids Metabolism in Colorectal Cancer
by Pedro Nuno Brandão, Lúcia Lacerda and Marisa D. Santos

Preface

Before the 1980s, surgery for colorectal cancer had a high mortality rate according to the incidence of side effects, including pelvic failure. In trials from the 1980s to the 1990s, the combination of chemotherapy and radiotherapy greatly contributed to overcoming the shortcomings of conventional treatment, which relied entirely on surgery and improved the survival rate, making it possible to routinely manage patients with advanced stages of colorectal cancer. In recent years, as the surgical experience in developed countries has increased, it has become possible to manage cancer through a delicate level of local control. Additionally, since chemo- and targeted agents, which are approved as new agents every year, can significantly improve the prognosis of patients with metastatic colorectal cancer, the approach to treating colorectal cancer using conventional therapies and new therapeutics in combination has been standardized worldwide. Unfortunately, however, the integration of these drugs reduces patient quality of life due to the induction of acute toxicity and thus alternatives are needed. Nevertheless, the use of these agents as radiosensitizers for the treatment of rectal cancer could potentially lead to reduced staging and increased rates of pathological complete response, so we must keep in mind that those therapies can be a double-edged sword. As such, it is important to improve our understanding of the various colorectal cancer treatments currently available. This book presents a comprehensive overview of the latest diagnostics, surgical technology, interventional radiology, and supportive care for colorectal cancer and highlights how conventional strategies are gradually being improved by the application of advanced science and technology. The information contained herein is presented from a multidisciplinary perspective, allowing for a broader discussion of colorectal cancer treatment.

I would like to express my deepest gratitude to the authors for their hard work and contributions.

Keun-Yeong Jeong
PearlsinMires,
Chief Executive Officer and Chief Technology Officer,
Seoul, Republic of Korea

Section 1

Introduction

Chapter 1

Introductory Chapter: Efforts to Conquer Colorectal Cancer from the Past to the Present

Keun-Yeong Jeong

1. Introduction

In the United States, the incidence rate of colon cancer increased by 0.5% to 2.4% annually since the mid-1980s in adults aged 20 to 54 years. Moreover, the rectal cancer incidence rate also increased faster by 3.2% annually since the 1970s in relatively younger ages (20–29 years) [1]. The recent global trend of colorectal cancer has been reported to have confirmed about 1.14 million, which accounts for about 6% of all newly diagnosed cancer patients, and the annual mortality is approaching about 580 K [2]. Such facts make it possible to recognize the high incidence rate and mortality of colorectal cancer, and it gives a continuous challenge to conquer colorectal cancer for physicians and basic researchers. Up to now, a variety of treatments have been developed as strategies responding to metical unmet needs while succeeding with existing therapeutic options targeting colorectal cancer, and those options are still effective. Therefore, a broad understanding of recent therapies including the past things will be essential to lay the groundwork for the step-by-step process of making innovations in colorectal cancer treatment.

2. Conventional options for colorectal cancer treatment

The treatment of colon cancer is mainly well-known in three types: surgery, chemotherapy, and radiation therapy, and appropriate options are selected according to the stage of colorectal cancer between these therapies [3]. The progression of colorectal cancer is divided into stages from 0 to 4. Most cases of stage 0 colorectal cancer are forming as polyps that do not grow beyond the inner lining of the colon or rectum, the local lesions are excised through a colonoscopy or transanal resection [3, 4]. Stage 1 colorectal cancer has grown deeper into the layer of the colon or rectal wall, but it means that the cancer cells do not spread outside of the colon or rectal wall or into the nearby lymph nodes [3, 4]. Complete removal of polyps is done during the colonoscopy, and if cancer cells are not found at the edge of lesions after removal, no other treatment may be needed [3, 5]. Stage 2 means that the cancer cells have grown into nearby tissues outside the walls of the colon or rectum but have not spread to the lymph nodes [3, 4]. Treatment may require partial colectomy, which removes the portion of the colon or rectum that contains cancer along with the surrounding lymph nodes. If the risk of cancer recurrence is high, adjuvant chemotherapy may be recommended according to the status of microsatellite instability or mismatch repair gene expression [3, 5]. The main options for chemotherapy include a combination of 5-FU and leucovorin with oxaliplatin (FOLFOX) or capecitabine (XELOX), but other combinations are also available including radiation followed by surgery [6–8]. Stages 3 and 4 are belonging to advanced, refractory colorectal cancer, which means that spreads to nearby lymph nodes or distant organs (mainly the liver or lungs) [3, 4]. At these stages of colon cancer, surgery to remove the cancerous portion of the colon along with nearby lymph nodes followed by adjuvant chemotherapy is the standard treatment for this stage. For rectal cancer, FOLFOX, XELOX, or capecitabine alone is given along with radiation therapy followed by surgery to remove rectal cancer and nearby lymph nodes, usually by low anterior resection, proctectomy with coloanal anastomosis, or abdominoperineal resection [5–7]. If primary or spread colorectal cancer cannot be completely removed with surgery, treatment options are likely to be selected with chemo or targeted therapies, such as 5-FU, oxaliplatin, irinotecan, capecitabine, bevacizumab, cetuximab, and/or regorafenib used alone or in combination [3, 6, 7]. A relatively wide range of treatment options depending on the stage of colorectal cancer may give hope to the patients for a cure, and providing a variety of options to physicians can also have important implications in terms of effective cancer management in clinical. However, it should not be overlooked that even in the presence of these known options, colorectal cancer has not yet been conquered. This is because even if these standard options are applied, there are still limitations in treatment. Briefly, recurrence after surgery, resistance to chemotherapies by mutations, and side effects of radiation therapy have been considered the main difficulties, therefore attempts to find bettered therapeutics to overcome these limitations are undergoing.

3. Finding better therapeutics

The recently developed robotic resection offers the clinical advantage of a more precise incision than laparoscopy in the narrow space where the rectum is located and these precision technologies are constantly being improved [9]. The development of immunotherapeutic agents such as programmed death-ligand 1 antibodies, therapeutic chimeric antigen receptor-T cells, and cancer vaccines is also believed to be a remarkable achievement in taking one step closer to conquering colorectal cancer [10]. In addition, the development of sotorasib also means a breakthrough in the treatment of intractable cancer by mutation, recent clinical trials reported a disease control rate of about 73.8% targeting $KRAS^{G12C}$ expressed colorectal cancer [11]. The case opens up the possibility that RAS mutations may no longer be defined as an area of an incurable disease. Along with these latest endeavors for the development of suitable therapies, several conditions that must be considered in order to develop better innovative therapies in the future or to overcome the limitations for the increase in therapeutic efficiency can be considered as follows: 1. Innovative diagnostic technologies such as proteomics, organoid culture, and virtual colonoscopy are encouraged to be included preferentially, and a developmental strategy reflecting characteristics of the target (eg. cancer stage, genetic predisposition, immune surveillance, and so on) is required. 2. Characteristics of the surrounding and internal microenvironment of the tumor, such as cancer-specific metabolism governing biochemical reaction by sphingolipids, characteristics of the tumor immune microenvironment, and the activity of microorganisms in the tumor, should be taken into account. 3. It would be important to select essential nutrients in consideration of the patient's health condition and to find a strategy that can optimize their supply or control methods. Of course, these three categories for better colorectal cancer treatment are handled in this book with interest.

4. Closing remarks

Strategies for targeting colorectal cancer based on existing treatments are gradually being developed, but they do not overcome the recognized limitations yet. Therefore, based on an understanding of various treatment methods from the past to the present, better and more innovative treatments should be proposed with the optimal diagnostic condition, cancer stage, tumor microenvironment, and nutrition should be considered. I hope that readers will be able to shape their ideas for the future of colorectal cancer treatment based on the content of this book.

Conflict of interest

No conflict of interest exists with the publication of this chapter.

Author details

Keun-Yeong Jeong
Metimedi Pharmaceuticals, Uiwang-si, Gyeonggi-do, Republic of Korea

*Address all correspondence to: alvirus@naver.com

References

[1] Siegel RL, Fedewa SA, Anderson WF, Miller KD, Ma J, Rosenberg PS, et al. Colorectal cancer incidence patterns in the United States, 1974-2013. Journal of the National Cancer Institute. 2017;**109**(8):djw322

[2] Sung H, Ferlay J, Siegel RL, Laversanne M, Soerjomataram I, Jemal A, et al. Global cancer statistics 2020: GLOBOCAN estimates of incidence and mortality worldwide for 36 cancers in 185 countries. CA: a Cancer Journal for Clinicians. 2021;**71**(3):209-249

[3] Nakayama G, Tanaka C, Kodera Y. Current options for the diagnosis, staging and therapeutic Management of Colorectal Cancer. Gastrointest Tumors. 2013;**1**(1):25-32

[4] Mahmoud NN. Colorectal cancer: Preoperative evaluation and staging. Surgical Oncology Clinics of North America. 2022;**31**(2):127-141

[5] Matsuda T, Yamashita K, Hasegawa H, Oshikiri T, Hosono M, Higashino N, et al. Recent updates in the surgical treatment of colorectal cancer. Annals of Gastroenterological Surgery. 2018;**2**(2):129-136

[6] Xie YH, Chen YX, Fang JY. Comprehensive review of targeted therapy for colorectal cancer. Signal Transduction and Targeted Therapy. 2020;**5**(1):22

[7] Nalli M, Puxeddu M, La Regina G, Gianni S, Silvestri R. Emerging therapeutic agents for colorectal cancer. Molecules. 2021;**26**(24):7463

[8] Hafner MF, Debus J. Radiotherapy for colorectal cancer: Current standards and future perspectives. Visceral Medicine. 2016;**32**(3):172-177

[9] Lee JL, Alsaleem HA, Kim JC. Robotic surgery for colorectal disease: Review of current port placement and future perspectives. Annals of Surgical Treatment and Research. 2020;**98**(1):31-43

[10] Golshani G, Zhang Y. Advances in immunotherapy for colorectal cancer: A review. Therapeutic Advances in Gastroenterology. 2020;**13**:1756284820917527

[11] Patelli G, Tosi F, Amatu A, Mauri G, Curaba A, Patane DA, et al. Strategies to tackle RAS-mutated metastatic colorectal cancer. ESMO Open. 2021;**6**(3):100156

Section 2

Diagnostics, Basic to Clinical

Chapter 2

Utilising Proteomics and Organoid Cultures for Predicting Treatment Response in Colorectal Cancer

Isaac Micallef and Byron Baron

Abstract

Colorectal cancer (CRC) remains one of the most frequently diagnosed tumours worldwide. Despite advances in surgical intervention and therapeutics, development of chemoresistance remains a challenge to treating CRC. Predicting treatment response in CRC has strongly relied on genomics, transcriptomics and epigenomics, combined with different cancer staging and classification systems. Despite being beneficial, these omics technologies fail to provide any assessment at a protein level. Thus, having high-throughput tools that assess tumour response to therapy at a protein level will definitely complement the current approaches. In this regard, the field of proteomics holds promise to understand treatment response in tumours. Additionally, patient-derived tumour organoids are replacing the traditional cell lines and xenograft models as the preferred *in vitro* models for predicting clinical response due to being a better representative model of typical tumour characteristics *in vivo*. Combining proteomics and tumour organoids can provide more personalised and optimal treatments for CRC in the coming years. This chapter aims to provide an overview of the progress made in proteomic research and use of organoids for understanding CRC treatment response, together with discussing the strengths and limitations of these two approaches when linked together. This overview will then be used to propose future perspectives.

Keywords: colorectal cancer, proteomics, organoids, treatment response, prediction

1. Introduction

Despite the methodological advancements made in cancer detection and treatment administration, colorectal cancer (CRC) remains one of the most common types of gastrointestinal malignancies diagnosed worldwide [1]. Development of this tumour involves genetic, histological and morphological changes which arise within the crypt cells of the colon or rectum. Hyperproliferation of these cells gives rise to benign polyps which protrude the surface of the epithelial cells within the intestinal lumen. Progression of pre-cancerous polyps can take a few years or decades to become malignant polyps, referred to as adenocarcinomas. This phenomenon is associated with different forms of inherited, acquired and epigenetic mutations in different proto-oncogenes and tumour suppressor genes, which accrue in several mechanisms [2, 3].

To deal with CRC progression and metastasis, different staging and classification systems together with different modes of treatment have been established throughout the years [4, 5]. Despite the advancements made in therapeutic strategies, CRC mortality rate remains high, and development of chemoresistance due to different circumstances remains a major constraint to patients being treated [6–8].

Current research and preclinical treatment development is centred around the traditional tumour biology research models of xenografts and two-dimensional (2D) cell culturing. Unfortunately, cell lines in particularly, do not always present an integrative microenvironment of cells living within a tissue, cannot replicate tumour heterogeneity and at times cannot retain all genetic information. Additionally, for xenografts, genetics and growth environment tend to differ from those of patients, have a lower success rate, are more time consuming and costly [9]. All in all, measures to evaluate the standardisation of CRC therapy are not well established, thus the urge to develop new tumour models and to identify accurate and substantiated predictive markers is required, so that clinicians can appropriately select which chemotherapy to administer.

Throughout the last decade, various research teams have taken the initiative to predict treatment response through different high-throughput methodologies, some of which in the coming years could potentially accompany the current staging and classification systems used. Proteomics, which is the study of proteomes and their functions in cells and tissues, is one of the fields that has stood out the most, due to the promising opportunities it has presented when it comes to understanding treatment response in various tumours, including CRC [10–12]. Additionally, three-dimensional (3D) culturing is another high-throughput technique which has made rapid progress in the fields of drug discovery and screening. This form of culturing is an advanced system in which cells from both healthy or tumour tissues are cultured as spheres in a scaffold or non-scaffold-based system. In turn, this approach provides a better representation of an *in vivo* environment when compared to the traditional 2D monolayered cell culturing system [13–15]. This model permits the development of either spheroids (through cell lines using a scaffold or non-scaffold system) or organoids (through tissue samples using a scaffold system). The two models have similar and distinctive purposes, however the preparation, time, and tumour cell sources needed to establish the respective model differs [15]. Patient derived organoids (PDOs), have shown potential in different research fields, including high throughput drug screening analysis and to analyse the efficacy of different treatments [13, 16]. However, their use in predicting treatment response in relation to proteomics is still fairly novel, thus further research is still ongoing.

The purpose of this chapter is to first provide an overview of the current CRC staging and classification systems and their involvement in predicting treatment administration. Then, the chapter will address the involvement and progress of proteomics and PDOs, in predicting therapy response in CRC. Based on this, it will end by discussing the strengths and limitations of these two approaches when linked together, as well as propose potential future perspectives in this field.

2. Colorectal cancer (CRC)

Like many cancers, CRC development involves multiple different mutations and is linked to various risk factors. Most of the diagnosed patients display alterations in a number of proto-oncogenes and tumour suppressors which result in the dysregulation of specific signalling pathways: mainly the Wingless-related integration site (WNT)/β-catenin pathway (mutations in the adenomatous polyposis coli (*APC*) gene), Rat Sarcoma Virus/Rapidly Accelerated Fibrosarcoma/Mitogen activated protein kinase/Extracellular signal regulated protein kinase (RAS-RAF-MEK-ERK) pathway (mutations in the *KRAS* gene), transforming growth factor-beta (TGF-β) pathway (mutations in the mothers against decapentaplegic homologue 2 and 4 (*SMAD2/4*) genes), p53 related pathways (mutations in the tumour protein 53 (*p53*) gene), phosphatidylinositol-3-kinase/Akt/mammalian target of rapamycin (PI3K/AKT/mTOR) pathway (mutations in the *PIK3CA* gene) and DNA mismatch repair system (several gene mutations), among others [2, 17].

CRC development is also dependent on three different pathways: (1) microsatellite instability (MSI) pathway (2) chromosomal instability (CIN) pathway and (3) CpG island methylator pathway (CIMP) [2, 3, 18]. MSI-tumours are linked to mutations and inactivation of the DNA mismatch repair system which arise from gene errors due to DNA polymerase slippage, giving rise to uneven microsatellite lengths [2]. The genes typically affected in these pathways include MutL homologue 1 or 3 (MLH1 or MLH3), MutS homologue 2 or 6 (MSH2 or MSH6) and post-meiotic segregation 2 (PMS2). Furthermore, CIN tumours account for the bulk of the cases, and these arise due to mutation build up in the *TP3*, *APC* and *KRAS* genes, among others which occur less frequently [3, 18]. As for CIMP tumours, these exhibit a high degree of promoter hypermethylation on tumour suppressor genes, giving rise to transcriptional inactivation [2, 3].

Considering the known mutations and pathways affected, the CRC carcinogenesis genetic model proposed by Fearon and Vogelstein [19] is at present the accepted model for CRC progression. Since CRC is considered as a heterogeneous disease, patients present unique genetic and epigenetic modifications; hence, the therapy administered, mortality and heterogeneity differ between patients [20]. Current CRC therapy options are limited, thus treatment selection for each patient is dependent on the classification (extent) of the tumour as will be explained in the coming sections.

2.1 Staging and classifications

As introduced previously, CRC is a heterogeneous disease comprised of different subtypes, which can be distinguished by the clinical and/or molecular features presented. Due to the different mutations and pathways that have been defined for CRC development, biologically distinct groups having their respective characteristics have been proposed. The currently available technologies have enabled the generation of large-scale sequencing data for the identification of genetic and epigenetic CRC alterations. To understand and classify CRCs into different subtypes that can be used to predict treatment response, prognosis and cancer relapse risk, different molecular biomarkers have been utilised, including: (1) CRC developmental pathways (CIN, MSI, CIMP), (2) polymerase ε (POLE) mutations, (3) LINE-1 Hypomethylation, (4) RAS, BRAF, and PIK3CA mutations in the MAPK/PIK3 pathway, (5) mutations in the WNT/APC/CTNNB1/TGF-β pathway, (6) TP53 mutations and (7) immune biomarkers and the microbiome [20].

Different classifications have been established and proposed to categorise CRC diagnosis by molecular subtype [20–30]. These CRC molecular subtypes consider different biological features, alterations and clinical behaviour. However, the currently most accepted CRC classification is that proposed by Guinney et al. [30], composed of four consensus molecular subtypes (CMS, CMS1-CMS4). These subtypes are based on different levels of immune infiltration, distinct mutations and altered somatic copy number alterations. In general, the CMS classification system is the most robust from the established classifications due to having a clear biological interpretability. Thus, it is expected to continue being used for future clinical stratification and subtype-based targeted interventions. All in all, despite the various classifications systems being useful for predicting treatment outcome in patients, such systems do not consider tumour heterogeneity which is typically the reason for therapy resistance.

Prior to the development of CRC classifications, categorisation of diagnosed CRC patients was based on clinical and pathological features, mainly the degree of differentiation, the stage of the tumour and the localisation of the tumour [21]. Various CRC staging systems were established by surgeons to categorise the four CRC stages (I–IV) for diagnosis and treatment. The preferred staging system is known as the American Joint Committee on Cancer (AJCC) tumour-node-metastasis (TNM) staging model, first implemented in 1977 [31]. Since then, this model has been continuously revised, with the latest being the eighth edition, released and implemented globally in 2018 [31]. Prior to this system, two other models were developed, the Dukes' staging system [32] and the Modified Astler-Coller (MAC) classification [33], implemented in 1932 and 1954, respectively. The limitation of these two models is that only tumour invasion depth and lymphatic metastasis is considered [32–35]. Thus, both have now been replaced with the TNM staging model, which is dependent on (1) tumour size and invasion (T), (2) regional lymph nodes involvement (N) and (3) metastasis (M) (**Table 1**) [31, 34]. Lastly, CRC histological grading is denoted as 'G' and this defines the state of cell differentiation when compared to a healthy cell (G1: well differentiated, G2: moderately differentiated, G3: poorly differentiated and G4: undifferentiated) [37].

Cell Type	**TNM Stages (AJCC-8)**				**Other Staging Methods**	
	Stage	**T**	**N**	**M**	**Dukes**	**MAC**
Healthy	0	Tis	N0	M0	—	—
Polyp	I	T1–T2	N0	M0	A	A–B1
Tumour	IIA–IIC	T3–T4b	N0	M0	B	B2–B3
Extended to Lymph Node	IIIA–IIIC	T1–T4b	N1c–N2b	M0	C	C1–C3
Metastasis	IVA-IVC	Any T	Any N	M1a–M1c	D	D

Roman numbers (I–IV) describe disease severity (least to most severe—I to IV). Stage 0 are carcinoma in situ, stage I cancers are small, less deeply invasive and have not reached the lymph nodes, stage II and III cancers refer to tumours which have increased in size and stage IV cancer refers to distant metastasis. Tis; tumour limited to mucosa, T1; tumour invaded submucosa, T2; tumour invaded muscalaris propria, T3; tumour invaded subserosa and beyond but not to other organs, T4; tumour invaded other organs (T4a: Invades visceral peritoneum, T4b: Invades or adheres to other organs or structures). N0; no regional lymph nodes (RNLs) metastasis, N1; metastasis to 1–3 RNLs (N1a: 1 RLN metastasis, N1b: 2–3 RLNs metastasis, N1c: metastasis into areas of fat near lymph nodes but not in the nodes), N2; metastasis to 4 or more RLNs (N2a: metastasis to 4–6 RLNs, N2b: metastasis to 7 or more RLNs). M0; no distant metastasis, M1; distant metastasis (M1a: metastasis to distant organ/site without peritoneal metastasis, M1b: metastasis to 2 or more organs/sites without peritoneal metastasis, M1c: metastasis to peritoneal surface with or without other organ/site metastases). Information summarised in this table was retrieved from: [4, 31, 34, 36].

Table 1.
A summarised classification for the different CRC staging systems.

2.2 Treatment administration

Different approaches are considered when treating CRC, starting with simple endoscopic polypectomy to remove any polyps which are benign or potentially malignant, to more sophisticated surgical interventions to eradicate non-metastatic primary tumours. Stage 0 to early-Stage II CRC are normally curative through surgery [4, 9], however nowadays some patients are inoperable due to bulky tumours. Thus, a range of therapy regimens are selected to shrink the metastatic lesion, which prolongs patient survival rates and reduces risk of metastatic spread due to microscopic tumour foci, distant from the primary tumour location [3, 9]. Nowadays, Stage I/II CRC patients can also receive neoadjuvant chemotherapy, while late III/IV stages CRC receive adjuvant treatment (**Table 2**), with the latter form of therapy at times also being administered to high risk stratified Stage II CRC patients [4, 5]. Cytotoxic agents [5, 8], administered as single agents or in combination, immunotherapy [38], targeted therapy [40] and sometimes radiotherapy [4], are the main treatment regimens for CRC (**Table 2**). Through these approaches, clinicians attempt to improve the response rate and overall survival of patients, especially those with metastatic CRC (mCRC). Despite the wide range of treatments available, it is estimated that around 90% of patients with late-stage CRC are resistant to the available frontline therapy [14]. Thus, combination therapy has been implemented to prevent the development of chemoresistance, to increase response rate and to reduce potential toxicity which arises when single cytotoxic agents are administered [5].

2.3 Current approaches for predicting treatment administration

Most registered CRC studies with targeted medicines in previous decades had no pre-planned biomarker analyses, apart from exploratory analysis, and did not stratify patients into biomarker-defined subgroups [29]. Significant advances being implemented have demonstrated slightly improved treatment predictions. Despite this, selecting which form of therapy to administer remains a complex process for each patient due to the lack of evidence for the CRC therapy existing, particularly chemotherapy [8]. Individual cancer patient therapy is presently dependent on clinical gene sequencing, however only 7% of the population benefits from personalised care established from next-generation sequencing (NGS) [9].

One of the initial advances arose from a retrospective correlative clinical trial analysis which focused on innate resistance to anti-EGFR treatment due to the KRAS mutations on exon 2. This biomarker stratification served as the first precision medicine CRC model ('one gene, one drug' paradigm), since patients harbouring KRAS mutations on exon 2 do not benefit from cetuximab and panitumumab [29, 40]. However, this concept had major limitations when it was employed to study potential predictive CRC markers [29]. Similar efficacy was obtained when administering BRAF inhibitors [41] or MEK inhibitors [42] to advanced CRC bearing specific *BRAF* or *KRAS* mutations, respectively. Other molecular biomarkers have shown to serve as predictive biomarkers in CRC, including miRNAs, Phosphatidylinositol 3-kinase catalytic subunit alpha (PI3KCA), VEGF and Human epidermal growth factor receptor 2 (HER2) [20, 43–45]. Furthermore, specific biomarkers for selected cytotoxic agents have served as biomarkers for predicating efficacy and toxicity of said agents [45, 46].

From the known classifications, CMS subtypes have shown to be of prognostic significance due to being suitable for the assessment of therapy responses and treatment choice [47–49]. For instance, Kwon et al. [50] used this classification to categories 101

Treatment	Class	Mechanism of action	Application
5-Fluorouracil (5FU) (cytotoxic agent)	Antimetabolite (pyrimidine analogue)	Inhibits thymidylate synthase (TS)	Alone or in combination for adjuvant or palliative care
Capecitabine (cytotoxic agent)	Antimetabolite (pyrimidine analogue)	Inhibits TS	Alone or in combination for adjuvant (Stage III) treatment
Irinotecan (cytotoxic agent)	Topoisomerase I (Topo I) inhibitor	Inhibits Topo I	Combined with FOLFOX, capecitabine or cetuximab for mCRC
Oxaliplatin (OXA) (cytotoxic agent)	Alkylating agent (platinum compound)	Inhibits DNA replication/ transcription	Combined with FOLFOX for adjuvant treatment and mCRC
Regorafenib (targeted therapy)	Kinase inhibitor	Tyrosine kinase inhibitor	Alone for mCRC
Cetuximab (targeted therapy)	Monoclonal antibody	EGFR inhibitor	Alone or combined with irinotecan or FOLFOX for mCRC
Bevacizumab (targeted therapy)	Monoclonal antibody	Vascular endothelial growth factor (VEGF) ligand inhibitor	Combined with FOLFIRI for mCRC
Panitumumab (targeted therapy)	Monoclonal antibody	EGFR inhibitor	Alone or combined with FOLFOX or FOLFIRI for mCRC
Pembrolizumab (immunotherapy)	Monoclonal antibody	Inhibits programmed cell death protein 1 (PD1)	mCRC
Nivolumab (immunotherapy)	Monoclonal antibody	Inhibits PD1	mCRC
Aflibercept (targeted therapy)	Recombinant fusion protein	VEGF-A and placental growth factor (PIGF) inhibitor	Alone or combined with FOLFIRI for mCRC
FOLFOX	Combination treatment (5-FU, leucovorin (LV) and OXA)		Adjuvant chemotherapy
FOLFIRI	Combination treatment (5-FU, LV and irinotecan)		Adjuvant chemotherapy
FOLFIRINOX	Combination treatment (5-FU, LV, irinotecan and OXA)		Adjuvant chemotherapy
XELOX	Combination treatment (OXA and capecitabine)		Adjuvant chemotherapy
Radiotherapy	At times combined with 5-FU or capecitabine		mCRC

Information summarised in this table was retrieved from: [4, 5, 8, 38, 39].

Table 2.
Current therapy used against colorectal cancer (CRC).

patients with stage III CRC which were treated with FOLFOX. However, despite the significant role shown by CMS subtypes in predicting treatment response throughout the last decade, this classification is not suitable for selecting patients for treatment with anti-VEGF or anti-EGFR agents [21].

The introduction of NGS with pre-screening approaches and clinical sample trials, together with the use of advanced preclinical models (organoids), are now being implemented to further characterise target agents in CRC [29]. This has helped in identifying and validating new predictive biomarkers, as well as gaining a better understanding of dynamic target inhibition so as to develop novel combination therapy which improves the overall patient outcome. Lastly, proteomics is another field which has slowly started to be implemented in treatment prediction throughout the last decade [10–12], however the advancements made will be discussed in the coming section.

3. Proteomics

Proteomics is generally defined as the comprehensive study of the proteins inside a cell, considering both their levels and distribution. Proteomes are dynamic and change in a spatial, temporal, or chemical manner, expanding the roles that the available complement of proteins can perform within a cell. One of the major aims of such investigations is to deduce the changes to biological pathways and cellular operations with the onset and progression of disease [51].

Similar to the expansion of genomic and transcriptomic information by inclusion of epigenetics (e.g. CpG promoter methylation), the acquisition of information from post-translational modifications (PTMs) can be considered as epiproteomics. The most common PTMs investigated are phosphorylation, acetylation and methylation, although proteins can undergo over 200 PTMs, which depend on cell type, cellular context, biological condition, and other parameters. Each PTM can alter protein properties, having some form of effect on protein function [51–54] and can also confer distinct biomarker properties to proteins [55]. Phosphorylation and acetylation are linked to protein activation, while methylation can alter the majority of the protein characteristics depending on the cellular conditions [54]. Throughout cancer development and the eventual therapy resistance, the aberrant signalling arising is not only due to an overall change in protein expression, but also due to changes in protein activity arising from the addition or removal of PTMs taking place on key proteins [52, 53, 56].

Proteomics incorporates numerous methods utilised for the measurement, large scale recognition, characterisation and analysis of proteins [53, 54]. With the continual development taking place in this field and its application in various diseases, including cancer, substantial improvement has been achieved in discovering clinically applicable biomarkers [57]. The main tool used for proteomics is mass spectrometry (MS), principally because it is sensitive, versatile, and can identify target proteins found in complex sample matrices. The approach most commonly used is known as bottom-up proteomics, also called "Shotgun Proteomics", in which the protein sample is enzymatically or chemically digested and then separated by liquid chromatography (LC) before being identified by tandem mass spectrometry (MS/MS), hence the name LC-MS/MS. On the contrary, the less popular, top-down approach analyses intact proteins, with the major advantage of the latter being the complete coverage of the protein sequence [58–60].

This omics approach permits the qualitative and quantitative profiling of several proteins within a sample. LC-MS/MS is the key approach to obtaining high-resolution spectra of mixed peptides, which in turn permit identification of sensitive and unique biomarkers [57, 58]. For accurate quantification analysis and minimal discrepancies, both label-based and label-free quantification approaches have been developed, both of which have been used in clinical research [57, 60–62]. Through label-based approaches, the tagged protein can be compared to the control proteins tagged with isotope-free markers in a qualitative or quantitative manner [57, 58]. Different forms of labels having been developed, including SILAC (stable isotope labelling by amino acids in cell culture), Heavy methyl-SILAC (hmSILAC), Tandem Mass Tag (TMT), Isotope-Coded Affinity Tag (ICAT) and isobaric Tag for Relative and Absolute Quantitation (iTRAQ) [57–63]. These labelling approaches permit multiplexing of several samples under different experiment conditions within the same run and reduce the experimental biases and time needed for analysis [59, 61]. As for label-free approaches, "Targeted Proteomics" is preferred due to its high sensitivity, accuracy and reproducibility [58, 61]. This technique allows the focus on a subset of proteins of interest and is possible through Multiple Reaction Monitoring-Mass Spectrometry (MRM-MS), Selected Reaction Monitoring-Mass Spectrometry (SRM-MS), or Sequential Window Acquisition of all Theoretical fragment ion spectra (SWATH) [11, 57, 61]. Through the MS analysis performed, proteins can be quantified based on the intensity of the signals or spectral counts obtained for the peptides of interest. Apart from MS-based approaches, the amount of protein within a sample can also be semi-quantitatively or quantitatively analysed through antibody arrays or enzyme-linked immunosorbent assays (ELISA) [11, 55, 57].

Different studies have applied proteomics to CRC using most of the aforementioned approaches to investigate either cell lines or patient tissues samples [12, 55, 58, 64, 65]. However, utilisation of proteomics and CRC PDOs to understand and predict treatment response in a clinical settings has been extremely limited, thus this will be the main focus in the next sections.

3.1 Clinical proteomics

Current clinical cancer testing relies heavily on genomics to identify and classify patient tumours based on known mutations in key genes within the regulatory biochemical pathways important for a specific cancer type. This is due to the ease and accessibility of genetic techniques. However, such genetic biomarkers for diagnosis, prognosis and therapeutic effectiveness fall short of their aim as they do not take into consideration all the downstream changes that the products of such genes undergo, until they come to perform their cellular roles as proteins. Furthermore, genomics gives no information related to protein localisation, turnover, PTMs or functional activity, all of which can impinge on the effectiveness of therapeutics [56, 57].

The primary purpose of clinical proteomics is to analyse the proteome and its modifications in body fluids, cells and tissues so as to ascertain distinctive or signature biomarkers which can be utilised in a clinical setting, so as to promote personalised medicine [61, 63]. This interdisciplinary field highlights the efforts and research needed to further move forward. Clinical proteomics translates the biochemical data generated in the lab related to tumour changes undergone throughout the process of carcinogenesis up to metastasis and therapeutic evasion into patient-specific data, which provides a useful tool in improving decision-making to define the steps that can be taken to better treat a patient in a targeted manner. Clinical proteomics thus adds a critical layer of information to the available genomic data such that while the genomics provides the complement of mutations that give the tumour growth advantages, metastatic properties and resistance to therapy, the proteomics

DOI: http://dx.doi.org/10.5772/intechopen.106028

provides an indication of any aberrant protein activity in the tumour, adding the functional consequences of the genomic data at the proteomic level [56].

Clinical proteomics can thus benefit patients with regards to cancer detection, treatment and management. As proteomic technologies improve and the potential of clinical proteomics grows, the applications and benefits for patients will improve. The application of serum proteomics could improve early cancer detection through non-invasive testing. The availability of reliable biomarkers for diagnosis and molecular classification at an early stage would increase the therapeutic options. The quantification of enzymatic activity using high-throughput array-based proteomics would allow more personalised therapeutic regimens targeting the most critically dysregulated pathways. Therapeutic efficacy and toxicity could then be assessed in real-time so as to adjust dosage or change treatment if resistance is detected [56].

3.2 Predictive biomarkers for clinical proteomics

In recent years, the search for protein biomarkers has become crucial. Biomarkers, as defined by the National Cancer Institute, are biological molecules found within the blood, other body fluids or tissues, which may be used as indicators for identifying signs of a normal/abnormal process, or of a pathological condition. Identifying biomarkers is of significant interest because these markers are suitable for: (1) evaluating clinical prognosis, (2) assessing and identifying risk of recurrence (diagnostic biomarkers), (3) following the development of disease or predicting relapse (prognostic biomarkers) and (4) determining and improving patients' response to therapy (predictive biomarkers) [11, 61]. Cancer biomarkers in the clinic are used to provide quantifiable information about the aberrant cellular processes arising in tumours and this information is critical for targeting the molecular mechanisms driving the cancer as well as determining the effectiveness of the therapeutic regimens administered to patients. While at a clinical level, diagnostic biomarkers assisting in histopathological tumour classification are the most commonly used, both prognostic and predictive biomarkers are needed for clinicians to determine a tumours level of malignancy and to exploit therapeutic sensitivities so as to provide more effective treatment regimens, respectively [66]. Through proteomics, one can examine several tumour proteins, thus hypothetically generating novel therapeutic targets and markers for CRC. Additionally, protein markers could be measured easily through routinely available body fluids, thus reducing the necessity for fresh or frozen tissue biopsies. Even though different research groups have shown that CRC leads to fluctuations in the blood proteome [67, 68], blood biomarkers specific to CRC have not been validated or approved for clinical uses.

As well reviewed by Chauvin and Boisvert [62] and Lee et al. [69], predictive biomarker discovery has proven to be quite a laborious process, with three stages being involved: (1) discovery/screening, (2) verification and (3) validation. The initial step is performed via shotgun proteomics, using small cohorts of patient tissue samples, whose proteins can be extracted and analysed through MS. The proteome is examined to monitor and identify any dysregulated proteins between different groups of patients (e.g. responsive vs. unresponsive). Different labelling techniques are applied to better quantify the proteins within samples. In the second stage, the proteins presenting the biggest changes between the different cohorts are selected for verification. Targeted proteomics is used here as it facilitates precise and accurate quantification of the selected proteins, across a slightly larger cohort. Thirdly, the validation stage involves the clinical assessment phase of the biomarkers which involves very large cohorts to validate the sensitivity and specificity of the putative biomarkers. The main drawback of the latter stage is that very few studies have been reported with regard to protein biomarker identification for predictive therapy response through the use of proteomics and human samples, especially for CRC [61]. Lastly, the ideal biomarker selected should be sensitive and precise for the proteins of interest in a cost-effective assay, which is fast and robust against both inter-operator and inter-institutional variability. For a biomarker to be reliable it has to be validated through a regulated clinical study having a variety of patients, utilising thorough standards for each step, from sample collection to result analysis, all of which should be reproducible by different laboratories [56].

It has become apparent that no single biomarker exists for a particular cancer type due to the substantial heterogeneity existing within the proteome of patients, together with the processes involved in the development of the disease or therapy resistance. Moreover, most biomarker breakthroughs employ laborious searchers for one or a small range of dysregulated proteins in cancer samples, through which a panel of biomarkers can be selected for clinical analysis [56]. Different proteomic approaches have been utilised to identify new CRC biomarkers to elucidate not only molecular mechanisms, but to also predict treatment response. However, the latter has only been slightly investigated, especially from a clinical perspective and through the use of PDOs. Despite being far from pathophysiological tumour conditions, cell lines have been used mostly to model and reveal predictive biomarkers through proteomics, due to being inexpensive and easy to manipulate to generate resistant cultures. Most studies that used cell lines have made use of both gel-based and gel-free approaches, in order to compare the differential protein expression profiles in cell lines pre- and post-treatment administration [70–72]. Even though PTMs have not being given that much importance in their potential use as predictive biomarkers, some research groups have or are currently investigating their potential through the use of 2D cell lines [73–75], 3D spheroid cultures [73, 76, 77] or patient samples [78, 79], with the majority focusing on phosphorylated proteins. Use of spheroids for proteomic studies provides more valuable data about how therapy might affect an *in vivo* tumour when compared to 2D cultured cell lines [80].

The different CRC-related proteins discovered from proteomic-based studies indicate that these might be novel predictive biomarkers for CRC. Thus, further proving that proteomics is an absolute, highly reliable and translatable research tool for identification of novel biomarkers in cancers. However, further investigation on current putative biomarkers, together with others yet to be discovered can result in the development of a panel of markers which have adequate sensitivity and specificity for CRC in a clinical and therapeutic setting. Apart from total protein levels, more research efforts are being put into quantifying protein activity and the levels of key PTMs in an effort to provide patients with more suitable therapy regimens [56].

3.3 Limitations in clinical proteomics

Protein and peptide level identification through different MS-based approaches can recognise and quantify hundreds to thousands of proteins within a biological sample, however this only depends on the complexity and amount of the starting material [64]. Despite this, even from simplified cancer models such as cell lines, where protein yield is generally high, there is very limited amount of information present on most detected proteins, and their potential use as clinical biomarkers. In comparison, protein yield from clinical samples is much lower, due to the complexity of the samples [64]. Even though studies reporting the detection and quantification of differentially expressed proteins in CRC through various approaches, a full understanding of the implications and functionality arising due to such dysregulations is required for a significant inference. Moreover, identifying the proteins of interest within a particular sample remains cumbersome at times. It is expected that the results derived from the different proteomic approaches will be combined with data collected from other omics approaches to further understand the significance of such dysregulation, as will be discussed in Section 5.

As for PTM-based research, identification and characterisation of PTMs is a challenging task, since these modifications are generally present in low (sub-stoichiometric) amounts and their existence is mostly transient, thus further making it difficult to analyse [64]. Sample preparation for PTM analysis through MS is laborious, requires a large amount of the starting material and contains several optimisation stages when compared to normal global proteome analysis. Additionally, we lack reliable tools and methods for studying PTMs and we lack enrichment techniques for specific PTMs, particularly those making use of antibodies. Commercially available antibodies that are capable of detecting and enriching PTMs are limited in availability, are of low quality and have low binding efficiency. Moreover, the production and application of antibodies is a long and costly process.

Most advancements made in order to (1) increase the number of modified protein or peptides identified and (2) to quantify the difference between modified and unmodified proteins or peptides have focused mostly on phosphorylation. Thus, it is expected that future advanced research will centre around other PTMs, particularly methylation, since this modification has been given the least importance when it comes to identification and quantification [59]. The implication and functional roles for most PTMs arising on proteins in CRC throughout cancer development and the eventual therapy resistance, remains unknown. Moreover, there are still several aspects of PTM biology that need to be defined such as their position, degree and the affector enzymes responsible for giving rise to the different PTMs.

Despite different labelling techniques currently available, the disadvantage of these approaches is the incorporation of a light or heavy amino acid to cells in culture in case of SILAC and hmSILAC [59], or the addition of chemically bonded mass labels to the peptides following preparation, as in the case of iTRAQ and TMT [58, 61], both of which complicate the sample preparation workflow. Consequently, this comes with additional disadvantages due to their high costs, and these techniques being scarcely or not used at all in shotgun proteomics on human samples since label-free quantification is preferred here. The problem with label-free approaches is that accuracy is much lower, the analysis system is quite complex since sophisticated software tools are needed, and multiplexing is not possible, when compared to the labelling approaches [57, 58]. Another limitation for SILAC and hmSILAC is that these two can only be applied to cell culturing samples, but not directly to patient tissue samples. Thus, for this reason, the better option would be to combine the generation of PDOs with these labelling approaches [59, 62]. Moreover, not all of these labelling techniques can be applied to all samples [11].

A common clinical limitation for cancer proteomics studies in general is the patient cohort size available, particularly when high resolution proteomics workflows are applied. Sample analysis for such workflows can take up to 24 h of instrument analysis time, thus limiting studies to either a handful of individual sample analysis or to pooled sample analysis [13]. This is slowly being overcome due to the development of multiplexed MS approaches and the decrease in instrument analysis time needed due to ongoing development in instrument speed, thus permitting for larger scale clinical proteomic analyses in the near future. Another drawback is the long process of clinical approval needed for the discovery of new biomarkers through proteomic approaches. This is obviously expected, since as explained in Section 3.2, the validation phase demands a lot of further work, to ensure the biomarker selected provides reproducible data. This is not only a limitation in this field but research in general and it is one of the reasons why most putative and candidate biomarkers do not go beyond the proof-of-concept phase [60].

Considering the current knowledge gained through clinical proteomics, these limitations, as well as others well reviewed by Maes et al. [81], will not hinder the discovery and the growing panel of potential biomarkers suitable for the analysis of CRC development, progression and treatment response. Significant scientific and technical limitations are yet to be overcome in the process of identifying putative biomarkers through proteomics, however the constant advancement being made in this field are expected to decrease or eliminate the current bottlenecks.

4. Organoids

Development of 'mini-gut' organoids were first pioneered by Sato et al. [82]. These 3D models are self-organised multicellular structures, primarily derived from adult multipotent stem cells (ASCs-organ specific), human pluripotent stem cells (hPSCs-can differentiate into multiple cell types), embryonic stem cells (ESCs) or cancer stem cells (CSCs) [17]. Recent advancements have enabled the development of these CRC models through different approaches, particularly using patient tumour samples, which in turn provide a better representation of *in vivo* tumours [83]. Organoids are established by culturing cells extracted from tumour tissues in a supportive extracellular matrix (ECM), such as matrigel or basement membrane extract, with collagen IV, laminin and entactin also being major components [14, 84]. The ECM enables long-term proliferation and differentiation capacities; however, these two factors are also dependent on a cocktail of growth factors, small molecules and inhibitors which are supplemented to the culturing medium [14, 84, 85]. Based on the conditions provided, the typical SC niches found within the intestinal crypts are produced, which permit proliferation and differentiation of cells which self-organise into 3D structures. Over the years, organoids have shown to be better models for research in different fields when compared to cell lines and xenografts. Of note, organoids have been implemented to study CRC from different perspectives, such as: initiation, progression and invasion of CRC [84], genetic mutations [83], intratumoral heterogeneity and tumour evolution [86], and drug screening or development [9, 14, 16, 83–86].

4.1 Use in predicting treatment response

Drug screening through PDOs has not been limited to only cancer therapies but has been utilised to screen drugs for a range of diseases, thus further proving the usefulness of these models. It is expected that therapy screening through organoids will further help in predicting treatment response in patients, thus the value of PDOs in predicting the response of cytotoxic agents, targeted therapy and radiotherapy has also started to be investigated. For years, compounds displaying cytotoxic activity on cultured cancer cell lines resulted in being unsuccessful in the beginning stages of clinical studies. This ineffectiveness is because of dissimilarity between genetically unstable immortal cell lines and patient tumours, and due to cell lines not representing the whole tumour. This has shown to not be the case with PDOs, since genetic and phenotypic characteristics are preserved over long-term culturing, the original features (heterogeneity) of the tumours they are derived from are recapitulated and cell-to-cell or cell-to-matrix interactions are maintained. Different research teams have demonstrated the benefit of using PDOs for drug screening in different settings, mainly; (1) drug innovation, (2) toxicity analysis and (3) precision medicine. Thus, PDOs are a unique system to test and predict drug effects within tumour tissues collected from a patient [17].

Recent reports which made use of intestinal organoids showed the adverse consequences of treatment [9, 86–90]. For instance, organoid cultures showed to be suitable for the detection of genotypes to drug association [86]. Through gene assessment, which revealed a number of altered genes, the authors designed a customised library to screen the sensitivity of a range of drugs, with the relationship between the two being detected through high throughput drug screening. For example, organoids harbouring *KRAS* mutations showed resistance to afatinib and cetuximab, while only two out of 10 *KRAS* wild-type organoid were insensitive to cetuximab [86]. In another study, therapy response of 23 CRCs in clinical trials was compared to that of PDOs. The group found 93% specificity, 100% sensitivity, 88% positive predictive value, and 100% negative predictive value in predicting response to targeted agents or chemotherapy in CRC patients [89]. Interestingly, PDOs have also been utilised to monitor the effect of radiotherapy, whereby PDOs are exposed to such treatment through an irradiator [91, 92]. It should be noted that there have also been times were patients who received PDOs informed therapy did not have any clinical benefit, as discussed in Ooft et al.'s [93] study. Considering all these studies, together with others also discussed in recent reviews by Furbo et al. [91] and Flood et al. [94], it is clearly evident that PDOs can be exploited for therapy analysis, to stimulate cancer behaviour *ex vivo* and incorporate molecular pathology in the verdict process of clinical trials.

4.2 Organoid limitations

Despite being among one of the most reliable models currently available to understand and predict treatment response, use of organoids also has its limitations.

The success rate of PDOs is not only affected by intrinsic experimental difficulties, including bacterial contamination and small tissue sample sizes, but it is also dependent on the culturing medium selected and the characteristics of the tumour (subtypes and mutations) [17]. Additionally, culturing of PDOs can at times be difficult, especially from patients having mucinous tumours, MSI tumours, poorly differentiated, and tumours bearing the BRAF gene mutation [95]. This suggests that patients having any of these characteristics are less prone to be contenders for *ex-vivo* drug testing under standard culturing conditions. No standardised culturing methodologies exist, and the culturing medium used can vary between one organoid and the next, thus experimental variation arises [94]. In addition to the culturing stages, preparation of these cultures is only possible when there is access to a hospital or 'tissue network' through which patient samples can be obtained, together with the required expertise needed to prepare and maintain organoids, which can be considered as additional limitations [86]. In fact, the success rates of organoid development, even with substantial experience, is estimated to be around 70% [83]. Additionally, the lack of easy and reproducible readout approaches limits their use in high-throughput drug screening studies.

Intratumour heterogeneity is another problem which has to be considered, since at the start of culturing, PDOs present genetic stability and heterogeneity [94]. However, throughout the course of duration this cannot be predicted. During therapy, tumours change over time, thus PDOs established during one interval only represent that specific tumour at the time of culturing [17]. Furthermore, some organoids cannot be expanded for a long period of time, thus improvement in the cell culturing medium should be considered. Since a number of different inhibitors are generally also added throughout the culturing period, these might have a significant effect on signalling pathways and gene expression but could also alter drug sensitivity. Considering all these limitations, further effort is still needed to address these drawbacks, however specific organoids can still be effective models for monitoring and predicting tumour response to different treatments.

5. Advancements in predicting treatment response

To better understand the complex mechanisms and processes involved in CRC, research teams have started to move beyond single omics approaches and have started to integrate multi-omics approaches. This approach involves comprehensive and integrated analyses which are produced from different omics methods, such as proteomics, genomics, metabolomics, epigenomics, and transcriptomics. This multi-analysis can generate much larger datasets compared to only single analysis, thus providing more significant information on the pathophysiology of diseases. In turn, this further supports disease diagnosis, treatment administration and development. Moreover, the implementation of combining omics approaches will most likely have a bigger impact on translational studies, including tumour biology and cancer therapy [57]. As will be discussed in Section 5.2, despite multi-omics proving to be a powerful approach for molecular characterisation and discovery of novel biomarkers, this approach is impeded due to the lack of a standard workflow which can be applied to different cancer types [69]. As this field continues to advance and mature, it is highly likely that combining these different approaches will lay out records of all omics-based data as a whole, which will help provide more significant information at a molecular level for discovering novel predictive biomarkers.

The past and ongoing advances in omics tools have allowed systematic and extensive identification of molecular markers in CRC [58, 69]. Moreover, the involvement of PDOs in both proteomics, and other omics techniques, has slowly started to be implemented throughout the last few years. In relation to CRC, use of PDOs together with the different omics techniques has only been slightly investigated, as will be discussed in the coming sections. A look into the challenges currently being faced in multi-omics in relation to treatment prediction, together with potential future ideas to be considered in this field will also be discussed.

5.1 Combining proteomics and organoids for treatment response

With the recent advancements made in culturing PDOs for use in precision medicine, combining organoids and proteomics together would become valuable for quantifying protein expression changes, thus identifying novel signalling pathways, and suitable biomarkers for better understanding therapeutic response [62]. As of yet, published data tackling the topic of 'PDOs and proteomics as tools for treatment prediction in CRC' has been very limited, as to our knowledge, only one study has been reported to date in relation to this matter. Schumacher et al. [96] made use of well-characterised CRC organoids and targeted proteomics to investigate the effect of tumour heterogeneity on the KRAS/MAPK-signalling pathway and the effects of treatment by inhibitors targeting EGFR and downstream effectors. Their data showed that heterogeneity presented variable response to EGFR inhibition. These findings could help in improving preclinical assessment of individual tumours by modelling heterogeneity in cultures, to better comprehend therapeutic failure in clinical situations and to improve therapy response prediction [96].

Despite only one study highlighting the potential of combining proteomics and PDOs for analysis of treatment response, this should further encourage other research groups to make use of such an approach in their research interest. This is because proteomic data will further facilitate the mechanistic understanding of differences observed in PDOs treated with various forms of therapy. As discussed in Section 3.2, proteomics together with cell lines have been used to investigate treatment response. However, it is time to replicate such analysis but through the use of PDOs to determine whether the same outcome can be reproduced or not, considering the differences between the two forms of culturing. Moreover, the data collected through PDOs should be of more significance since they provide a better representation of the atypical *in vivo* environment. Another benefit which comes with utilising organoids for treatment response through proteomic analysis is that non-cancerous organoids can also be established. This permits comparison between healthy and tumour proteomes, something which is not possible with either spheroid cultures, or 2D cell cultures [80]. However, it also provides information on whether the therapy being tested is harmful to healthy organoids as well.

Analysis can also be slightly hindered when combining PDOs and proteomics together. One of the main issues is the supporting medium in which the PDOs are generally cultured, that being Matrigel. As discussed in Section 4, since this matrix is composed of several growth factors which are needed to maintain the organoids in culture, this can hamper LC-MS/MS identification of peptides through ion suppression effects [97]. Furthermore, since the matrix is also composed of several proteins, the MS data collected contains a higher background of unwanted peptides within the sample, thus resulting in less identification of organoid proteins [98]. To eliminate such background, one would have to run a sample of matrigel on its own.

Apart from PDOs and proteomics being combined together to understand and predict CRC treatment response, these two approaches have previously been applied to study other biological characteristics, such as protein abundance, signalling pathway analysis, heterogeneity, PTMs, protein localisation and protein–protein interactions [62, 96, 99–101]. Overall, collection of proteomics data from CRC PDOs has been limited and has not been explored enough yet, thus this opens avenues for more novel development in the coming future, especially with respect to predicting treatment response.

5.2 Challenges and future prospects

Further understanding CRC progression, as well as identifying potential predictive biomarkers can refine therapy administration and patient care. The ongoing advancements being made through the different omics approaches will enable a more precise treatment prediction, especially if the use of PDOs is further implemented in this field. Logically, when comparing the different omics approaches, particularly transcriptomics and proteomics, the latter is more suitable for novel therapy strategies since most protein-based biomarkers depend on the dysregulated protein signalling pathways and their respective PTMs. The proteome provides much more information on the functional state of the cells and tissues over a longer period of time. Proteome profiling of several dysregulated cell signalling cascades are anticipated to provide a better prediction on the behaviour of the disease when compared to single pathway investigations. Further implementing multi-omics studies will improve our understanding of not only treatment outcomes, but cancer related research as a whole. Ideally, different omics approaches should also start being implemented together when using CRC PDOs to understand and predict treatment response. Utilising more than one omics approach and PDOs to understand specific biological characteristics has slowly started being introduced, based on current published data [96, 100, 101].

Another way by which treatment response could be studied is through the use of array-based proteomic platforms, such as the use of peptide or protein arrays. Similar to MS approaches, this technique can provide multiplexing and sensitive analysis, however through the use of lower amounts of sample. Using minimal amounts of patient samples would be of significant benefit in a clinical setting. Additionally, such techniques can be advantageous in situations where MS analysis is not readily available, since these offer a cheaper yet reliable alternative. The use of protein and peptide arrays has shown promising results in disease biomarker discovery with different platforms [56, 69] being readily available for screening aberrant protein expression, including enzymes. In fact, such arrays have shown potential in monitoring treatment response by targeting specific PTMs and monitoring enzyme activity, with most of the currently published studies focusing on phosphorylation and kinase enzymes [102–104]. Most of these studies made use of either cell lines or patient tissues samples, however to our knowledge there have not been any published reports which made use of this technique to predict treatment in CRC through PTMs or enzyme activity. Moreover, the enzyme activity analysis of cell lysates collected from pre- and post-treated PDOs has not been reported, thus it could be a possible investigation in the coming future. Considering the positive results obtained it is expected that this same approach is to be applied to other PTMs and enzymes such as methylation and methyltransferase enzymes, which is something currently being investigated by our group.

Ideally, more focus is given to precision oncology or precision medicine, whose objective is to make use of molecular features and markers within an individual tumour to guide in therapy selection [63, 105]. This field focuses on selecting therapy based on genomic alterations, however the patient generally does not respond to the treatment selected based on genomics or responds throughout the early stages but then leads to relapse and resistance. By now, it has become evident that biological complexities which control drug response do not only depend on genomics data alone, but additional evidence is needed to fully unlock the potential of this field in predicting treatment response. As discussed in this chapter, proteomics-based data has been underutilised in this field, however the National Cancer Institute's Clinical Proteomic Tumour Analysis Consortium (CPTAC) have now started to combine proteomics data with information retrieved through transcriptomics profiling and genomics [70, 105, 106]. This is referred to proteogenomics, which provides functional contexts to explain and compare genomic and transcriptomic alterations in relation to proteomics data collected from MS, which in turn also improves the detection of proteins variants within a sample [59, 105, 107]. Moreover, the benefits arising through this field are manifold, as well reviewed by Sheynkman et al. [107]. Despite these advantages, drawbacks are also inherently present, mainly because of false positives and false negatives, difficulty in detecting low abundance or novel peptides and the need for bioinformatics tools to analyse such large data sets [107]. Protein variants discovered through proteogenomics might be potential biomarkers for specific cancer types, which can assist in identifying therapeutic targets [59]. Incorporating proteogenomic analysis will open up new avenues for biological discoveries and it will most certainly lead to a vast range of opportunities for the identification of novel therapeutic targets. In the context of CRC, proteogenomics has been reported to have been utilised to characterise and subtype this tumour [108, 109] and to predicting treatment sensitivity [63, 106].

One of the main problems with applying multi-omics approaches to PDO-based investigations, is the need for a substantial amount of cellular material, which is not always possible due to minimal patient samples. Besides, the general challenge for researchers performing omics analyses for therapeutic application is the large data sets which arise from any of the omics approaches. Proper data mining tools are needed to analyse not only proteomics data but combined omics data as a whole, since this a challenge for everyone. As more data is collected from different (1) sample types, (2) time points, (3) drugs, (4) patients, and so forth, integrating all this data together will continue to be challenging and remains the limiting step when it comes to understanding biomarkers and their potential in predicting treatment response in patients. Thus, computational technologies (Bioinformatics) are strongly needed in order to combine proteomics data with that derived from other omics techniques. Such bioinformatic tools can be considered a major backbone in generating a biologically relevant output. The problem with these tools is that high false discovery rates are generally obtained, especially when PTMs are involved, since high specificity and sensitivity is difficult to achieve. Some research groups have opted to design in-house prediction tools to verify the data analysis collected through the use of positive data sets, however these tools generally treat any other datasets as negative tools, thus reducing the prediction accuracy [59]. Furthermore, real-time analysis of proteomics data is required in order to increase the clinical applicability of proteomics and improve patient outcome. Moreover, combining and integrating proteomic real-time analysis with other omics technologies will further improve the clinical application of advanced technologies and improve patient outcome. Combining multi-omics data is not an easy feat, but nevertheless the goals are: (1) to develop new and improve current bioinformatic tools to combine such data, and (2) to maintain and continually update the available open access resources, such as the Human Protein Atlas [110] and the Reactome Project [111].

There have been various reports which made use of proteomics or multi-omics to analyse the drug response relationship in CRC cell lines, and there is enough evidence which demonstrates the benefits and limitations of cell lines as models of primary diseases [70]. However, controversy persists since cell lines are not a good representative for primary tumours, thus more research teams should implement the use of PDOs for not only CRC therapy prediction, but cancer treatment prediction in general. Additionally, it is still unclear whether cell lines are representative of primary tumours at a proteomic level, and to what degree molecular programs and proteogenomic connections are sustained under *in vitro* conditions. The significance of proteomic data as a predictor of anti-cancer therapy response in contrast to transcriptomics and genomics has not been systematically studied [70].

It is worth mentioning that development of sensitive and powerful methods in the field of proteomics are constantly being pioneered so as to overcome the challenges faced when analysing lesser amounts of specific protein markers of interest. It is strongly believed that these advancements will continue to promote proteomic studies on predictive biomarkers in CRC. In turn, any future data collected can further support the current approaches for predicting treatment support.

6. Conclusions

Survival rate of patients with advanced CRC has significantly improved throughout the years due to the introduction of chemotherapeutics, targeted therapies, and the combination of multidisciplinary techniques. Even though CRC molecular subtypes and classifications have assisted in the selection of the proper therapy to improve the overall patient outcome, the downside is that tumour heterogeneity is not considered. Despite the drawbacks and limitations encountered with these subtypes and classifications, more advanced approaches have now started to be implemented to overcome such difficulties.

PDOs have shown to be a more reliable and suitable model to study CRC treatment response, when compared to the commonly used cell lines. However, given the small number of studies conducted and published, many issues remain unanswered. The accumulation of studies regarding the predictive potential of PDOs in personalised medicine will definitely determine their ultimate relevance in the near future.

The ongoing progress of proteomics has presented new insights to the therapeutic field. New technologies and different approaches which are being developed have offered a different alternative through which the search for predictive biomarkers in CRC can be achieved. With further advances in proteomic technologies and a greater push for their application in clinical proteomics, the prospective benefits for cancer patients will concomitantly increase. Proteomics, along with other omics approaches have ushered CRC PDOs research into a new era, generating loads of novel information, which is sometimes at a pace too fast for proper validation and evaluation. The development of computational technologies through which data from different omics approached can be combined, validated and analysed will hopefully further strengthen our understanding of CRC, which will in turn help in better predicting and selecting the right treatment to administer.

Acknowledgements

This research was financed by the Malta Council for Science & Technology, for and on behalf of the Foundation for Science and Technology, through the FUSION: R&I Technology Development Programme.

Conflict of interest

"The authors declare no conflict of interest."

Author details

Isaac Micallef and Byron Baron*
Centre for Molecular Medicine and Biobanking, University of Malta, Msida, Malta

*Address all correspondence to: byron.baron@um.edu.mt

References

[1] Sung H, Ferlay J, Siegel RL, Laversanne M, Soerjomataram I, Jemal A, et al. Global cancer statistics 2020: GLOBOCAN estimates of incidence and mortality worldwide for 36 cancers in 185 countries. CA: A Cancer Journal for Clinicians. 2021;**71**(3): 209-249. DOI: 10.3322/caac.21660

[2] Nguyen HT, Duong HQ. The molecular characteristics of colorectal cancer: Implications for diagnosis and therapy. Oncology Letters. 2018;**16**(1): 9-18. DOI: 10.3892/ol.2018.8679

[3] Centelles JJ. General aspects of colorectal cancer. ISRN Oncology. 2012;**2012**:139268. DOI: 10.5402/2012/139268

[4] Daaboul HE, El-Sibai M. Treatment strategies in colorectal cancer. In: Chen J, editor. Colorectal Cancer—Diagnosis, Screening and Management [Internet]. London: IntechOpen; 2017. DOI: 10.5772/intechopen.71620

[5] Briffa R, Langdon SP, Grech G, Harrison DJ. Acquired and intrinsic resistance to colorectal cancer treatment. In: Chen J, editor. Colorectal Cancer—Diagnosis, Screening and Management [Internet]. London: IntechOpen; 2017. pp. 57-81. DOI: 10.5772/intechopen.70781

[6] Micallef I, Baron B. The mechanistic roles of ncRNAs in promoting and supporting chemoresistance of colorectal cancer. Non-coding RNA. 2021;**7**(2):24. DOI: 10.3390/ncrna7020024

[7] Kurter H, Yeşil J, Daskin E, Koçal GC, Ellidokuz H, Başbinar Y. Drug resistance mechanisms on colorectal cancer. Journal of Basic and Clinical Health Sciences. 2021;**5**(1):88-93. DOI: 10.30621/jbachs.869310

[8] Ivanov K, Kolev N, Shterev I, Tonev A, ValentinIgnatov V, Bojkov V, et al. Adjuvant treatment in colorectal cancer. In: Khan J, editor. Colorectal Cancer—Surgery, Diagnostics and Treatment [Internet]. London: IntechOpen; 2014. pp. 305-328. DOI: 10.5772/56914

[9] Luo L, Ma Y, Zheng Y, Su J, Huang G. Application progress of organoids in colorectal cancer. Frontiers in Cell and Developmental Biology. 2022;**10**:815067. DOI: 10.3389/fcell.2022.815067

[10] Martins BA, De Bulhões GF, Cavalcanti IN, Martins MM, De Oliveira PG, Martins AM. Biomarkers in colorectal cancer: The role of translational proteomics research. Frontiers in Oncology. 2019;**9**:1284. DOI: 10.3389/fonc.2019.01284

[11] Corbo C, Cevenini A, Salvatore F. Biomarker discovery by proteomics-based approaches for early detection and personalized medicine in colorectal cancer. PROTEOMICS–Clinical Applications. 2017;**11**(5-6):1600072. DOI: 10.1002/prca.201600072

[12] de Wit M, Fijneman RJ, Verheul HM, Meijer GA, Jimenez CR. Proteomics in colorectal cancer translational research: Biomarker discovery for clinical applications. Clinical Biochemistry. 2013;**46**(6):466-479. DOI: 10.1016/j.clinbiochem.2012.10.039

[13] Langhans SA. Three-dimensional in vitro cell culture models in drug discovery and drug repositioning. Frontiers in Pharmacology. 2018;**23**(9):6. DOI: 10.3389/fphar.2018.00006

[14] Reidy E, Leonard NA, Treacy O, Ryan AE. A 3D view of colorectal cancer

models in predicting therapeutic responses and resistance. Cancers. 2021;**13**(2):227. DOI: 10.3390/cancers13020227

[15] Gunti S, Hoke AT, Vu KP, London NR. Organoid and spheroid tumor models: Techniques and applications. Cancers. 2021;**13**(4):874. DOI: 10.3390/cancers13040874

[16] Ji DB, Wu AW. Organoid in colorectal cancer: Progress and challenges. Chinese Medical Journal. 2020;**133**(16):1971-1977. DOI: 10.1097/CM9.0000000000000882

[17] Barbáchano A, Fernández-Barral A, Bustamante-Madrid P, Prieto I, Rodríguez-Salas N, Larriba MJ, et al. Organoids and colorectal cancer. Cancers. 2021;**13**(11):2657. DOI: 10.3390/cancers13112657

[18] Baran B, Ozupek NM, Tetik NY, Acar E, Bekcioglu O, Baskin Y. Difference between left-sided and right-sided colorectal cancer: A focused review of literature. Gastroenterology Research. 2018;**11**(4):264. DOI: 10.14740/gr1062w

[19] Fearon ER, Vogelstein B. A genetic model for colorectal tumorigenesis. Cell. 1990;**61**(5):759-767. DOI: 10.1016/0092-8674(90)90186-i

[20] Inamura K. Colorectal cancers: An update on their molecular pathology. Cancers. 2018;**10**(1):26. DOI: 10.3390/cancers10010026

[21] Cervena K, Siskova A, Buchler T, Vodicka P, Vymetalkova V. Methylation-based therapies for colorectal cancer. Cell. 2020;**9**(6):1540. DOI: 10.3390/cells9061540

[22] Hong SN. Genetic and epigenetic alterations of colorectal cancer. Intestinal Research. 2018;**16**(3):327-337. DOI: 10.5217/ir.2018.16.3.327

[23] Jass JR. Classification of colorectal cancer based on correlation of clinical, morphological and molecular features. Histopathology. 2007;**50**(1):113-130. DOI: 10.1111/j.1365-2559.2006.02549.x

[24] Ogino S, Goel A. Molecular classification and correlates in colorectal cancer. The Journal of Molecular Diagnostics. 2008;**10**(1):13-27. DOI: 10.2353/jmoldx.2008.070082

[25] Cancer Genome Atlas Network. Comprehensive molecular characterization of human colon and rectal cancer. Nature. 2012;**487**(7407):330-337. DOI: 10.1038/nature11252

[26] Sadanandam A, Lyssiotis CA, Homicsko K, Collisson EA, Gibb WJ, Wullschleger S, et al. A colorectal cancer classification system that associates cellular phenotype and responses to therapy. Nature Medicine. 2013;**19**(5):619-625. DOI: 10.1038/nm.3175

[27] Phipps AI, Limburg PJ, Baron JA, Burnett-Hartman AN, Weisenberger DJ, Laird PW, et al. Association between molecular subtypes of colorectal cancer and patient survival. Gastroenterology. 2015;**148**(1):77-87. DOI: 10.1053/j.gastro.2014.09.038

[28] Fennell L, Dumenil T, Wockner L, Hartel G, Nones K, Bond C, et al. Integrative genome-scale DNA methylation analysis of a large and unselected cohort reveals 5 distinct subtypes of colorectal adenocarcinomas. Cellular and Molecular Gastroenterology and Hepatology. 2019;**8**(2):269-290. DOI: 10.1016/j.jcmgh.2019.04.002

[29] Dienstmann R, Vermeulen L, Guinney J, Kopetz S, Tejpar S, Tabernero J. Consensus molecular subtypes and the evolution of precision medicine in

colorectal cancer. Nature Reviews Cancer. 2017;**17**(2):79-92. DOI: 10.1038/nrc.2016.126

[30] Guinney J, Dienstmann R, Wang X, De Reynies A, Schlicker A, Soneson C, et al. The consensus molecular subtypes of colorectal cancer. Nature Medicine. 2015;**21**(11):1350-1356. DOI: 10.1038/nm.3967

[31] Tong GJ, Zhang GY, Liu J, Zheng ZZ, Chen Y, Niu PP, et al. Comparison of the eighth version of the American Joint Committee on Cancer manual to the seventh version for colorectal cancer: A retrospective review of our data. World Journal of Clinical Oncology. 2018;**9**(7):148-161. DOI: 10.5306/wjco.v9.i7.148

[32] Dukes CE. The classification of cancer of the rectum. The Journal of Pathology and Bacteriology. 1932;**35**(3):323-332. DOI: 10.1002/path.1700350303

[33] Marzouk O, Schofield J. Review of histopathological and molecular prognostic features in colorectal cancer. Cancers. 2011;**3**(2):2767-2810. DOI: 10.3390/cancers3022767

[34] Akkoca AN, Yanık S, Özdemir ZT, Cihan FG, Sayar S, Cincin TG, et al. TNM and modified Dukes staging along with the demographic characteristics of patients with colorectal carcinoma. International Journal of Clinical and Experimental Medicine. 2014;**7**(9):2828-2835

[35] Tian Y, Xu T, Huang J, Zhang L, Xu S, Xiong B, et al. Tissue metabonomic phenotyping for diagnosis and prognosis of human colorectal cancer. Scientific Reports. 2016;**6**:20790. DOI: 10.1038/srep20790

[36] Weisenberg E. Staging-Carcinoma [Internet]. 2022. Available from: https://www.pathologyoutlines.com/topic/colontumorstaging8ed.html. [Accessed: April 30, 2022]

[37] Barresi V, Bonetti LR, Leni A, Caruso RA, Tuccari G. Histological grading in colorectal cancer: New insights and perspectives. Histology and Histopathology. 2015;**30**(9):1059-1067. DOI: 10.14670/HH-11-633

[38] Golshani G, Zhang Y. Advances in immunotherapy for colorectal cancer: A review. Therapeutic Advances in Gastroenterology. 2020;**13**:1756284820917527. DOI: 10.1177/1756284820917527

[39] Khanal N, Upadhyay S, Silberstein PT. Colorectal carcinoma and emerging targeted therapies. Federal Practitioner. 2015;**32**(Suppl 7):27S-31S

[40] Dienstmann R, Salazar R, Tabernero J. Overcoming resistance to anti-EGFR therapy in colorectal cancer. American Society of Clinical Oncology Educational Book. 2015;**35**(1):e149-e156. DOI: 10.14694/EdBook_AM.2015.35.e149

[41] Kopetz S, Desai J, Chan E, Hecht JR, O'Dwyer PJ, Maru D, et al. Phase II pilot study of vemurafenib in patients with metastatic BRAF-mutated colorectal cancer. Journal of Clinical Oncology. 2015;**33**(34):4032-4038. DOI: 10.1200/JCO.2015.63.2497

[42] Zimmer L, Barlesi F, Martinez-Garcia M, Dieras V, Schellens JH, Spano JP, et al. Phase I expansion and pharmacodynamic study of the oral MEK inhibitor RO4987655 (CH4987655) in selected patients with advanced cancer with RAS-RAF mutations. Clinical Cancer Research. 2014;**20**(16):4251-4261. DOI: 10.1158/1078-0432.CCR-14-0341

[43] Gherman A, Balacescu L, Gheorghe-Cetean S, Vlad C,

Balacescu O, Irimie A, et al. Current and new predictors for treatment response in metastatic colorectal cancer. The role of circulating miRNAs as biomarkers. International journal of molecular sciences. 2020;**21**(6):2089. DOI: 10.3390/ijms21062089

[44] Shuford RA, Cairns AL, Moaven O. Precision approaches in the management of colorectal cancer: Current evidence and latest advancements towards individualizing the treatment. Cancers. 2020;**12**(11):3481. DOI: 10.3390/cancers12113481

[45] Ross JS, Torres-Mora J, Wagle N, Jennings TA, Jones DM. Biomarker-based prediction of response to therapy for colorectal cancer: Current perspective. American Journal of Clinical Pathology. 2010;**134**(3):478-490. DOI: 10.1309/AJCP2Y8KTDPOAORH

[46] Rodrigues D, Longatto-Filho A, Martins SF. Predictive biomarkers in colorectal cancer: From the single therapeutic target to a plethora of options. BioMed Research International. 2016;**2016**:6896024. DOI: 10.1155/2016/6896024

[47] Lenz HJ, Ou FS, Venook AP, Hochster HS, Niedzwiecki D, Goldberg RM, et al. Impact of consensus molecular subtype on survival in patients with metastatic colorectal cancer: Results from CALGB/SWOG 80405 (Alliance). Journal of Clinical Oncology. 2019;**37**(22):1876-1885. DOI: 10.1200/JCO.18.02258

[48] Del Rio M, Mollevi C, Bibeau F, Vie N, Selves J, Emile JF, et al. Molecular subtypes of metastatic colorectal cancer are associated with patient response to irinotecan-based therapies. European Journal of Cancer. 2017;**76**:68-75. DOI: 10.1016/j.ejca.2017.02.003

[49] Okita A, Takahashi S, Ouchi K, Inoue M, Watanabe M, Endo M, et al. Consensus molecular subtypes classification of colorectal cancer as a predictive factor for chemotherapeutic efficacy against metastatic colorectal cancer. Oncotarget. 2018;**9**(27):18698-18711. DOI: 10.18632/oncotarget.24617

[50] Kwon Y, Park M, Jang M, Yun S, Kim WK, Kim S, et al. Prognosis of stage III colorectal carcinomas with FOLFOX adjuvant chemotherapy can be predicted by molecular subtype. Oncotarget. 2017;**8**(24):39367-39381. DOI: 10.18632/oncotarget.17023

[51] Baron B. Lysine methylation of non-histone proteins. Biochemistry and Modern Applications. 2015;**1**(1):1-2. DOI: 10.33805/2638-7735.e101

[52] Hermann J, Schurgers L, Jankowski V. Identification and characterization of post-translational modifications: Clinical implications. Molecular Aspects of Medicine. 2022;**86**:101066. DOI: 10.1016/j.mam.2022.101066

[53] Zhu G, Jin L, Sun W, Wang S, Liu N. Proteomics of post-translational modifications in colorectal cancer: Discovery of new biomarkers. Biochimica et Biophysica Acta (BBA)-Reviews on Cancer. 2022;**1877**(4):188735. DOI: 10.1016/j.bbcan.2022.188735

[54] Nanni P, Gehrig P, Schlapbach R. Mass spectrometry in proteomics: Technologies, methods, and research applications for the life sciences. Chimia. 2022;**76**(1-2). DOI: 10.2533/chimia.2022.73

[55] Ikonomou G, Samiotaki M, Panayotou G. Proteomic methodologies and their application in colorectal cancer research. Critical Reviews in Clinical Laboratory Sciences. 2009;**46**(5-6):319-342. DOI: 10.3109/10408360903375277

[56] Baron B. Application of Proteomics to Cancer Therapy. SMGEBooks; 2016

[57] Kwon YW, Jo HS, Bae S, Seo Y, Song P, Song M, et al. Application of proteomics in cancer: Recent trends and approaches for biomarkers discovery. Frontiers in Medicine. 2021;**8**:747333. DOI: 10.3389/fmed.2021.747333

[58] Wang K, Huang C, Nice EC. Proteomics, genomics and transcriptomics: Their emerging roles in the discovery and validation of colorectal cancer biomarkers. Expert Review of Proteomics. 2014;**11**(2):179-205. DOI: 10.1586/14789450.2014.894466

[59] Baron B. Comprehensive mass spectrometric investigation strategies of the human methylproteome. Journal of Proteome Data and Methods. 2021;**3**:1. DOI: 10.14889/jpdm.2021.0001

[60] Ma H, Chen G, Guo M. Mass spectrometry based translational proteomics for biomarker discovery and application in colorectal cancer. PROTEOMICS–Clinical Applications. 2016;**10**(4):503-515. DOI: 10.1002/prca.201500082

[61] Chauvin A, Boisvert FM. Clinical proteomics in colorectal cancer, a promising tool for improving personalised medicine. Proteomes. 2018;**6**(4):49. DOI: 10.3390/proteomes6040049

[62] Gonneaud A, Asselin C, Boudreau F, Boisvert FM. Phenotypic analysis of organoids by proteomics. Proteomics. 2017;**17**(20):1700023. DOI: 10.1002/pmic.201700023

[63] Zhou L, Wang K, Li Q, Nice EC, Zhang H, Huang C. Clinical proteomics-driven precision medicine for targeted cancer therapy: Current overview and future perspectives. Expert Review of Proteomics. 2016;**13**(4):367-381. DOI: 10.1586/14789450.2016.1159959

[64] Jimenez CR, Knol JC, Meijer GA, Fijneman RJ. Proteomics of colorectal cancer: Overview of discovery studies and identification of commonly identified cancer-associated proteins and candidate CRC serum markers. Journal of Proteomics. 2010;**73**(10):1873-1895. DOI: 10.1016/j.jprot.2010.06.004

[65] Barderas R, Babel I, Casal JI. Colorectal cancer proteomics, molecular characterization and biomarker discovery. PROTEOMICS–Clinical Applications. 2010;**4**(2):159-178. DOI: 10.1002/prca.200900131

[66] Baron B. The unsuccessful hunt for pancreatic cancer biomarkers—Time to search deeper in the proteome. Asian Journal of Science and Technology. 2014;**5**(12):883-891

[67] Ahn SB, Sharma S, Mohamedali A, Mahboob S, Redmond WJ, Pascovici D, et al. Potential early clinical stage colorectal cancer diagnosis using a proteomics blood test panel. Clinical Proteomics. 2019;**16**:34. DOI: 10.1186/s12014-019-9255-z

[68] Fayazfar S, Zali H, Oskouie AA, Aghdaei HA, Tavirani MR, Mojarad EN. Early diagnosis of colorectal cancer via plasma proteomic analysis of CRC and advanced adenomatous polyp. Gastroenterology and Hepatology from Bed to Bench. 2019;**12**(4):328-339

[69] Lee PY, Chin SF, Low TY, Jamal R. Probing the colorectal cancer proteome for biomarkers: Current status and perspectives. Journal of Proteomics. 2018;**187**:93-105. DOI: 10.1016/j.jprot.2018.06.014

[70] Wang J, Mouradov D, Wang X, Jorissen RN, Chambers MC,

Zimmerman LJ, et al. Colorectal cancer cell line proteomes are representative of primary tumors and predict drug sensitivity. Gastroenterology. 2017;**153**(4):1082-1095. DOI: 10.1053/j.gastro.2017.06.008

[71] Gong FM, Peng XC, Tan BX, Ge J, Chen X, Chen Y, et al. Comparative proteomic analysis of irinotecan-sensitive colorectal carcinoma cell line and its chemoresistant counterpart. Anti-Cancer Drugs. 2011;**22**(6):500-506. DOI: 10.1097/CAD.0b013e3283408596

[72] Guo J, Zhu C, Yang K, Li J, Du N, Zong M, et al. Poly (C)-binding protein 1 mediates drug resistance in colorectal cancer. Oncotarget. 2017;**8**(8):13312-13319. DOI: 10.18632/oncotarget.14516

[73] Katsila T, Juliachs M, Gregori J, Macarulla T, Villarreal L, Bardelli A, et al. Circulating pEGFR is a candidate response biomarker of cetuximab therapy in colorectal cancer. Clinical Cancer Research. 2014;**20**(24):6346-6356. DOI: 10.1158/1078-0432.CCR-14-0361

[74] Sakai A, Otani M, Miyamoto A, Yoshida H, Furuya E, Tanigawa N. Identification of phosphorylated serine-15 and-82 residues of HSPB1 in 5-fluorouracil-resistant colorectal cancer cells by proteomics. Journal of Proteomics. 2012;**75**(3):806-818. DOI: 10.1016/j.jprot.2011.09.023

[75] Li H, Lan J, Wang G, Guo K, Han C, Li X, et al. KDM4B facilitates colorectal cancer growth and glucose metabolism by stimulating TRAF6-mediated AKT activation. Journal of Experimental & Clinical Cancer Research. 2020;**39**(1):12. DOI: 10.1186/s13046-020-1522-3

[76] LaBonia GJ, Ludwig KR, Mousseau CB, Hummon AB. iTRAQ quantitative proteomic profiling and MALDI–MSI of colon cancer spheroids treated with combination chemotherapies in a 3D printed fluidic device. Analytical Chemistry. 2018;**90**(2):1423-1430. DOI: 10.1021/acs.analchem.7b04969

[77] Feist PE, Sidoli S, Liu X, Schroll MM, Rahmy S, Fujiwara R, et al. Multicellular tumor spheroids combined with mass spectrometric histone analysis to evaluate epigenetic drugs. Analytical Chemistry. 2017;**89**(5):2773-2781. DOI: 10.1021/acs.analchem.6b03602

[78] Dobi E, Monnien F, Kim S, Ivanaj A, N'Guyen T, Demarchi M, et al. Impact of STAT3 phosphorylation on the clinical effectiveness of anti-EGFR–based therapy in patients with metastatic colorectal cancer. Clinical Colorectal Cancer. 2013;**12**(1):28-36. DOI: 10.1016/j.clcc.2012.09.002

[79] Zulato E, Bergamo F, De Paoli A, Griguolo G, Esposito G, De Salvo GL, et al. Prognostic significance of AMPK activation in advanced stage colorectal cancer treated with chemotherapy plus bevacizumab. British Journal of Cancer. 2014;**111**(1):25-32. DOI: 10.1038/bjc.2014.274

[80] Lindhorst PH, Hummon AB. Proteomics of colorectal cancer: Tumors, organoids, and cell cultures—A minireview. Frontiers in Molecular Biosciences. 2020;**7**:604492. DOI: 10.3389/fmolb.2020.604492

[81] Maes E, Mertens I, Valkenborg D, Pauwels P, Rolfo C, Baggerman G. Proteomics in cancer research: Are we ready for clinical practice? Critical Reviews in Oncology/Hematology. 2015;**96**(3):437-448. DOI: 10.1016/j.critrevonc.2015.07.006

[82] Sato T, Vries RG, Snippert HJ, Van De Wetering M, Barker N, Stange DE,

et al. Single Lgr5 stem cells build crypt-villus structures in vitro without a mesenchymal niche. Nature. 2009;**459**(7244):262-265. DOI: 10.1038/nature07935

[83] Weeber F, van de Wetering M, Hoogstraat M, Dijkstra KK, Krijgsman O, Kuilman T, et al. Preserved genetic diversity in organoids cultured from biopsies of human colorectal cancer metastases. Proceedings of the National Academy of Sciences. 2015;**112**(43):13308-13311. DOI: 10.1073/pnas.1516689112

[84] Seidlitz T, Stange DE. Gastrointestinal cancer organoids—Applications in basic and translational cancer research. Experimental & Molecular Medicine. 2021;**53**(10):1459-1470. DOI: 10.1038/s12276-021-00654-3

[85] Sato T, Stange DE, Ferrante M, Vries RG, Van Es JH, Van Den Brink S, et al. Long-term expansion of epithelial organoids from human colon, adenoma, adenocarcinoma, and Barrett's epithelium. Gastroenterology. 2011;**141**(5):1762-1772. DOI: 10.1053/j.gastro.2011.07.050

[86] Van de Wetering M, Francies HE, Francis JM, Bounova G, Iorio F, Pronk A, et al. Prospective derivation of a living organoid biobank of colorectal cancer patients. Cell. 2015;**161**(4):933-945. DOI: 10.1016/j.cell.2015.03.053

[87] Cho YH, Ro EJ, Yoon JS, Mizutani T, Kang DW, Park JC, et al. 5-FU promotes stemness of colorectal cancer via p53-mediated WNT/β-catenin pathway activation. Nature Communications. 2020;**11**:5321. DOI: 10.1038/s41467-020-19173-2

[88] Engel RM, Chan WH, Nickless D, Hlavca S, Richards E, Kerr G, et al. Patient-derived colorectal cancer organoids upregulate revival stem cell marker genes following chemotherapeutic treatment. Journal of Clinical Medicine. 2020;**9**:128. DOI: 10.3390/jcm9010128

[89] Vlachogiannis G, Hedayat S, Vatsiou A, Jamin Y, Fernández-Mateos J, Khan K, et al. Patient-derived organoids model treatment response of metastatic gastrointestinal cancers. Science. 2018;**359**(6378):920-926. DOI: 10.1126/science.aao2774

[90] Narasimhan V, Wright JA, Churchill M, Wang T, Rosati R, Lannagan TR, et al. Medium-throughput drug screening of patient-derived organoids from colorectal peritoneal metastases to direct personalized therapy. Clinical Cancer Research. 2020;**26**(14):3662-3670. DOI: 10.1158/1078-0432.CCR-20-0073

[91] Furbo S, Urbano PC, Raskov HH, Troelsen JT, Kanstrup Fiehn AM, Gögenur I. Use of patient-derived organoids as a treatment selection model for colorectal cancer: A narrative review. Cancers. 2022;**14**(4):1069. DOI: 10.3390/cancers14041069

[92] Pasch CA, Favreau PF, Yueh AE, Babiarz CP, Gillette AA, Sharick JT, et al. Patient-derived cancer organoid cultures to predict sensitivity to chemotherapy and radiation. Clinical Cancer Research. 2019;**25**(17):5376-5387. DOI: 10.1158/1078-0432.CCR-18-3590

[93] Ooft SN, Weeber F, Schipper L, Dijkstra KK, McLean CM, Kaing S, et al. Prospective experimental treatment of colorectal cancer patients based on organoid drug responses. ESMO Open. 2021;**6**(3):100103. DOI: 10.1016/j.esmoop.2021.100103

[94] Flood M, Narasimhan V, Wilson K, Lim WM, Ramsay R, Michael M, et al.

Organoids as a robust preclinical model for precision medicine in colorectal cancer: A systematic review. Annals of Surgical Oncology. 2022;**29**(1):47-59. DOI: 10.1245/s10434-021-10829-x

[95] Li X, Larsson P, Ljuslinder I, Öhlund D, Myte R, Löfgren-Burström A, et al. Ex vivo organoid cultures reveal the importance of the tumor microenvironment for maintenance of colorectal cancer stem cells. Cancers. 2020;**12**(4):923. DOI: 10.3390/cancers12040923

[96] Schumacher D, Andrieux G, Boehnke K, Keil M, Silvestri A, Silvestrov M, et al. Heterogeneous pathway activation and drug response modelled in colorectal-tumor-derived 3D cultures. PLoS Genetics. 2019;**15**(3):e1008076. DOI: 10.1371/journal.pgen.1008076

[97] Abe Y, Tada A, Isoyama J, Nagayama S, Yao R, Adachi J, et al. Improved phosphoproteomic analysis for phosphosignaling and active-kinome profiling in matrigel-embedded spheroids and patient-derived organoids. Scientific Reports. 2018;**8**(1):11401. DOI: 10.1038/s41598-018-29837-1

[98] Wang M, Yu H, Zhang T, Cao L, Du Y, Xie Y, et al. In-depth comparison of matrigel dissolving methods on proteomic profiling of organoids. Molecular & Cellular Proteomics. 2022;**21**(1):100181. DOI: 10.1016/j.mcpro.2021.100181

[99] Meissner F, Geddes-McAlister J, Mann M, Bantscheff M. The emerging role of mass spectrometry-based proteomics in drug discovery. Nature Reviews Drug Discovery. 2022:1-18. DOI: 10.1038/s41573-022-00409-3

[100] Michels BE, Mosa MH, Grebbin BM, Yepes D, Darvishi T, Hausmann J, et al. Human colon organoids reveal distinct physiologic and oncogenic Wnt responses. Journal of Experimental Medicine. 2019;**216**(3):704-720. DOI: 10.1084/jem.20180823

[101] Codrich M, Dalla E, Mio C, Antoniali G, Malfatti MC, Marzinotto S, et al. Integrated multi-omics analyses on patient-derived CRC organoids highlight altered molecular pathways in colorectal cancer progression involving PTEN. Journal of Experimental & Clinical Cancer Research. 2021;**40**(1):198. DOI: 10.1186/s13046-021-01986-8

[102] Wu D, Sylvester JE, Parker LL, Zhou G, Kron SJ. Peptide reporters of kinase activity in whole cell lysates. Peptide Science. 2010;**94**(4):475-486. DOI: 10.1002/bip.21401

[103] Shigaki S, Yamaji T, Han X, Yamanouchi G, Sonoda T, Okitsu O, et al. A peptide microarray for the detection of protein kinase activity in cell lysate. Analytical Sciences. 2007;**23**(3):271-275. DOI: 10.2116/analsci.23.271

[104] Hilhorst R, Schaake E, van Pel R, Nederlof PM, Houkes L, Mommersteeg M, et al. Blind prediction of response to erlotinib in early-stage non-small cell lung cancer (NSCLC) in a neoadjuvant setting based on kinase activity profiles. Journal of Clinical Oncology. 2011;**29**(15_suppl):10521-10521. DOI: 10.1200/jco.2011.29.15_suppl.10521

[105] Lei JT, Zhang B. Proteogenomics drives therapeutic hypothesis generation for precision oncology. British Journal of Cancer. 2021;**125**(1):1-3. DOI: 10.1038/s41416-021-01346-5

[106] Vasaikar S, Huang C, Wang X, Petyuk VA, Savage SR, Wen B, et al. Proteogenomic analysis of human colon cancer reveals new therapeutic

opportunities. Cell. 2019;**177**(4): 1035-1049. DOI: 10.1016/j.cell.2019.03.030.4

[107] Sheynkman GM, Shortreed MR, Cesnik AJ, Smith LM. Proteogenomics: Integrating next-generation sequencing and mass spectrometry to characterize human proteomic variation. Annual Review of Analytical Chemistry. 2016;**9**(1):521-545. DOI: 10.1146/annurev-anchem-071015-041722

[108] Yang W, Shi J, Zhou Y, Liu T, Zhan F, Zhang K, et al. Integrating proteomics and transcriptomics for the identification of potential targets in early colorectal cancer. International Journal of Oncology. 2019;**55**(2):439-450. DOI: 10.3892/ijo.2019.4833

[109] Zhang B, Wang J, Wang X, Zhu J, Liu Q, Shi Z, et al. Proteogenomic characterization of human colon and rectal cancer. Nature. 2014;**513**:382-387. DOI: 10.1038/nature13438

[110] Uhlen M, Oksvold P, Fagerberg L, Lundberg E, Jonasson K, Forsberg M, et al. Towards a knowledge-based human protein atlas. Nature Biotechnology. 2010;**28**(12):1248-1250. DOI: 10.1038/nbt1210-1248

[111] Gillespie M, Jassal B, Stephan R, Milacic M, Rothfels K, Senff-Ribeiro A, et al. The reactome pathway knowledgebase 2022. Nucleic Acids Research. 2022;**50**(D1):D687-D692. DOI: 10.1093/nar/gkab1028

Chapter 3

Simple and Fast DNA-Based Tool to Investigate Topoisomerase 1 Activity, a Biomarker for Drug Susceptibility in Colorectal Cancer

Josephine Geertsen Keller, Kamilla Vandsø Petersen, Birgitta R. Knudsen and Cinzia Tesauro

Abstract

With the increased effort for identification of anticancer compounds, there is a growing need for tools to investigate the activity of enzyme biomarkers. Human topoisomerase 1 is the only target of the camptothecin derivatives, and the cellular drug response depends on the enzyme activity. Here we use the colon cancer cell line Caco2 to investigate the topoisomerase 1 activity using a simple and improved version of our rolling circle enhanced enzyme activity detection, the REEAD assay. We present two fast readout methods that do not require the use of specialized training or equipment. In this setup, topoisomerase 1 converts specific DNA substrates to closed circles. The circles are amplified by rolling circle amplification in the presence of biotinylated nucleotides allowing for the detection of the products using horse radish peroxidase conjugated anti-biotin antibodies. The visualization occurs by either ECL or by color development through the precipitation of the TMB onto the surface. The presented readouts allow for fast and sensitive screening of topoisomerase 1 activity in extracts from Caco2 cells, potentially enabling the patients' stratification and the prediction of the chemotherapeutic response for individualized treatment. For these reasons, we believe that the presented method would be easily adaptable to the clinical settings.

Keywords: topoisomerase 1 activity, rolling circle amplification, colorimetric readout, drug response, colon cancer

1. Introduction

Colorectal cancer is the third most common cancer worldwide with more than 1.9 million new cases in 2020 [1]. Camptothecin (CPT) is the mother compound of a class of molecules that specifically targets the Topoisomerase 1 enzyme (TOP1) [2–4]. Currently, derivatives of the camptothecin (CPTs) family such as irinotecan are in clinical use for treatment of advanced stage of colorectal malignancies [5–7].

However, despite promising results [5], only a subset of the patients respond well to CPTs-based treatment and the development of chemoresistance remains a major issue [4, 8–10]. Tumor cells are characterized by a high degree of heterogeneity not only in morphology, but also in the functionality of the cells, including the activity of intracellular enzymes [11, 12]. Hence, investigation of TOP1 activity is a good biomarker for determining the response to CPTs-based anticancer treatment.

TOP1 maintains the genomic DNA integrity by regulating the DNA topology during replication and transcription. This is achieved by introducing a transient nick in the double-stranded DNA and the formation of a DNA-TOP1 cleavage complex (TOP1cc). The TOP1 enzyme becomes covalently attached to the 3′end of the DNA, and this is followed by a rapid religation of the scissile strand. These cleavage and ligation reactions allow for the relaxation of the supercoiling state of the DNA [13]. Although the cleavage-ligation reactions are fast, CPTs are able to reversibly bind to the interface of TOP1cc and selectively inhibit the religation step of the TOP1 catalysis, thereby prolonging the half-life of TOP1cc [14]. Upon collision with the replication- or transcription machinery, TOP1cc is converted to permanent double-stranded breaks resulting in genome fragmentation, which potentially can cause cell death [15, 16]. Hence, CPTs convert the activity of TOP1 into a cell poison, explaining the direct correlation between TOP1 activity and the TOP1 susceptibility to CPTs [17–20]. Consistent with the cytotoxic effect of CPTs, high level of TOP1 activity is associated with high CPTs' sensitivity, and these drugs are indeed particularly effective on fast dividing cells, such as cancer cells, where TOP1 is generally upregulated to manage the increased number of S-phase cycles [15, 21, 22]. Therefore, common mechanisms behind chemoresistance toward CPTs include downregulation of TOP1 level [17, 19, 20, 23–28] or mutations in the TOP1 gene leaving the enzyme insensitive toward CPTs [8, 29–32]. Cancer cells are frequently observed to have an upregulated activity of TOP1 [33–35], and enzyme activity can be regulated posttranslationally and not necessarily correlate to the TOP1 protein levels in the cells [36, 37]. Hence, a central aspect in investigating biomarkers for drug resistance is the measurement of enzymatic activity rather than RNA level or protein amount alone.

Over the years, a number of assays have been developed to investigate the activity of the TOP1 enzyme [38] to allow for the enzyme mechanism to be dissected [39], to investigate the inhibition of potential new small-molecule compounds [40], or to validate TOP1 as a cancer biomarker in cell lines [41, 42]. Among the most used assays, we have the gold standard relaxation assay [43], the DNA suicide cleavage-ligation assay [44, 45], the electrophoretic mobility shift assay [46], and the *in vivo* complex of enzymes (ICE) assay [47]. These assays have been extensively used to dissect the steps of the TOP1 catalytic cycle, but they have a lot of limitations. They require either gel electrophoresis, which involves DNA intercalating agents, or highly specialized expertise and training, and they all usually perform optimally when using a large amount of purified TOP1 enzyme or cell extract. For all these reasons, these assays have been used only in research settings, making the potential of investigating TOP1 as a predictive marker for anticancer response very limited.

We have previously developed a rolling circle enhanced enzyme activity detection (REEAD) assay [48] that enables the specific detection of TOP1 activity at the single catalytic event level [49]. In the REEAD assay, the cleavage and ligation reaction of TOP1 converts a specifically designed DNA substrate to a closed circle. This reaction can either be performed in solution, where the generated DNA circles are hybridized to a glass-slide-anchored primer or directly onto the glass slide upon hybridization of the DNA substrate to the primer-coupled slide (On-slide REEAD) [50, 51]. In either case, each closed circle acts as a template for isothermal rolling circle amplification (RCA) generating ~10^3 tandem repeat rolling circle products (RCPs). These RCPs can then be detected in a fluorescent microscope at the single molecule level by hybridization to a fluorescently labeled DNA probe or by the incorporation of fluorescently labeled nucleotides during the RCA step. Using this setup, the assay proved to be highly sensitive, as each TOP1-mediated cleavage-ligation generates one closed DNA circle that results in one detectable product in the microscope, and thereby the assay is directly quantitative. For these reasons, REEAD is a powerful tool that allows the investigation of TOP1 activity in crude extract from small biological samples. Indeed, using the described REEAD setup, we have been able to measure the activity of TOP1 in biopsies from cancer patients [52], and in single cells [50, 51] and to predict the CPT cytotoxicity in cancer cell lines [42]. Moreover, REEAD allowed to measure the activity and CPT sensitivity of rare subpopulation of colon cancer cell lines, showing a high degree of chemoresistance [42, 50, 51]. Finally, we have recently developed a new REEAD-based assay, called REEAD C/L that allows for the cleavage and ligation steps of the catalytic cycle to be investigated separately [53]. This enables the identification of new small-molecule compounds as potential TOP1 poisons, which specifically inhibit the relegation step or as TOP1 catalytic inhibitors, which inhibit the DNA binding/cleavage of the enzyme catalysis.

However, both the basic REEAD setup and the REEAD C/L have some limitations. Using a fluorescently labeled probe or fluorescently labeled nucleotides requires a fluorescent microscope for the detection of the RCPs, and to use such a microscope requires specialized training. Moreover, this setup is not well adaptable to non-specialized laboratories or clinical settings. Therefore, the development of other readout methods is highly relevant.

In this chapter, we present two newly developed simple and fast readout methods for the REEAD assay that do not require the use of a fluorescent microscope. In these setups, TOP1 converts a specific DNA substrate to a closed circle, and the RCA is performed in the presence of biotinylated nucleotides. This allows for the detection *via* the two readouts, by enhanced chemiluminescence (ECL) or by color development directly onto the slide. In this way the assay becomes easy adaptable to all laboratory settings, including clinics, where a screening for the patient response to treatment can be performed with results in only few hours.

2. Results and discussion

2.1 Detection of TOP1 activity using REEAD with easy-to-perform readout formats

Here, we present alternative readout methods for the quantitative and sensitive detection of TOP1 activity using the previously described REEAD assay [48]. In the new assay setup, the fluorescent detection of TOP1 generated products has been substituted with either chemiluminescent or a colorimetric readout. The original and the modified REEAD assays are schematically depicted in **Figure 1**. The setup uses a specially designed dumbbell-shaped DNA substrate that contains a double-stranded stem and two single-stranded loops. The stem contains a TOP1 preferred cleavage site three bases upstream from the 3′ end (**Figure 1, I**). Cleavage of the substrate results in temporary covalent binding of TOP1 to the 3′-end and diffusion of the three-base fragment, allowing the 5′ hydroxyl overhang to anneal to the

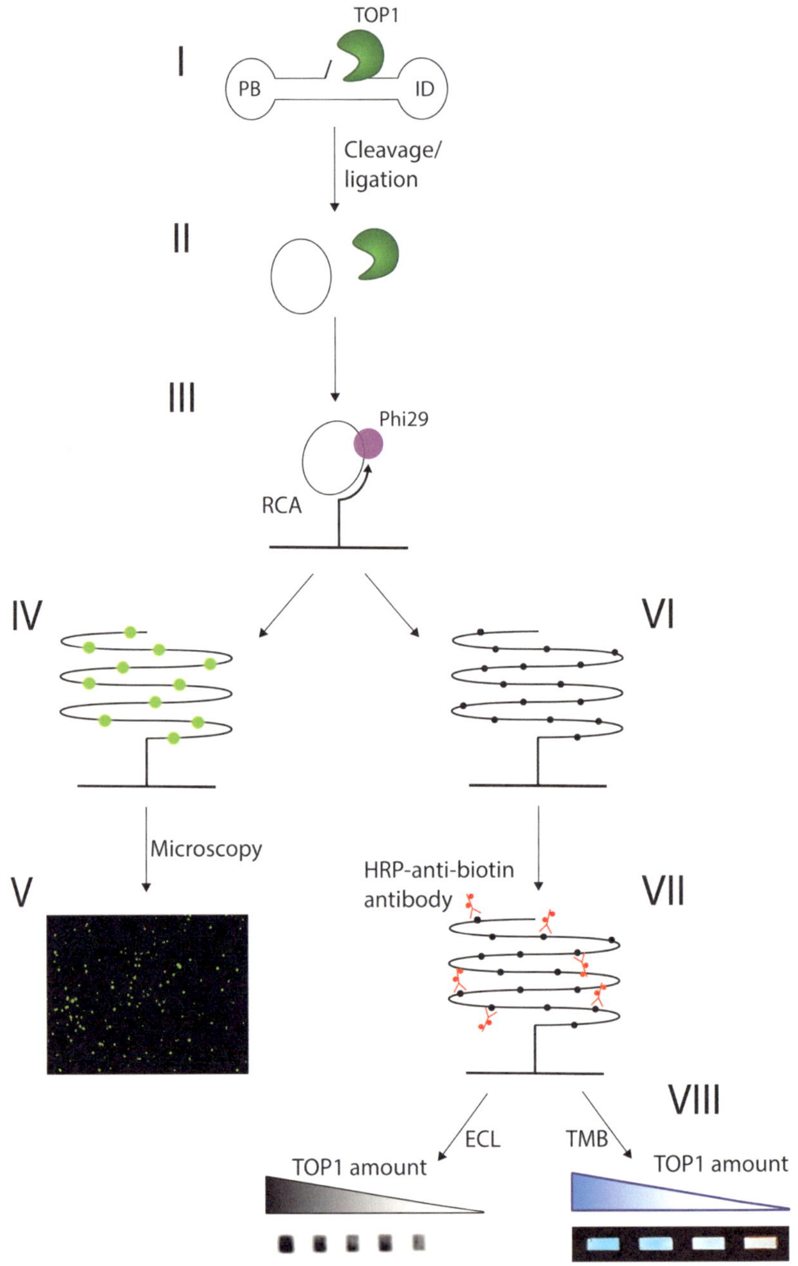

Figure 1.
Schematic representation of the REEAD assay. (I) The dumbbell-shaped substrate contains a preferred TOP1 cleavage site in the double-stranded stem, as well as a primer binding (PB) sequence and an identifier (ID) element in the two single-stranded loops. The substrate acts as a specific template for TOP1 and is upon the TOP1 cleavage and ligation reaction converted into a closed circle (II). (III) The anchored circles are amplified by rolling circle amplification (RCA) initiated by Phi29 polymerase. The RCA can be performed either by incorporation of fluorescent nucleotides (IV) or biotinylated nucleotides (VI). The fluorescent rolling circle products are visualized using a fluorescent microscope (V). The biotinylated rolling circle products are incubated with an anti-biotin antibody conjugated with horse radish peroxidase (HRP) (VII), which binds specifically to the incorporated biotin molecules. The signal development is mediated by the HRP enzyme bound to the rolling circle products. The signals are then visualized by enhanced chemiluminescence (ECL) (VIII, left) and detected in a CCD camera or using Kodak films. Alternatively, HRP catalyzes the conversion of a chromogenic substrate TMB into a blue color for a colorimetric visualization of the signals (VIII, right).

substrate, thus positioning itself for TOP1 mediated ligation. The religation reaction results in the conversion of the dumbbell substrate from an open conformation to a closed DNA molecule, named circle in the following (**Figure 1**, **II**). The closed DNA circle is hybridized to a surface-anchored oligonucleotide, which is complementary to the region in one of the single-stranded loops of the TOP1 substrate (loop PB, **Figure 1**, **I**). RCA is initiated from this surface-anchored oligonucleotide using the phi29 polymerase, which is able to perform RCA with a high degree of strand displacement (**Figure 1**, **III**). RCA generates a long tandem repeat product complementary to the initial DNA circle. In the original REEAD assay, after RCA is performed, a fluorescent probe, complementary to the other loop of the dumbbell substrate (loop ID, **Figure 1**, **I**), is hybridized to the RCPs, thus allowing for the visualization in the fluorescence microscope. Alternatively, the RCA can be carried out in the presence of fluorescently labeled nucleotides (**Figure 1**, **IV**) generating bright fluorescent dots as a product that can be visualized in the microscope. In both cases, the RCPs will appear as fluorescent dots, and given the sensitivity of the assay, each dot will correspond to one cleavage-religation reaction (**Figure 1**, **V**). Upon taking pictures of the fluorescent RCPs coupled to the slide, these dots can be counted using a software and plotted as a direct measure of the number of the TOP1-mediated cleavage-religation reactions.

To enable the visualization of the RCPs to be performed without the use of a big, expensive, and not easy to use instrument, and without the time-consuming image analysis, the RCA can be performed in the presence of biotinylated nucleotides (**Figure 1**, **VI**). This generates long tandem repeat products with several incorporated biotins. The detection of the products can then be achieved by incubation with horse radish peroxidase (HRP)-conjugated anti-biotin antibodies that will bind the biotin molecule on the RCPs (**Figure 1**, **VII**). This enables visualization in two ways by adding specific substrates for HRP. The substrate can be the components of an ECL kit resulting in a chemiluminescence readout. Alternatively, the substrate can be 3,3′,5,5′-Tetramethylbenidine (TMB) that is oxidized by HRP and converted from colorless to blue giving a colorimetric readout (**Figure 1**, **VIII**). Both detection methods enable a fast, simple, and quantitative detection of TOP1 activity.

2.2 Detection of TOP1 activity in the Caco2 colon cancer cells: direct comparison of the fluorescent, chemiluminescent, and colorimetric readouts of the REEAD assay

The well-defined colorectal cancer derived cell line Caco2 was used as a model cell line to demonstrate the functionality of the modified colorimetric/ECL REEAD assay and to investigate whether this readout method can be used instead of the fluorescence-microscope-based readout. Nuclear extract from increasing number of Caco2 cells (as indicated in **Figure 2**) was incubated with the TOP1-specific substrate and, upon hybridization to the surface-anchored primer on a glass slide, the generated closed DNA circles were amplified by RCA in the presence of fluorescently labeled nucleotides. The fluorescent RCPs were visualized using 60× magnification in a fluorescence microscope. Fifteen pictures per sample were taken and the number of RCPs was estimated by using Image J software [54]. **Figure 2A** and **B** show the results of such analysis. **Figure 2A** depicts representative microscopic images of the observed fluorescent signals in extracts from 0 to 10,000 Caco2 cells. Note that due to the high sensitivity of the assay, it was not possible to quantify the signals obtained

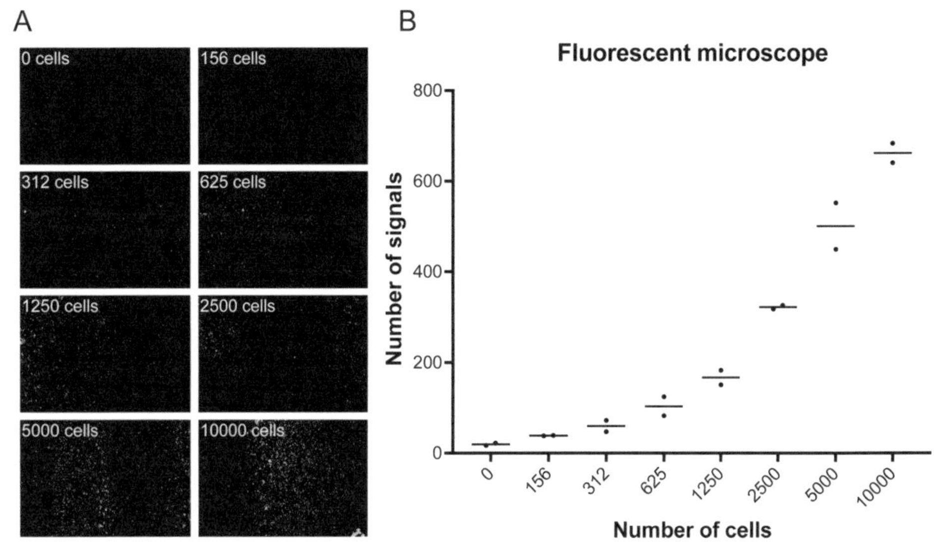

Figure 2.
Analyses of TOP1 activity using a fluorescence microscopic readout. (A) Representative microscopic images obtained when analyzing TOP1 activity in cell extracts from 156, 312, 625, 1250, 2500, 5000, or 10,000 Caco2 cells. Each green dot corresponds to a single TOP1 cleavage-ligation reaction. (B) Graphical depiction of the results obtained when analyzing the TOP1 activity from 156 to 10,000 Caco2 cells as indicated on the figure. A negative control without cell extract was included. Plotted data represent average from two independent experiments.

when using extract from >10,000 Caco2 cells, due to the abundance of signals that hinders the discrimination between the single RCPs in the image frame. **Figure 2B** shows a graphical depiction resulting from the quantification of the REEAD signals obtained from two independent experiments. As evident from the graphical depiction, the TOP1 activity increased as the amount of Caco2 cells increased. Hence, with this REEAD setup, it was possible to get a quantitative measure of the TOP1 activity in even a small number of cells, as low as 150–350 Caco2 cells. This high sensitivity of the assay, when performed in bulk, already proved the relevance of using the REEAD assay in the cancer research field as well as in cancer diagnostics and treatment-outcome prediction, where often the amount of cells in a biological sample is very limited [42, 52]. However, as described previously using the fluorescent readout requires time, training, and the use of an advanced fluorescence microscope.

To overcome the disadvantages of using a fluorescent readout in the REEAD assay, two new readout methods, chemiluminescent or colorimetric, were introduced (as schematically depicted in **Figure 1**). The closed DNA circles were obtained by incubating nuclear extracts from Caco2 cells with the TOP1-specific substrate, as described under **Figure 2**. The circles were hybridized into separated wells created onto the surface of a glass slide in a multi-well system, called Wellmaker in the following. In addition, two more sets of nuclear extraction from 0 to 40,000 Caco2 cells were included, and the TOP1 activity was then measured in four independent experiments. **Figure 3A**, left panel shows a representative image of the intensities of the biotin-containing RCPs when visualized using ECL. The quantitative depiction in **Figure 3A**, right panel, indicates a linear relationship between TOP1 activity and the increasing number of Caco2 cells. Similar results were obtained using the colorimetric readout with a TMB substrate that can be converted into an insoluble form that precipitates onto the slide upon HRP-mediated oxidation, as shown in **Figure 3B**.

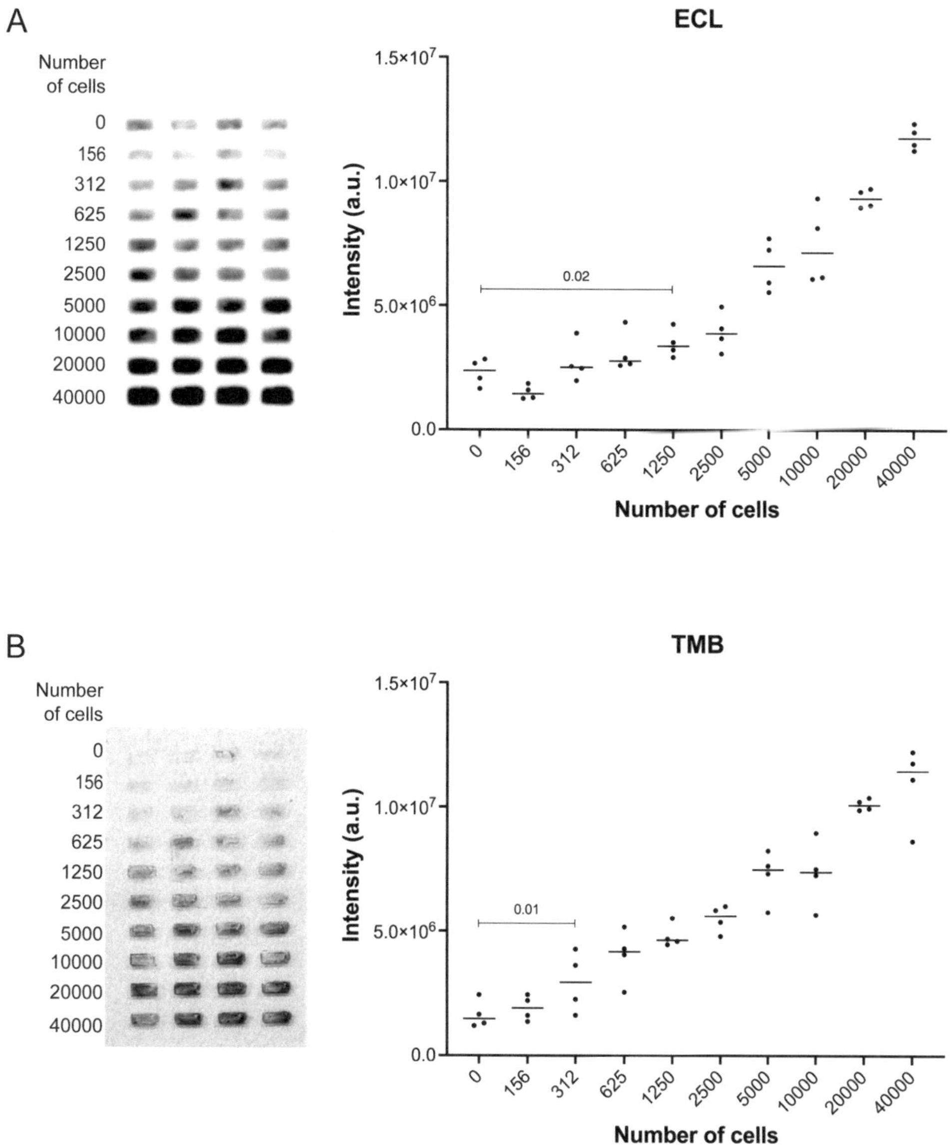

Figure 3.
Analyses of TOP1 activity using the chemiluminescent and colorimetric readout. (A) Left panel: Image obtained after measuring TOP1 activity in Caco2 cells using the ECL readout REEAD. The number of cells in each sample is indicated to the left of the image. Right panel: Graphical depiction of the results obtained when analyzing the TOP1 activity from 156 to 40,000 Caco2 cells as indicated on the figure. A negative control without cell extract was included. Plotted data represent average from three independent experiments. Welch's t-test, $p = 0.02$. a.u: arbitrary units. (B) Same as A, except that TMB was used instead of ECL. Plotted data represent average from three independent experiments. Welch's t-test, $p = 0.01$. a.u: arbitrary units.

This makes the RCPs permanently colored and visible to the naked eye. In both the ECL and the TMB readouts, the quantification can easily be performed by acquiring a picture with a CCD or a smartphone camera. Then, the Image J software can be used to determine the intensity of the rectangular-shaped areas of the slide, which correlate with the number of RCPs and in turn with the cleavage-ligation activity of

TOP1 in the cell extracts. As evident form **Figure 3**, both readouts allowed detection of TOP1 activity with a detection limit around 1000 cells for the ECL and around 300 cells for the TMB. When using the ECL-based readout (**Figure 3A**), it is evident that a higher number of cells is required to be able to detect the TOP1 activity as compared with the fluorescent readout (**Figure 2**). However, the ECL-based readout can easily be developed using chemiluminescent developer solutions and detected either by a CCD camera or by using X-rays films (such as Kodak) in a darkroom. Strikingly, the TMB-based readout resembled that of the fluorescence microscope-based readout, with a comparable detection limit of 312 Caco2 cells, as indicated in **Figure 3B**. Another advantage of the TMB-based readout is that it does not require any specific equipment, and it can hence be implicated in any relevant setting. In conclusion, both the colorimetric and chemiluminescent readout methods are excellent alternatives to fluorescence in the detection of TOP1 activity using the REEAD assay. Furthermore, these readout methods make the REEAD assay usable to any relevant setting.

3. Conclusion

Chemotherapy is currently one of the most common treatment methods for colorectal cancers [55]. Frequently, treatment fails because of chemoresistance onset or due to poor prediction of the chemotherapy response. Especially for the most advanced stage of colorectal cancer, TOP1 has proved to be one of the best biomarkers and targets of chemotherapy [7, 56] thanks to the well-known and clinically used TOP1 poisons, CPTs. For instance, a study reported a borderline association between increased TOP1 gene-copy number and objective response to irinotecan [57]. This is in agreement with a previous clinical trial (FOCUS) where a significant association between immune-histochemistry-based assessment of TOP1 protein level and response to Irinotecan was reported [58]. However, a subsequent study from the same group (FOCUS3) and a large prospective trial (CAIRO) failed to confirm this findings [59, 60]. Indeed, in the clinical settings often it is the level of DNA-RNA or amount of the TOP1 that is measured, even though it is the TOP1 activity that determines the effect of an inhibitor.

In the case of TOP1, multiple factors can influence the activity and the drug sensitivity in the patients, and for this reason there is an increasing need of tools that allow the measure of TOP1 activity in samples with few hundreds of cells.

In this chapter, we described two alternative readout formats of the highly sensitive and fast, fluorescence-microscope-based REEAD assay, which has single-event sensitivity and recently proved to allow measurement of TOP1 activity in few cells, even a single cell [50, 51]. Even with such a great detection limit, the REEAD has the limitation of the need for skilled personnel and time-consuming image acquisition and analysis. For these reasons, the presented ECL and colorimetric readouts provide excellent alternatives. Both methods are fast, simple, and do not require expensive equipment or trained technicians. Especially the TMB-based method provides an excellent alternative as the limit of detection even resembles the very sensitive fluorescent readout. This modified REEAD assay provides a great platform for a fast and simple detection of TOP1 activity and for using TOP1 as a biomarker for drug susceptibility in cancer cells isolated from colorectal cancer patients. We believe that the presented results may pave the road for the use of the REEAD assay in the clinical setting for the identification of the best outcome for colon cancer patient treatment with CPTs.

4. Material and methods

4.1 Materials

4.1.1 Oligonucleotides

All oligonucleotides for construction of the TOP1-specific REEAD substate and the REEAD primer were synthesized by Merck Life Science A/S, Søborg, Denmark. The sequences of the oligonucleotides were as follows:

5′-amine REEAD primer: 5′-/5AmMC6/CCAACCAACCAACCAAGGAGCCAAA CATGTGCATTGAGG

TOP1 dumbbell substrate:
5′-AGAAAAATTTTTAAAAAAACTGTGAAGATCGCTTATTTTTTTAAAAATTTTTCT AAGTCTTTTAGATCCCTCAATGCACATGTTTGGCTCCGATCTAAAAGACTTAGA

4.1.2 Reagents

CodeLink HD Activated slides (#DHD1-0023) and BioFX TMB enhanced one compound HRP (ESPM-0100-01) were from SurModics and the custom silicon isolator grids were from Grace-Biolabs. Vectashield without DAPI (#H-1000) was from Vector Laboratories. ATTO-488 dUTP (#95387) and biotin-16-dCTP (NU-809-BIO16L) were from Jena Bioscience. Anti-Biotin HRP conjugated antibody (#A4541) was from Merck, and ECL mixture (#RPN2236) was from Cytiva. The synthetic gene of the phi29 polymerase was from GenScript, and the GST Gravitrap columns (#28952360) were from GE Healthcare.

4.2 Methods

4.2.1 Cell culture

Caco2 cells were cultured in MEM supplemented with 20% FBS, 1% non-essential amino acids, 1% penicillin-streptomycin. Cells were incubated in a humidified incubator (5% CO_2/95% air atmosphere) at 37°C and harvested by trypsin treatment. Fresh cell pellets were used for all analyses.

4.2.2 Phi29 purification

The synthetic gene of the phi29 polymerase was purchased from GenScript and cloned into the pGEX vector resulting in a recombinant N-term GST-tagged phi29 Polymerase expression plasmid. *E. coli* competent cells BL21 (Promega) were transformed with the plasmid and grown in 2xTY media supplemented with 100 μg/ml of ampicillin. Expression of the fusion protein was induced in log phase cells at OD_{600} = 0.8, by addition of 1 mM isopropyl b-D-1-thiogalactopyranoside at 37°C for 2 h. Cells were harvested after induction and resuspended in sonication buffer (50 mM Tris-HCL pH 7.5, 2.5 M NaCl, 1 mM EDTA, 1 mM DTT, 10 mg/ml of Lysozyme). Following 1 h of incubation on ice, the cells were then lysed by freezing and thawing in liquid N_2 followed by sonication. After centrifugation, the lysate was mixed with 4% Streptomycin Sulfate for 1 h at 4°C. The insoluble particles were removed by centrifugation and the lysate was filtered by using a 0.45 μm filter. The lysate was loaded onto a pre-equilibrated GST Gravitrap column (GE Healthcare) following manufacturer's instructions. The column was washed in 10-time volumes of sonication buffer. Protein was eluted in 10-time column volumes of elution buffer (10 mM Tris-HCl pH 8, 5 mM Glutathione, 500 mM NaCl) and collected in fractions. The fractions were analyzed on a protein gel. The fractions were then adjusted to 50% glycerol, 0.5% Tween20, 1 mM DTT, and 0.5% NP40 and stored at −20°C.

4.2.3 Preparation of slides

A custom-designed silicone isolator grid, the Wellmaker (Grace-bio lab, USA), was attached to the CodeLink HD slides (Surmodics, USA). The 5′-amine REEAD primer was coupled to the slides in print buffer (300 mM Na_3PO_4, pH 8) and incubated overnight in a humidity chamber with saturated NaCl. The slides were blocked in 50 mM Tris, 50 mM Tris-HCl, 50 mM Ethanolamine, pH 9 for 30 min at 50°C, and subsequently washed in 4xSSC, 0.1% SDS for 30 min at 50°C.

4.2.4 Circularization and rolling circle amplification

The circularization of the TOP1-specific dumbbell substrate was carried out by incubating a serial dilution of cell extract from Caco2 cells with 0.1 μM substrate in 10 mM Tris-HCl, pH 7.5, 5 mM EDTA, and 50 mM NaCl for 1 h at 37°C in a humidifier chamber. The circularization reaction was terminated by heat inactivation for 5 min at 95°C. Subsequently, the circles were hybridized to the primer-coupled slides for 1 h at 37°C in a humidifier chamber. The slides were washed for 1 min at room temperature in wash buffer 1 (100 mM Tris-HCl, pH 7.5, 150 mM NaCl, 0.3% SDS) followed by 1 min wash at room temperature in wash buffer 2 (100 mM Tris-HCl, pH 7.5, 150 mM NaCl, 0.05% Tween-20). Finally, the slides were dehydrated for 1 min in 70% ethanol and air-dried.

Rolling circle amplification was carried out for 2 h at 37°C in a humidifier chamber in 1× Phi29 buffer (50 mM Tris-HCl, pH 7.5, 10 mM $MgCl_2$, 10 mM $(NH_4)_2SO_4$, 4 mM DTT) supplemented with 0.2 μg/μL BSA, 100 μM dATP, 100 μM dTTP, 100 μM dGTP, 90 μM dCTP, 10 μM biotin-dCTP, and 1 unit/μL Phi29 polymerase for colorimetric readout. Alternatively, the rolling circle amplification was carried out in 1× Phi29 buffer supplemented with 0.2 μg/μL BSA, 100 μM dATP, 100 μM dCTP, 100 μM dGTP, 90 μM dTTP, 10 μM ATTO-488-dUTP, and 1 unit/μL Phi29 polymerase for fluorescent readout. The reaction was stopped by washing the slide in wash buffer 1 and 2 for 5 min, dehydrated in 70% ethanol, and air-dried.

4.2.5 Detection of rolling circle products

For the fluorescent readout, the slide was mounted with Vectashield without DAPI and visualized using a 60x objective in a fluorescent microscope (Olympus IX73). The signals detected in an average of 12 images were counted in ImageJ and plotted as mean.

Alternatively, the slide was blocked in 1xTBST (20 mM Tris-HCl pH 9, 150 mM NaCl, 0.05% Tween-20) supplemented with 5% nonfat dry milk and 5% BSA for 30 min at room temperature followed by a 2-min wash in 1xTBST. This was repeated before an incubation with 1:300 HRP conjugated anti-Biotin antibody in a 1xTBST supplemented with 5% nonfat dry milk and 5% BSA buffer for 50 min at room temperature in a humidifier chamber. The slide was washed three times for 3 min in 1xTBST buffer. The chemiluminescent detection was performed by adding 2 μL

1:1 ECL mixture and visualized in a CCD camera. The colorimetric detection was performed by incubation with 2 μL TMB for 30 min followed by 1 min wash in 70% EtOH. The slide was air-dried, and a picture of the color development was taken using the camera of a smartphone.

4.2.6 Statistical analysis

Data were analyzed using GraphPad Prism software and expressed as mean ± standard deviation.

Statistical significance between two groups was assessed with a two-tailed unpaired Student's t-test, applying Welch correction.

Acknowledgements

The authors would like to thank laboratory technician Noriko Y. Hansen (Department of Molecular Biology and Genetics, Aarhus University, 8000 Aarhus, Denmark) for technical assistance in relation to Phi29 enzyme purifications. We like to acknowledge the support from Food & Bio Cluster Denmark.

Conflicts of interests

The authors C.T. and B.R.K. declare that they are named inventors on the patent EP2022/057172 filed in the name of VPCIR Biosciences ApS. The author C.T. is employee of VPCIR Biosciences ApS. C.T. and B.R.K. are shareholders and/or share option holders. The other authors declare that they have no competing interests.

List of abbreviations

CPT	camptothecin
CPTs	CPT derivatives
ECL	enhanced chemiluminescence
HRP	horse radish peroxidase
RCA	rolling circle amplification
RCPs	rolling circle products
REEAD	rolling circle enhanced enzyme activity detection
TMB	3,3′,5,5′-Tetramethylbenidine
TOP1	topoisomerase 1
TOP1cc	topoisomerase 1-DNA cleavage complex

Author details

Josephine Geertsen Keller[1,2†], Kamilla Vandsø Petersen[1,2†], Birgitta R. Knudsen[1,3] and Cinzia Tesauro[3*]

1 Department of Molecular Biology and Genetics, Aarhus University, Aarhus C, Denmark

2 Department of Clinical Medicine, Aarhus University, Aarhus C, Denmark

3 VPCIR Bioscience ApS, Aarhus C, Denmark

*Address all correspondence to: ct@vpcir.com

† These authors contributed equally.

References

[1] WCRF International. Colorectal cancer statistics. Available from: https://www.wcrf.org/cancer-trends/colorectal-cancer-statistics.

[2] Eng WK, Faucette L, Johnson RK, Sternglanz R. Evidence that DNA topoisomerase I is necessary for the cytotoxic effects of camptothecin. Molecular Pharmacology. 1988;**34**:755-760

[3] Soret J, Gabut M, Dupon C, Kohlhagen G, Stévenin J, Pommier Y, et al. Altered serine/arginine-rich protein phosphorylation and exonic enhancer-dependent splicing in mammalian cells lacking topoisomerase I. Cancer Research. 2003;**63**(23):8203-8211

[4] Beretta GL, Gatti L, Perego P, Zaffaroni N. Camptothecin resistance in cancer: Insights into the molecular mechanisms of a DNA-damaging drug. Current Medicinal Chemistry. 2013;**20**(12):1541-1565

[5] Wolpin BM, Mayer RJ. Systemic treatment of colorectal cancer. Gastroenterology. 2008;**134**(5):1296-1310

[6] Kuipers EJ, Grady WM, Lieberman D, Seufferlein T, Sung JJ, Boelens PG, et al. Colorectal cancer. Nature Reviews. Disease Primers. 2015;**1**:15065

[7] Bailly C. Irinotecan: 25 years of cancer treatment. Pharmacological Research. 2019;**148**:104398

[8] Beretta GL, Perego P, Zunino F. Mechanisms of cellular resistance to camptothecins. Current Medicinal Chemistry. 2006;**13**(27):3191-3305

[9] Goldberg RM, Sargent DJ, Morton RF, Fuchs CS, Ramanathan RK, Williamson SK, et al. A randomized controlled trial of fluorouracil plus leucovorin, irinotecan, and oxaliplatin combinations in patients with previously untreated metastatic colorectal cancer. Journal of Clinical Oncology. 2004;**22**(1):23-30

[10] Douillard J, Cunningham D, Roth A, Navarro M, James R, Karasek P, et al. Irinotecan combined with fluorouracil compared with fluorouracil alone as first-line treatment for metastatic colorectal cancer: A multicentre randomised trial. Lancet. 2000;**355**(9209):1041-1047

[11] Hanahan D, Weinberg R, a. Hallmarks of cancer: The next generation. Cell. 2011;**144**(5):646-674

[12] Meacham CE, Morrison SJ. Tumour heterogeneity and cancer cell plasticity. Nature. 2013;**501**(7467):328-337

[13] Champoux JJ. DNA topoisomerases: Structure, function, and mechanism. Annual Review of Biochemistry. 2001;**70**(1):369-413

[14] Pommier Y. Drugging topoisomerases: Lessons and challenges. ACS Chemical Biology. 2013;**8**:82-95

[15] Pommier Y. Topoisomerase I inhibitors: Camptothecins and beyond. Nature Reviews. Cancer. 2006;**6**(10):789-802

[16] Pommier Y. DNA topoisomerase I inhibitors: Chemistry, biology, and interfacial inhibition. Chemical Reviews. 2009;**109**(7):2894-2902

[17] Roy A, Tesauro C, Frøhlich R, Hede MS, Nielsen MJ, Kjeldsen E, et al. Decreased camptothecin sensitivity of the stem-cell-like fraction of

Caco2 cells correlates with an altered phosphorylation pattern of topoisomerase I. Leng F, editor. PLoS One. 2014;**9**(6):e99628

[18] Bendixen C, Thomsen B, Alsner J, Westergaard O. Camptothecin-stabilized topoisomerase I-DNA adducts cause premature termination of transcription. Biochemistry. 1990;**29**(23):5613-5619

[19] Sugimoto Y, Tsukahara S, Oh-hara T, Isoe T, Tsuruo T. Decreased expression of DNA topoisomerase I in camptothecin-resistant tumor cell lines as determined by a monoclonal antibody. Cancer Research. 1990;**50**(21):6925-6930

[20] Burgess DJ, Doles J, Zender L, Xue W, Ma B, McCombie WR, et al. Topoisomerase levels determine chemotherapy response *in vitro* and *in vivo*. Proceedings of the National Academy of Sciences. 2008;**105**(26):9053-9058

[21] Pommier Y. DNA Topoisomerases and Cancer. Book. 2012:1-443

[22] Tesauro C, Simonsen AK, Andersen MB, Petersen KW, Kristoffersen EL, Algreen L, et al. Topoisomerase I activity and sensitivity to camptothecin in breast cancer-derived cells: A comparative study. BMC Cancer. 2019;**19**:1158

[23] Bandyopadhyay K, Gjerset RA. Protein kinase CK2 is a central regulator of topoisomerase I hyperphosphorylation and camptothecin sensitivity in cancer cell lines. Biochemistry. 2011;**50**(5):704-714

[24] Desai SD, Li TK, Rodriguez-Bauman A, Liu LF, Rubin EH. Ubiquitin/26s proteasome-mediated degradation of topoisomerase I as a resistance mechanism to camptothecin in tumor cells. Cancer Research. 2001;**61**(15):5926-5932

[25] Pommier Y. DNA topoisomerase I and II in cancer chemotherapy: Update and perspectives. Cancer Chemotherapy and Pharmacology. 1993;**32**(2):103-108

[26] Jansen WJM, Zwart B, Hulscher STM, Giaccone G, Pinedo HM, Boven E. CPT-11 in human colon-cancer cell lines and xenografts: Characterization of cellular sensitivity determinants. International Journal of Cancer. 1997;**70**(3):335-340

[27] Sorensen M, Sehested M, Jensen P. Characterisation of a human small-cell lung cancer cell line resistant to the DNA topoisomerase I-directed drug topotecan. British Journal of Cancer. 1995;**72**(2):399-404

[28] Madelaine I, Prost S, Naudin A, Riou G, Lavelle F, Riou J-F. Sequential modifications of topoisomerase I activity in a camptothecin-resistant cell line established by progressive adaptation. Biochemical Pharmacology. 1993;**45**(2):339-348

[29] Gongora C, Vezzio-Vie N, Tuduri S, Denis V, Causse A, Auzanneau C, et al. New Topoisomerase I mutations are associated with resistance to camptothecin. Molecular Cancer. 2011;**10**(1):64

[30] Tesauro C, Morozzo Della Rocca B, Ottaviani A, Coletta A, Zuccaro L, Arnò B, et al. Molecular mechanism of the camptothecin resistance of Glu710Gly topoisomerase IB mutant analyzed in vitro and in silico. Molecular Cancer. 2013;**12**(1):100

[31] Pommier Y, Pourquier P, Urasaki Y, Wu J, Laco GS. Topoisomerase I inhibitors: Selectivity and cellular resistance. Drug Resistance Updates. 1999;**2**(5):307-318

[32] Kjeldsen E, Bonven BJ, Andoh T, Ishii K, Okada K, Bolund L, et al. Characterization of a camptothecin-resistant human DNA topoisomerase I. The Journal of Biological Chemistry. 1988;**263**(8):3912-3916

[33] Gaillard H, García-Muse T, Aguilera A. Replication stress and cancer. Nature Reviews. Cancer. 2015;**15**:276-280

[34] Macheret M, Halazonetis TD. DNA replication stress as a hallmark of cancer. Annual Review of Pathology: Mechanisms of Disease. 2015;**10**:425-448

[35] Kotsantis P, Silva LM, Irmscher S, Jones RM, Folkes L, Gromak N, et al. Increased global transcription activity as a mechanism of replication stress in cancer. Nature Communications. 2016;**7**:13087

[36] Kowalska-Loth B, Girstun A, Derlacz R, Staroń K. Activation of human topoisomerase I by protein kinase CK2. Molecular Biology Reports. 2003 Jun;**30**(2):107-111

[37] Seet BT, Dikic I, Zhou MM, Pawson T. Reading protein modifications with interaction domains. Nature Reviews. Molecular Cell Biology. 2006;**7**(7):473-83

[38] Nitiss JL, Kiianitsa K, Sun Y, Nitiss KC, Maizels N. Topoisomerase assays. Current Protocols. 2021;**1**:10

[39] Frøhlich RF, Andersen FF, Westergaard O, Andersen AH, Knudsen BR. Regions within the N-terminal domain of human topoisomerase I exert important functions during strand rotation and DNA binding. Journal of Molecular Biology. 2004;**336**(1):93-103

[40] Martín-Encinas E, Selas A, Tesauro C, Rubiales G, Knudsen BR, Palacios F, et al. Synthesis of novel hybrid quinolino[4,3-b][1,5] naphthyridines and quinolino[4,3-b][1,5]naphthyridin-6(5H)-one derivatives and biological evaluation as topoisomerase I inhibitors and antiproliferatives. European Journal of Medicinal Chemistry. 2020;**195**:112292

[41] Jensen NF, Agama K, Roy A, Smith DH, Pfister TD, Rømer MU, et al. Characterization of DNA topoisomerase I in three SN-38 resistant human colon cancer cell lines reveals a new pair of resistance-associated mutations. Journal of Experimental & Clinical Cancer Research. 2016;**35**(1):56

[42] Tesauro C, Keller JG, Gromova I, Gromov P, Frohlich R, Erlandsen JU, et al. Different camptothecin sensitivities in subpopulations of colon cancer cells correlate with expression of different phospho-isoforms of Topoisomerase I with different activities. Cancers (Basel). 2020;**12**(5):1240

[43] Nitiss JL, Soans E, Rogojina A, Seth A, Mishina M. Topoisomerase assays. Current Protocol Pharmacology. 2012. Chapter 3

[44] Christiansen K, Westergaard O. Characterization of intra- and intermolecular DNA ligation mediated by eukaryotic topoisomerase I. Role of bipartite DNA interaction in the ligation process. The Journal of Biological Chemistry. 1994;**269**(1):721-729

[45] Svejstrup JQ, Christiansen K, Andersen AH, Lund K, Westergaard O. Minimal DNA duplex requirements for topoisomerase I-mediated cleavage in vitro. The Journal of Biological Chemistry. 1990;**265**(21):12529-12535

[46] Tesauro C, Fiorani P, D'Annessa I, Chillemi G, Turchi G, Desideri A. Erybraedin C, a natural compound from the plant Bituminaria bituminosa, inhibits both the cleavage and religation activities of human

topoisomerase I. The Biochemical Journal. 2010;**425**(3):531-539

[47] Anand J, Sun Y, Zhao Y, Nitiss KC, Nitiss JL. Detection of topoisomerase covalent complexes in eukaryotic cells. Methods in Molecular Biology. 2018;**1703**:283-299

[48] Stougaard M, Lohmann JS, Mancino A, Celik S, Andersen FF, Koch J, et al. Single-molecule detection of human topoisomerase I cleavage-ligation activity. ACS Nano. 2009;**3**(1):223-233

[49] Proszek J, Roy A, Jakobsen AK, Frøhlich R, Knudsen BR, Stougaard M. Topoisomerase I as a biomarker: Detection of activity at the single molecule level. Sensors (Switzerland). 2014;**14**(1):1195-1207

[50] Keller JG, Tesauro C, Coletta A, Graversen AD, Ho Y-P, Kristensen P, et al. On-slide detection of enzymatic activities in selected single cells. Nanoscale. 2017;**9**(36):13546-13553

[51] Keller JG, Stougaard M, Knudsen BR. Enzymatic activity in single cells. Methods in Enzymology. 2019;**628**:43-57

[52] Jakobsen AK, Lauridsen KL, Samuel EB, Proszek J, Knudsen BR, Hager H, et al. Correlation between topoisomerase I and tyrosyl-DNA phosphodiesterase 1 activities in non-small cell lung cancer tissue. Experimental and Molecular Pathology. 2015;**99**(1):56-64

[53] Petersen KV, Selas A, Hymøller KM, Mizielinski K, Thorsager M, Stougaard M, et al. Simple and fast dna based sensor system for screening of small-molecule compounds targeting eukaryotic topoisomerase 1. Pharmaceutics. 2021;**1**:13(8)

[54] Rasband WS. ImageJ [Software]. Bethesda, Maryland, USA: U S National Institute of Health; 2015

[55] Colorectal Cancer Chemotherapy. Chemo for Colon & Rectal Cancer. Available from: https://www.cancer.org/cancer/colon-rectal-cancer/treating/chemotherapy.html

[56] Gilbert DC, Chalmers AJ, El-Khamisy SF. Topoisomerase i inhibition in colorectal cancer: Biomarkers and therapeutic targets. British Journal of Cancer. 2012;**106**(1):18-24

[57] Palshof JA, Høgdall EVS, Poulsen TS, Linnemann D, Jensen BV, Pfeiffer P, et al. Topoisomerase I copy number alterations as biomarker for irinotecan efficacy in metastatic colorectal cancer. BMC Cancer. 2017;**17**(1):48

[58] Braun MS, Richman SD, Quirke P, Daly C, Adlard JW, Elliott F, et al. Predictive biomarkers of chemotherapy efficacy in colorectal cancer: Results from the UK MRC FOCUS Trial. Journal of Clinical Oncology. 2008;**26**(16)

[59] Maughan TS, Meade AM, Adams RA, Richman SD, Butler R, Fisher D, et al. A feasibility study testing four hypotheses with phase II outcomes in advanced colorectal cancer (MRC FOCUS3): A model for randomised controlled trials in the era of personalised medicine? British Journal of Cancer. 2014;**110**(9):2178-2186

[60] Koopman M, Knijn N, Richman S, Seymour M, Quirke P, Van TH, et al. The correlation between Topoisomerase-I (Topo1) expression and outcome of treatment with capecitabine and irinotecan in advanced colorectal cancer (ACC) patients (pts) treated in the CAIRO study of the Dutch Colorectal Cancer Group (DCCG). European Journal of Cancer Supplements. 2009;**7**(2):321-322

Chapter 4

Colorectal Cancer Stages, Progress, Genetic Predisposition, and Immune Surveillance

Samaa Abdullah

Abstract

Colon cancer (CC) is highly malignant and is considered the second cause of death worldwide. However, the overall CC survival rate is improving due to the rapid development of screening tools and improved treatment options. This raised the need to develop effective approaches for medical intervention. Moreover, CC is classified into four stages: stages I, II, III, and IV. On the other hand, the driver genes played vital regulatory roles in essential pathways for cellular division, cell survival, fate, and genome stability. For example, the RAS mitogen-activated protein kinase is essential for cellular division. Additionally, carcinogenesis is linked to the mutations, which are reported in the Kirsten rat sarcoma viral oncogene homolog gene, Adenomatous Polyposis Coli gene, Tumor Protein 53 gene, and SMAD family member 4 genes, Mothers against decapentaplegic homolog 4 gene. In addition, the immune system reactions have different impacts on CC growth and management. The inflammation process is described as one of the innate responses. The inflammation process is initiated and exacerbated by various types of immune cells included the macrophages, and neutrophils for their activation, margination, extravasation, and migration to the damaged tissue. The preferred role of inflammation against cancer is at stages I and II.

Keywords: colorectal cancer, genetic predisposition, immune surveillance, oncogene, tumor suppressor gene, immunostimulatory cytokines, immune inhibitory cytokines

1. Introduction

Colon cancer (CC) is highly malignant and is considered the second cause of death worldwide. For 2018 new cases, 10% of the newly recorded cases were dead [1]. However, the overall CC survival rate is improving due to the rapid development of screening tools and improved treatment options. This raised the need to develop effective approaches for medical intervention [2]. Moreover, CC is classified into four stages: stages I, II, III, and IV (**Figure 1**). Stage I includes the cancer growth through the mucosa, invasion of the muscular, and development through the colon or rectum wall, which is not infused into nearby tissue or lymph nodes. For stage II, cancer has infused through the colon or rectum wall and grown into nearby structures. In stage III, the cancer of the colon has spread to four or more lymph nodes, which may be

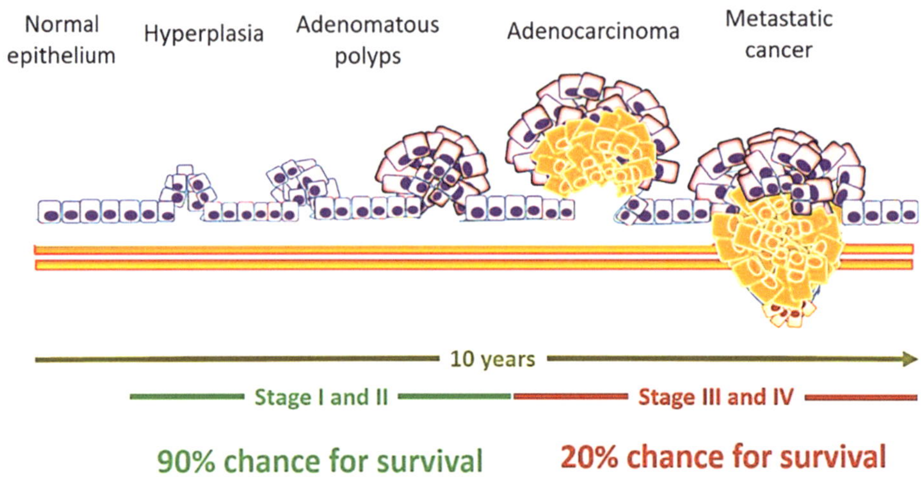

Figure 1.
Colon cancer stages, development, and survival rates [3].

metastasized to adjacent organs. Finally, cancer has spread to one or more distant organs in stage IV and may be diffused to the peritoneum [4].

According to the American Cancer Society, surgery may be the sole therapy for stage 0–I colon cancer. In most situations, this is accomplished by removing the polyp or eliminating the cancerous region with a colonoscope. However, if the malignancy is too big to be treated with local excision, a portion of the colon must be removed (partial colectomy) [5].

In stage I–II CC, on the other hand, surgery is a viable option for removing malignant tissue and adjacent lymph nodes, and it may be the only treatment required. Adjuvant chemotherapy is also suggested after surgery if the malignancy is at high risk of recurrence. 5-Fluorouracil with leucovorin, oxaliplatin, and capecitabine are the most common chemotherapeutic treatments. However, additional combinations may be employed. The typical treatment for stage II–III is a partial colectomy to remove the area of the colon with cancer as well as adjacent lymph nodes, followed by adjuvant chemotherapy. The FOLFOX (5-fluorouracil, leucovorin, and oxaliplatin), and CapeOx (capecitabine and oxaliplatin) regimens are the most often utilized adjuvant chemotherapy regimens. However, depending on their age and medical conditions, some people may be able to receive 5-Flourouracil in combination with leucovorin or capecitabine alone [6].

In stage IV, CC most commonly spreads to the liver, but it can also extend to the lungs, brain, peritoneum (the lining of the abdominal cavity), or distant lymph nodes. Surgery is usually unlikely to cure certain tumors. This will entail surgery to remove the piece of the colon harboring cancer, adjacent lymph nodes, and any regions of cancer metastasis. Following that, chemotherapy is usually administered. If the malignancy has progressed to the liver, hepatic artery infusion may be utilized in some circumstances. If the metastasis cannot be eliminated because the tumorous tissues are too big or numerous, chemotherapy may be administered prior to surgery (neoadjuvant). If the tumors diminish, surgery to remove them may be attempted. Chemotherapy may be administered again following surgery. Ablation and embolization are two alternative options for destroying liver tumors. Furthermore, chemotherapy is the primary treatment if the disease has gone too far for surgery to be effective [7].

To manage the malignancy, most stage IV patients will get chemotherapy and/or targeted treatments such as FOLFOX (leucovorin, 5-fluorouracil, and oxaliplatin "Eloxatin"), FOLFIRI (leucovorin, 5-fluorouracil, and irinotecan "Camptosar"), CAPEOX or CAPOX (capecitabine (Xeloda) and oxaliplatin), and FOLFOXIRI (leucovorin, 5-fluorouracil (leucovorin, 5-Fluorouracil, oxaliplatin, and irinotecan) [8].

Targeting medicines can be coupled with the regimens listed earlier. Bevacizumab (Avastin), ziv-aflibercept (Zaltrap), and ramucirumab (Cyramza) are drugs that target vascular endothelial growth factor (VEGF). On the other hand, cetuximab (Erbitux) and panitumumab (Vectibix) are drugs that target EGFR. 5-Fluorouracil and leucovorin with a targeted medication, capecitabine with a targeted drug, irinotecan with a targeted drug, cetuximab alone, and panitumumab alone are examples of the targeted regimens combinations with the chemotherapy. Several variables influence regimen selection, including past treatments [6].

After all, CC genetic predisposition and the host's immune responses influencing cancer growth were discussed and illustrated to understand the best management approach depending on the CC stage and pathogenesis.

2. Genetic predisposition of colon cancer

2.1 Genes involved in colon cancer expansion and prognosis

The driver genes played vital regulatory roles in essential pathways for cellular division, cell survival, fate, and genome stability. For example, the RAS mitogen-activated protein kinase (MAPK) is essential for cellular division. Additionally, carcinogenesis is linked to the mutations, which are reported in the Kirsten rat sarcoma viral oncogene homolog gene (KRAS), Adenomatous Polyposis Coli gene (APC), Tumor Protein 53 gene (P53), and SMAD family member 4 genes, Mothers against decapentaplegic homolog 4 gene (SMAD4). Additionally, epigenetics in conjunction with intestinal dysbiosis, bacterial drivers, and persistent mucosal inflammation are all contributing factors to CC [9, 10].

On the other hand, KRAS, nuclear factor-κB gene (NF-κB), signal transducer and activator of the transcription-3 gene (STAT-3), B-cell lymphoma type-2 gene (BCL-2), BCL-2-associated protein X gene (BAX), and the transforming growth factor-β gene (TGF-β) were selected in the molecular testing for their correlation in the CC predisposition and progression [9–11].

2.2 Kirsten rat sarcoma viral oncogene (KRAS)

Regarding CC, genes enrolled in cancer development are proto-oncogene (KRAS), tumor suppressor gene (P53 and APC), antiapoptotic gene (BCL-2), and proapoptotic gene (BAX) [10]. Mutations in the KRAS oncogene are common in human malignancies, notably those of the pancreas, gallbladder, bile duct, thyroid gland, and non-small cell lung cancer with CC. These mutations may influence prognosis and medication responsiveness to anticancer agents targeting the KRAS protein pathway [12].

KRAS mutations are considered an early influencer in CC that happened in 30 to 40% of patients. On the other hand, the KRAS gene activates NF-κB signaling in cancerous cells and triggers several proinflammatory mediators [9, 10, 12, 13].

The conventional first-line treatment for advanced CC is chemotherapy based on 5-fluorouracil, leucovorin, and oxaliplatin (FOLFOX). KRAS mutations, particularly

G12D, are associated with a poor response to the conventional treatment and a significant risk of recurrence. Furthermore, KRAS mutations are strong indicators of EGFR inhibitor therapy success in individuals with CC. Monoclonal antibodies targeting EGFR have been shown to assist CC patients who had failed previous treatments. Cetuximab and panitumumab are EGFR-targeting drugs used to treat KRAS mutations. LUMAKRAS™ (sotorasib), also known as AMG 510, recently received accelerated approval from the US Food and Drug Administration (FDA) for the treatment of adult patients with KRAS-G12C mutations who have received at least one prior systemic therapy [14, 15].

2.3 Adenomatous polyposis coli gene (APC)

For carcinogenesis to develop, the Adenomatous Polyposis Coli gene (APC) mutation has to occur before the KRAS mutation. Therefore, the adenoma would not progress to carcinoma if one of the previous mutations happened without the other. APC, KRAS, and P53 are considered the CC driver genes (**Figure 2**). APC and KRAS mutated as an early event in the transition from normal epithelium to adenoma. However, after mutations or epigenetic silencing, the loss of P53 function can happen as late events. Moreover, P53 mutation makes cancer cells able to invade surrounding tissues and metastasize. As a result, SMAD4 and P53 loss of functions aid for the transformation of adenoma into a carcinoma (**Figures 2** and **3**) [16, 17].

Moreover, the APC gene is the gatekeeper gene for CC. The APC mutation is considered a frameshift mutation that causes truncation of the APC protein. The APC mutation hinders it from binding β-catenin to the membrane E-cadherin complex's cytoplasmic domain. As a result, cellular damage occurs [10, 16]. The free cytoplasmic β-catenin molecules, on the other hand, migrate to the nucleus to elicit the Wnt signaling pathway and cancer cell survival. Moreover, TGF-β and β-catenin are indeed cancer resistance indicators [16, 18].

TASIN-1 (Truncated APC Selective INhibitor) is a small chemical that has just been discovered to preferentially destroy cancer cells having APC truncations. TASIN-1 can reduce tumor development of APC shortened CC cells with low toxicity in both xenograft models and a genetically modified CC animal model [19].

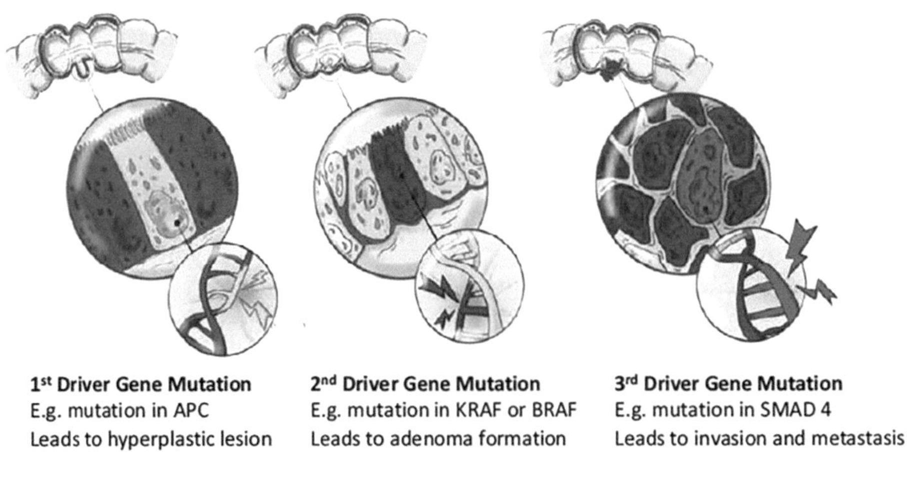

Figure 2.
Driver genes mutations of CC and the histopathological impacts [10].

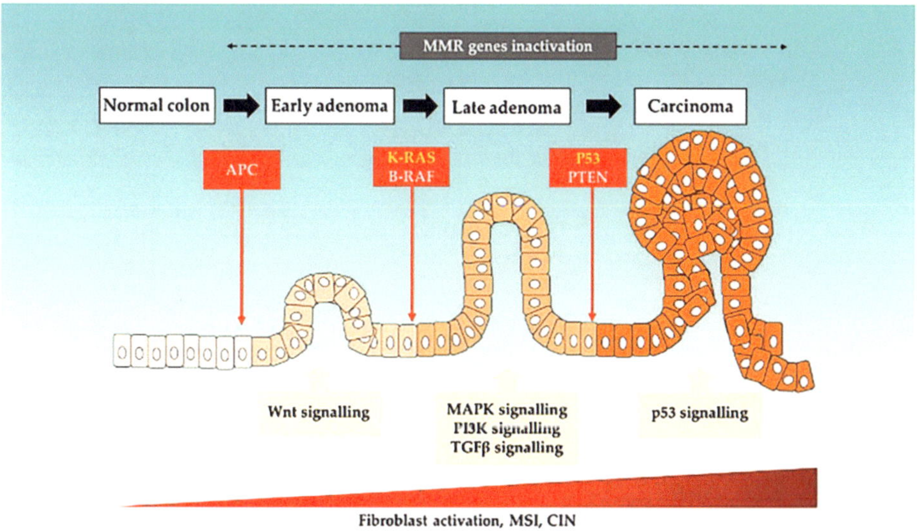

Figure 3.
Stages for CC development and the driver genetic mutation [15].

One of the most common events leading to CC transformation, as well as its aggressive and metastatic properties, is P53 tumor suppressor gene dysregulation. P53 reactivator mutant (PRIMA-1^{MET}) has been studied in Phase I/II clinical trials and has shown promising results [15, 20].

2.4 B-cell lymphoma (BCL-2) and BCL-2-associated X protein genes (BAX)

Mutations in genes controlling cell cycle checkpoint proteins (i.e. P53, BCL-2, and BAX) are the genetic drivers of CC and several types of cancers. The low level of BCL-2 expression and high level of BAX expression are correlated for better CC survival and control of cancer. The low BCL-2/BAX expression ratio leads to Cytochrome c (Cyto c) activation after external or internal stimuli. Cyto c is responsible for the Caspase family activation to trigger different cancer cells' apoptosis and phagocytosis (**Figure 4**). On the other hand, BCL-2 protein inhibits the action of the BAX protein that triggers the cancer cells' growth [21–23].

3. The influence of the host's immune responses on colon cancer growth

3.1 Cellular immune rejoinders

The immune system reactions, as innate and adaptive, have different impacts on CC growth and management. The inflammation process is described as one of the innate responses. The inflammation process is initiated and exacerbated by various types of immune cells including macrophages, neutrophils, and mast cells, for their activation, margination, extravasation, and migration to the damaged tissue [24]. The preferred role of inflammation against cancer is at stages I and II. Moreover, the inflammation role was to activate the adaptive immune cells by activating the innate system's antigen-presenting cells, such as dendritic cells. Additionally, natural killer

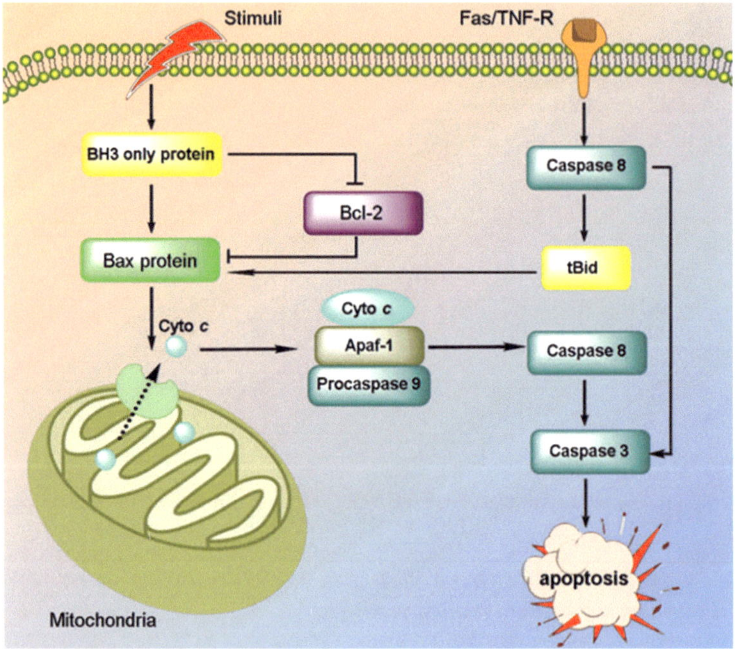

Figure 4.
The proapoptotic BAX protein and antiapoptotic BCL-2 protein signaling effects [21].

(NK) cells and macrophages of the innate system help capturing the cancer cells and releasing immunostimulatory cytokines to activate the adaptive system [25].

On the other hand, cancer is addicted to proliferative and survival signals in the cancer microenvironment as inflammation. Soluble factors, cytokines, and chemokines influence inflammation. They are secreted by cancerous cells with the innate cells recruited to the microenvironment, such as macrophages and mast cells. The depletion of mast cells or macrophages prevented the APC from mutating and preventing intestinal polyps' initiation. This confirms the role of immune cells and their soluble factors in intestinal cancer initiation and progression [22, 24, 26].

Moreover, T-lymphocytes, T-helper (TH or CD4), NK cells, and dendritic cells are associated with CC survival enhancement regarding the adaptive immune system's role in controlling CC. Additionally, cytotoxic T-lymphocytes (CTL or CD8) and TH cells enhance the cancer cells' apoptosis, engulfment, detection, and antibody production against cancer cells. Furthermore, B-cells' antibodies that target specific surface antigens are limited by the presence of the tumor-specific antigens, such as the carcinoembryonic antigen, to capture it by the antibodies and enhance the cancer cells removal [27].

In terms of CC immunotherapies, numerous FDA-approved vaccinations defend against viruses known to cause certain forms of cancer. Vaccination against human papillomavirus (HPV), for example, can protect against six forms of cancer, while a vaccine against hepatitis B virus (HBV) helps protect against some types of liver cancer. Unfortunately, however, there is no colorectal cancer vaccination available [28].

On the other hand, chimeric antigen receptor-T (CAR-T) cell immunotherapy is a unique technique that is genetically designed to recruit T-cells against malignant illness. CAR-T cell therapy has led to success in hematological malignancies, and it has long been advocated for solid tumors such as colorectal cancer (CC). However, this strategy did not meet expectations given solid tumors' intrinsic obstacles provided to CAR-T cells, owing to a lack of tumor-restricted antigens and undesirable adverse effects. New techniques, such as designing T-cells with immune-activating molecules, localized delivery of T-cell, bispecific T-cell engager, and combinatorial target-antigen recognition, are proposed to overcome many hurdles to ameliorate the challenging conditions of CAR-T cells in CC [29].

Furthermore, CAR-natural killer (NK) cells have received widespread interest due to their safety in clinical applications, the method for identifying cancer cells, and the quantity of clinical specimens. CAR-NK cells have been shown in preclinical and clinical trials to be capable of combating hematological malignancies as well as solid tumors such as CC. However, the use of CAR-NK cell therapy in solid tumors presents unique challenges, such as the expansion and activation of primary NK cells in vitro, the selection of CAR targets, the survival time of CAR-NK cells in vivo, NK cell storage and transportation, and the efficiency of NK cell transduction [30].

3.2 Cytokines and chemokines

Cytokines are classified into proinflammatory, immunostimulatory, and immunoinhibitory cytokines. For proinflammatory cytokines, the, interleukin (IL)-8 (chemokine), IL-1, IL-6, tumor necrosis factor (TNF)-α, and vascular endothelial growth factor (VEGF) serum levels are associated with cancer development and considered as predictive tools. Moreover, macrophages release IL-1, which contributes to fever and T-cell and macrophage activations. Furthermore, IL-6 is released by macrophages, endothelial cells, and T-cells. IL-6 inhibits the production of acute-phase proteins in the liver and promotes the proliferation of antibody-producing cells. On the other hand, IL-8 is a chemoattractant generated by macrophages that attracts immune system cells and phagocytes to the site of inflammation. Finally, TNF-α is mainly secreted from macrophages and TH cells, which has a cytotoxic reaction against cancer cells and enhances the activity of phagocytic cells. As a result, TNF-α and IL-1β are emerging as potential targets for drug candidates in anticancer therapy [24]. Furthermore, TNF-α antagonists are well studied in the rheumatoid arthritis, and IL-1β antagonists are used for inflammatory disorders characterized by excessive IL-1β production [27]. On the other hand, VEGF is secreted by the cancer cells to improve cancer cell vasculature (angiogenesis) [12].

For immune system stimulation, IL-2, IL-4, IL-5, IL-12, IL-18, and interferon (IFN)-Υ are immune-stimulatory cytokines. The immune-stimulatory cytokines activate the growth, differentiation, and maturation of CTL, TH cells, NK cells, and dendritic cells. Additionally, macrophages, lymphocytes, and NK cells produce IFN-Υ, in which IFN-Υ is significant macrophage and NK cells activator. As a result, IFN-Υ enhances major histocompatibility class I expression to activate CTLs. Moreover, IL-2 is secreted by TH cells and co-stimulates the proliferation of TH cells, CTLs, and B-cells, which activates NK cells. Additionally, IL-18 is primarily secreted by macrophages and promotes NK cells cytotoxicity as well as T-cell's IFN-Υ production. Furthermore, dendritic cells and macrophages release IL-12, which contributed to the TH-1 cell differentiation, NK cell, and T-cell activations. On the other hand, the lymphocytes and macrophages produce IL-4, which is involved in B-cell activation, differentiation of TH-2 cells, and TH-1 cells suppression. Finally, IL-5 is released by TH cells and mast cells and has the primary activity of activating and chemoattracting eosinophils [22, 31].

The immune regulatory system is activated by the secretion of IL-10 and TGF-β from the cancerous cells, tumor-associated macrophages, or immune cells, such as TH-2 cells. In addition, it enhances the activation and expression of the immune checkpoint molecules, such as cytotoxic T-lymphocyte antigen-4 and programmed cell death protein-1, which can inhibit the immune stimulatory signals activation between antigen-presenting cells and the CTLs to capture the cancer cells [31]. Moreover, IL-10 is involved in suppressing macrophage phagocytosis and B-cells' activation [11, 12, 27]. To summarize the role of cytokines and chemokines in the CC angiogenesis or immune system recognition, **Figure 5** illustrates the recently found relation between the CC and the cytokines [32].

3.3 Inflammatory signaling molecules

Proinflammatory cytokines are like TNF-α, IL-1, and IL-6, and their cell membrane receptors association influences downstream signaling factors activation. Moreover, colon cancer-associated inflammatory molecules are NF-κB and STAT-3, activated by binding the lipopolysaccharides to the toll-like receptor (TLR)-II and IV. NF-κB and STAT-3 actions enhance apoptosis of the cells and increase the expression of TNF-α, IL-1, and IL-6. However, STAT-3 and NF-κB are negatively correlated with the TGF-β release from cancer cells or with the TGF-β receptor expression on cancer cells, especially colon cancer [2, 24].

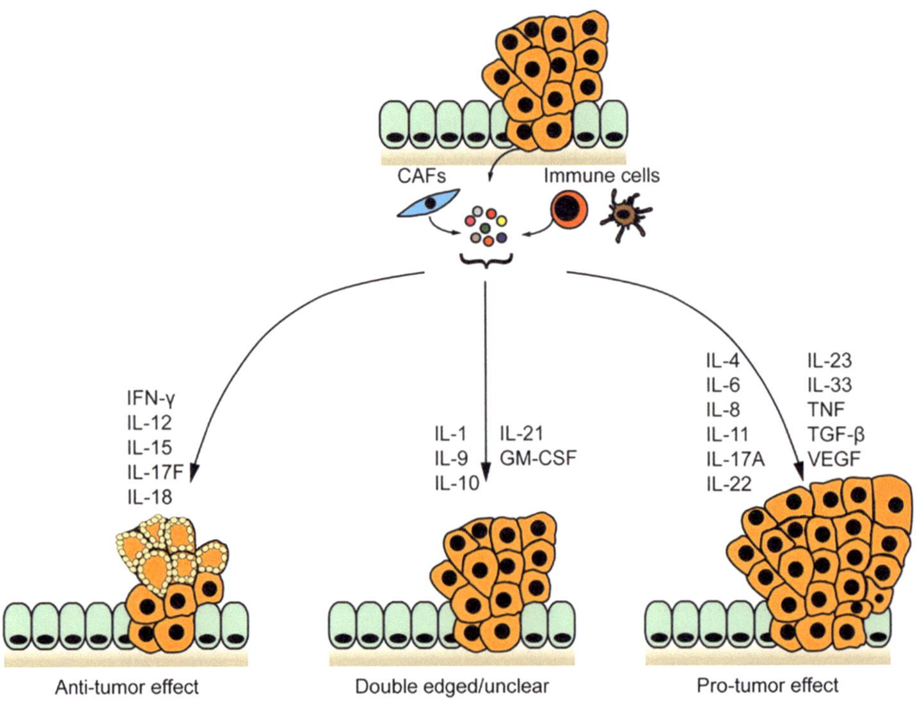

Figure 5.
The chemokines and cytokines and colorectal cancer growth interrelations [32].

3.3.1 NF-κB and STAT-3

The proinflammatory signaling molecules NF-κB and STAT-3 were associated with multiple types of hyper-inflammatory diseases or hyper-inflammatory foundations, such as inflammatory bowel syndrome, CC, lung cancer, and many other types of cancer. The higher levels of NF-κB and STAT-3 in the long term were correlated with CC angiogenesis and invasiveness. The activation of NF-κB mediator by TNF-α and IL-1β and the activation of STAT-3 mediator by IL-6 have led to cancer growth through the oncogenic signaling pathways activation in cancer cells (i.e. KRAS overexpression). On the other hand, their short-term secretions were reported to induce cancer cell apoptosis (proapoptotic) [13, 23].

3.3.2 TGF-β

The high levels of the immune-inhibitory cytokine (TGF-β) are associated with multiple types of immune deficiency diseases, resistant, and metastatic types of cancer (i.e. CC). This cytokine can be secreted from the tumor-associated macrophages and resistant cancer cells to induce the T-regulatory cells that will inhibit the activation of the CTL and TH cells. As a result, the CTL and TH cells cannot recognize cancer cells to induce apoptosis or their engulfment by the phagocytic cells [2, 18, 22, 33].

On the other hand, TGF-β enhances the VEGF secretions from the cancer cells. The VEGF amplifies the vasculature, the proinflammatory status, and the wound healing environment around the cancerous tissue. As a result, this can promote the cancer growth, metastasis, and activation of the tumor-associated macrophages to escape the immune surveillance for cancerous tissue [22, 25, 34].

Author details

Samaa Abdullah
Center of Excellence in Drug Research and Industrial Pharmacy, King Abdulaziz University, Jeddah, Saudi Arabia

*Address all correspondence to: stheebabdallah@stu.kau.edu.sa

References

[1] Bray F, Ferlay J, Soerjomataram I, Siegel RL, Torre LA, Jemal A. Global cancer statistics: GLOBOCAN estimates of incidence and mortality worldwide for 36 cancers in 185 countries. CA: A Cancer Journal for Clinicians. 2018;**68**:394-424. DOI: 10.3322/caac.21492

[2] Dekker E, Tanis PJ, Vleugels JLA, Kasi PM, Wallace MB. Colorectal cancer. The Lancet. 2019;**394**:1467-1480. DOI: 10.1016/s0140-6736(19)32319-0

[3] Siegel RL, Miller KD, Jemal A. Cancer statistics, 2019. CA: A Cancer Journal for Clinicians. 2019;**69**:7-34. DOI: 10.3322/caac.21551

[4] Karamchandani DM, Chetty R, King TS, Liu X, Westerhoff M, Yang Z, et al. Challenges with colorectal cancer staging: Results of an international study. Modern Pathology. 2020;**33**:153-163. DOI: 10.1038/s41379-019-0344-3

[5] Chakrabarti S, Peterson CY, Sriram D, Mahipal A. Early stage colon cancer: Current treatment standards, evolving paradigms, and future directions. World Journal of Gastrointestinal Oncology. 2020;**12**:808-832. DOI: 10.4251/wjgo.v12.i8.808

[6] Forman WB. The role of chemotherapy and adjuvant therapy in the management of colorectal cancer. Cancer. 1994;**74**:2151-2153

[7] Florescu-Țenea RM, Kamal AM, Mitruț P, Mitruț R, Ilie DS, Nicolaescu AC, et al. Colorectal cancer: An update on treatment options and future perspectives. Current Health Science Journal. 2019;**45**:134-141

[8] Chapelle N, Martel M, Toes-Zoutendijk E, Barkun AN, Bardou M. Recent advances in clinical practice: Colorectal cancer chemoprevention in the average-risk population. Gut. 2020;**69**:2244. DOI: 10.1136/gutjnl-2020-320990

[9] Kobunai T, Watanabe T, Yamamoto Y, Eshima K. The frequency of KRAS mutation detection in human colon carcinoma is influenced by the sensitivity of assay methodology: A comparison between direct sequencing and real-time PCR. Biochemical and Biophysical Research Communications. 2010;**395**:158-162. DOI: 10.1016/j.bbrc.2010.03.167

[10] Raskov H, Soby JH, Troelsen J, Bojesen RD, Gogenur I. Driver gene mutations and epigenetics in colorectal cancer. Annals of Surgery. 2020;**271**:75-85. DOI: 10.1097/SLA.0000000000003393

[11] Shou X, Li Y, Hu W, Ye T, Wang G, Xu F, et al. Six-gene Assay as a new biomarker in the blood of patients with colorectal cancer: Establishment and clinical validation. Molecular Oncology. 2019;**13**:781-791. DOI: 10.1002/1878-0261.12427

[12] Roseweir AK, Powell A, Horstman SL, Inthagard J, Park JH, McMillan DC, et al. Src family kinases, HCK and FGR, associate with local inflammation and tumour progression in colorectal cancer. Cellular Signalling. 2019;**56**:15-22. DOI: 10.1016/j.cellsig.2019.01.007

[13] Orlandi A, Di Salvatore M, Bagala C, Basso M, Strippoli A, Plastino F, et al. ERCC1 induction after oxaliplatin exposure may depend on KRAS mutational status in colorectal cancer cell

line: In Vitro Veritas. Journal of Cancer. 2015;**6**:70-81. DOI: 10.7150/jca.10478

[14] Zhu G, Pei L, Xia H, Tang Q, Bi F. Role of oncogenic KRAS in the prognosis, diagnosis and treatment of colorectal cancer. Molecular Cancer. 2021;**20**:143. DOI: 10.1186/s12943-021-01441-4

[15] Hasbullah HH, Musa M. Gene therapy targeting p53 and KRAS for colorectal cancer treatment: A myth or the way forward? International Journal of Molecular Sciences. 2021;**22**:11941. DOI: 10.3390/ijms222111941

[16] Chen L, Lu D, Sun K, Xu Y, Hu P, Li X, et al. Identification of biomarkers associated with diagnosis and prognosis of colorectal cancer patients based on integrated bioinformatics analysis. Gene. 2019;**692**:119-125. DOI: 10.1016/j.gene.2019.01.001

[17] Liu X, Cui Y, Zhang Y, Liu Z, Zhang Q, Wu W, et al. A comprehensive study of immunology repertoires in both preoperative stage and postoperative stage in patients with colorectal cancer. Molecular Genetics & Genomic Medicine. 2019;**7**:e504. DOI: 10.1002/mgg3.504

[18] Gmeiner WH. Fluoropyrimidine modulation of the anti-tumor immune response-prospects for improved colorectal cancer treatment. Cancers (Basel). 2020;**2020**:12. DOI: 10.3390/cancers12061641

[19] Zhang L, Shay JW. Multiple roles of APC and its therapeutic implications in colorectal cancer. Journal of the National Cancer Institute. 2017;**2017**:109

[20] Li X-L, Zhou J, Chen Z-R, Chng W-J. P53 mutations in colorectal cancer—Molecular pathogenesis and pharmacological reactivation. World Journal of Gastroenterology. 2015;**21**:84-93. DOI: 10.3748/wjg.v21.i1.84

[21] Bamehr H, Saidijam M, Dastan D, Amini R, Pourjafar M, Najafi R. Ferula pseudalliacea induces apoptosis in human colorectal cancer HCT-116 cells via mitochondria-dependent pathway. Archives of Physiology and Biochemistry. 2019;**125**:284-291. DOI: 10.1080/13813455.2018.1455710

[22] Mager LF, Wasmer MH, Rau TT, Krebs P. Cytokine-induced modulation of colorectal cancer. Frontiers in Oncology. 2016;**6**:96. DOI: 10.3389/fonc.2016.00096

[23] Suo H, Song JL, Zhou Y, Liu Z, Yi R, Zhu K, et al. Induction of apoptosis in HCT-116 colon cancer cells by polysaccharide of Larimichthys crocea swim bladder. Oncology Letters. 2015;**9**:972-978. DOI: 10.3892/ol.2014.2756

[24] Sondel PM, Gillies SD. Current and potential uses of immunocytokines as cancer immunotherapy. Antibodies (Basel). 2012;**1**:149-171. DOI: 10.3390/antib1020149

[25] Abdullah S, Aldahlawi A. Dendritic cell-based immunotherapies and their potential use in colorectal cancer immunotherapy. Journal of Microscopy and Ultrastructure. 2021;**0**:01-07. DOI: 10.4103/jmau.jmau_20_21

[26] Leman JK, Sandford SK, Rhodes JL, Kemp RA. Multiparametric analysis of colorectal cancer immune responses. World Journal of Gastroenterology. 2018;**24**:2995-3005. DOI: 10.3748/wjg.v24.i27.2995

[27] Xie YH, Chen YX, Fang JY. Comprehensive review of targeted therapy for colorectal cancer. Signal Transduction and Targeted Therapy. 2020;**5**:22. DOI: 10.1038/s41392-020-0116-z

[28] Corulli LR, Cecil DL, Gad E, Koehnlein M, Coveler AL, Childs JS, Lubet RA, Disis ML, Multi-Epitope-Based Vaccines for Colon Cancer Treatment and Prevention. 2021

[29] Li H, Yang C, Cheng H, Huang S, Zheng Y. CAR-T cells for colorectal cancer: Target-selection and strategies for improved activity and safety. Journal of Cancer. 2021;**12**:12, 1804-1814. DOI: 10.7150/jca.50509

[30] Peng X, Chen L, Chen L, Wang B, Wang Y, Zhan X. Chimeric antigen receptor-natural killer cells: Novel insight into immunotherapy for solid tumors (Review). Experimental and Therapeutic Medicine. 2021;**21**:340-340. DOI: 10.3892/etm.2021.9771

[31] Kuppusamy P, Govindan N, Yusoff MM, Ichwan SJA. Proteins are potent biomarkers to detect colon cancer progression. Saudi Journal of Biological Science. 2017;**24**:1212-1221. DOI: 10.1016/j.sjbs.2014.09.017

[32] Mager LF, Wasmer MH, Rau TT, Krebs P. Cytokine-Induced Modulation of Colorectal Cancer. 2016;**6**:01-19. DOI: 10.3389/fonc.2016.00096

[33] Gajjar KK, Vora HH, Kobawala TP, Trivedi TI, Ghosh NR. Deciphering the potential value of 5-fluorouracil metabolic enzymes in predicting prognosis and treatment response of colorectal cancer patients. The International Journal of Biological Markers. 2018;**33**:180-188. DOI: 10.1177/1724600817748539

[34] Chang DT, Pai RK, Rybicki LA, Dimaio MA, Limaye M, Jayachandran P, et al. Clinicopathologic and molecular features of sporadic early-onset colorectal adenocarcinoma: An adenocarcinoma with frequent signet ring cell differentiation, rectal and sigmoid involvement, and adverse morphologic features. Modern Pathology. 2012;**25**:1128-1139. DOI: 10.1038/modpathol.2012.61

Section 3

Surgical Care by Robotics

Chapter 5

Robotic Rectal Resection for Rectal Cancer: State of the Art

Francesca De Stefano, Gianfrancesco Intini, Giulia Costantini, Carlo Gennaro, Ali Chahrour and Igor Monsellato

Abstract

Surgical resection with total mesorectal excision (TME) represents a crucial milestone in the treatment of rectal cancer. Conventional open procedures have been gradually replaced by minimally invasive techniques. To date, laparoscopic and robotic resection associated with neoadjuvant chemo-radiotherapy, represent the gold standard for rectal malignancies. Robotic surgery, when performed by an experienced surgeon, can offer advantages in case of difficult anatomical conditions, such as in male patients with a narrow pelvis. Higher costs remain a matter of debate in the diffusion of robotic platforms in general surgery. However, encouraging surgical outcomes and a shorter learning curve for the surgeon counterbalance the associated expense. Different surgical approaches are available for rectal cancer, according to the extension of the tumor and its location. The cornerstone of the different approaches is represented by TME, both transabdominally and transanally. Adequate TME, associated with neoadjuvant therapy, is pivotal in the success of the oncological treatment, in terms of curative results and reduced recurrence. Current different approaches are low anterior resection, abdominoperineal resection, and intersphincteric resection. They can all be performed with the robotic system and their surgical steps are described in this chapter.

Keywords: rectal cancer, robotic surgery, total mesorectal excision, low anterior resection, abdomino-perineal resection, intersphincteric resection

1. Introduction

In the multimodal approach to rectal cancer, surgical resection is the gold standard for curative therapy. Early-stage rectal cancer, which does not spread further than the mucosa, can be treated by curative endoluminal resection. When rectal tumor spreads beyond the mucosa and the submucosa into the perirectal tissue, the transanal endoscopic resection is not curative and a multimodal approach with systemic and local therapies associated with surgical resection is required [1]. The initially proposed regimen was combined chemo-radiotherapy following surgical resection, as adjuvant therapy [2]. The German Rectal Trial in 2004 demonstrated, however, that chemo-radiotherapy is associated not only with improved compliance of patients but also with reduced toxicity and a potential preoperative downstaging of the tumor that can increase the number of sphincter-preserving resections in patients with low rectal tumors when administered preoperatively [3]. This trial analyzed about 800 patients and changed the systemic approach to locally advanced rectal cancer, thus making neoadjuvant radio-chemotherapy the standard of care. The optimal time of surgery after neoadjuvant radio-chemotherapy is still under debate. Many studies have been published on the topic, often reporting controversial results and no consensus has been reached yet. Historically, a time interval of 6–8 weeks was related to good oncological results and an increased rate of sphincter-preserving procedures [4]. After the publication of the results of the research by Habr-Gama in 2004, this time interval was revised, and the opportunity to consider longer intervals before surgery became a field of interest [5]. The attention of most researchers, indeed, focused on the optimization of the time interval and obtaining the highest pathological complete response. A recently published study from a high-volume center in China identifies a longer period of 10 weeks as the ideal time interval between neoadjuvant radio-chemotherapy and surgery, in terms of longer recurrence-free survival in 5-year follow-up [6]. Moreover, a time interval beyond eight weeks has been reported as protective for anastomotic dehiscence [7]. The most important limitation of these studies is their retrospective design. To date, several randomized trials, some unpublished, are ongoing to better define the optimal time interval in the search for tailored multimodal treatment for those patients suffering from local-advanced rectal cancer [8, 9].

Introduction of total mesorectal excision (TME) in the 1980s by Heald et al. represents the most relevant development in rectal cancer surgery [10]. And the standard procedure in the case of mid-to-low rectal cancer. TME addresses the mesorectum including the vascular and lymphatic structures, that are removed en-bloc with the involved rectum. Mesorectal and inferior mesenteric artery nodes are removed, which are the most common site of node metastasis. The dissection occurs along embryological planes, preserving the autonomic nerves involved in urinary and sexual function. Heald described the dissection plane as the avascular interface between the mesorectum and the surrounding somatic structures, identified as the "holy plane". Surgical plane and completeness of TME remain the most important prognostic factors. Dissection is performed circumferentially, until reaching the plane of the levator ani muscles. The gross appearance of the specimen, with a bilobed tissue block together with the involved rectum, is accurate proof of a proper TME. For mid-to-low rectal cancer, low anterior resection (LAR) with TME reduces locoregional recurrences. For tumors located at a distance >10 cms from the anal verge, whether a distal margin of 5 cm can be achieved, the mesorectum can be safely sectioned at the same level as the rectum, with outcomes similar to TME [11].

The advantages of laparoscopic TME versus open surgery have been demonstrated in several studies. In 2013, the COLOR II trial demonstrated that laparoscopic rectal surgery resulted in comparable oncologic outcomes, with the well-known advantages of laparoscopic surgery, in terms of faster recovery and decreased postoperative pain [12]. Valid oncologic outcomes were also confirmed in long-term follow-up, in terms of overall survival, disease-free survival, and local recurrence [13]. Nevertheless, laparoscopic surgery has different limitations and technical difficulties, especially in challenging anatomical conditions. A narrow pelvis, obese male patients, as well as bulky low tumors, represent a continuous challenge for the laparoscopic surgeon. In addition to the anatomical characteristics, specific drawbacks of laparoscopic procedures have been spotted such as a two-dimensional visualization, a restricted range of movement with instruments, suboptimal field exposure, and the amplification of hand tremor. Hence, with the development of robotic surgical platforms, several studies have been conducted to explore the potential benefits of robotic-assisted rectal surgery versus the laparoscopic approach. The robotic surgical platform offers the surgeon an increased range of motion, a stable surgical view, a three-dimensional visualization, and a more comfortable procedure. Short-term advantages have been widely demonstrated. Robotic rectal resection versus laparoscopic approach leads to less blood loss, inferior conversion rate, and reduced overall complication rate [14]. Moreover, recent meta-analysis on seven studies including more than 2500 patients, demonstrated the non-inferiority of long-term oncologic outcomes of robotic TME versus laparoscopic TME [15]. The ROLARR trial, showed that Robotic TME was beneficial for men and patients with low rectal tumors [16]. Despite the encouraging findings, two main concerns against robotic rectal surgery have been raised: the longer operative time and the elevated costs. Being the latter the most relevant limitation to the diffusion of the robotic surgical platforms in surgical departments, more recent data does not support the former one. It has been demonstrated that when robotic TME is performed by an experienced surgeon, the operative time is not higher than the laparoscopic procedure, especially when docking time is excluded. In addition, robotic TME may reduce the rate of diverting ileostomy, likely thanks to the option to reinforce the anastomosis or make a robot-assisted hand-sewn anastomosis, and postoperative pain, granted by the small dimensions and the wide range of motion of the robotic instruments and by the reduction of the fulcrum effect [17]. Robotic TME presents a shorter learning curve than laparoscopy, from about 30–50 cases per surgeon in laparoscopy to about 20 cases for robotic procedures. According to these data, fewer cases are needed for the surgeon to acquire the experience needed [18].

In conclusion, robotic surgical platforms are expanding and promising tools for TME and oncologic rectal surgery, with demonstrated advantages for the surgeon and for the patients compared to open surgery and laparoscopic approach. High costs are still the most relevant limitation that hampers its diffusion worldwide.

1.1 The da Vinci surgical platform

The da Vinci robot is currently the most widespread robotic surgical system, with thousands of units sold worldwide and thousands of peer-reviewed publications [19]. The first model of the da Vinci surgical platform was released in 1999 and since then, four different generations have been developed. In 2009 the daVinci Si surgical platform was released, consisting of four arms, while in 2014 Intuitive Surgical (Sunnyvale, CA, USA) developed and promoted the da Vinci Xi surgical platform, the current versinoe fo this robotic platform, which provides easier docking, as well as a wider range of motion with smaller arms on a rotating beam [20].

Numerous studies have been published after the introduction of the da Vinci Xi Surgical Platform, which was compared to the da Vinci Si Surgical Platform in colorectal surgery, in terms of surgical outcomes and surgeon's preference. In 2021, a meta-analysis including six studies for a total of 610 patients found that operative times significantly decreased using the da Vinci Xi, while no differences resulted in terms of conversion and complication rates compared to the daVinci Si [21]. Similar results were described more recently, confirming the advantages of the latest generation of the da Vinci platform, which present a more user-friendly design [22]. Interestingly, the reduction of the operating time when performing sphincter-saving TME in mid-low rectal cancer patients with the da Vinci Xi system has been correlated to a decrease in general costs. Lower operative room hours and shorter interventions, indeed, can be translated into lower expenses [23].

At the beginning of 2022, another retrospective analysis has been published, comparing the perioperative and postoperative outcomes of the third (da Vinci Si) and the fourth (da Vinci Xi) generation platforms on a single surgeon experience. This study confirmed significantly shorter operation time with the Xi system compared to Si system when performing sphincter-saving TME in mid-low rectal cancer patients [24].

Regardless of the different advantages that the da Vinci Xi shows over the Si, surgical steps and procedures are equivalent, except for trocar placement. Therefore, no difference in the description of the surgery itself nor any preference is reported. Trocar positioning is differently described according to the robotic platform.

2. Low anterior resection (LAR): surgical procedure

Low Anterior Resection is the most common surgical approach for rectal cancer. It is indicated for rectal cancer from distal to very low localization. In case of tumor invasion of the mesorectum, neoadjuvant chemo-radiotherapy is recommended to decrease long-term recurrence [25]. In the preoperative setting, the site of the diverting ileostomy is marked.

2.1 Surgical steps of robotic LAR with the daVinci robotic system for low or ultra-low rectal tumor

The procedure is performed under general anesthesia. Patient is in supine modified lithotomy position. A nasogastric tube is inserted before surgery.

Induction of pneumoperitoneum is performed, with the preferred technique. In our institution, the Veress needle technique is carried out, inserting the needle in the left hypochondrium (Palmer's point). Then, the trocars are placed accordingly to the type of robotic system available.

Exploratory laparoscopy is firstly performed to exclude carcinosis or undetected metastases. Cytologic examination is carried out in case of peritoneal effusion in searching for malignant cells. The small bowel is displaced with laparoscopic forceps to expose the left colon and the neoplasia.

When the daVinci Xi Surgical Platform (Intuitive Surgical Inc., Sunnyvale, CA, USA) is used, trocars are placed following the Universal Port Placement Guidelines provided by Intuitive Surgical for left lower abdominal procedures: an 8-mm port in the right iliac fossa, a 12-mm assistant trocar in the right flank, and two 8-mm robotic ports in the periumbilical region and the left hypochondrial space, in a line joining the right hip joint and the left subcostal margin at the level of the mid-clavicular line, at a distance of 6–8 cm from one another. Alternatively, the trocar line can be totally on the right side of the patient, being more vertical than in the first scenario, with Arm 1 in epigastrium up to Arm 4 in right iliac fossa. The daVinci Xi robotic system is targeted toward the left iliac fossa at the level of the sacral promontory. With the use of the laser pointer, the overhead boom is centered on the camera port. The boom is rotated to grant a better exposition of the robotic arms and instruments. A 12 mm-AirSeal-trocar system is placed on the right flank, for assistance.

The monopolar scissors are inserted through Arm 4, and placed in the right iliac fossa. A bipolar forceps is inserted through Arm 2, placed cranially and laterally off of the umbilicus on its left. A ProGrasp grasper is inserted through Arm 1 at the left hypochondriac space and is used for counter-traction and lifting. The endoscope is inserted through Arm 3 positioned between the umbilicus and the lower trocar (in the right iliac fossa). For performing the TME, the camera can be placed in a different arm or change its anatomical target. Alternatively, instruments' position and types can be the same as for the first phase.

The Xi robotic platform provides several "technical" advantages: torpedo-shaped robotic arm that are mounted on a rotating beam, universal arms where camera can be docked onto any arm, longer instruments, a new vision architecture with chip-at-the-tip technology and camera, endoscope, and cable integrated into one handheld design, an adapted user interface offering more assistance with robotic setup and installation, integrated energy with a single device for mono- and bipolar energy, a standard integration of Firefly Fluorescence Imaging. All these features help the surgeon to better perform the procedure and to access a greater field of surgery without the need to reinstall the robotic system (single docking approach).

When the daVinci Si Surgical Platform (Intuitive Surgical Inc., Sunnyvale, CA, USA) is used, four robotic trocars and one laparoscopic trocar for the assistant are used (AirSeal). The robotic trocar for the camera is placed 3 cm upward and 2 cm rightward to the umbilicus. Two robotic trocars are placed at the intersection of the midclavicular line and the spinoumbilical line, on both sides. The other two robotic trocars are positioned at the level of the midclavicular line in right and left hypochondrium. On the right flank, laterally to and between the two robotic trocars, the laparoscopic trocar for the assistant is placed (**Figure 1**).

The robotic docking is performed with the robot on the left side of the patient placed following an imaginary line connecting the left anterosuperior iliac spine of the patient, the umbilical scar, and the shoulder of the patient. The robotic camera is placed in the umbilical trocar. The first arm with monopolar scissor (Arm 1) is introduced through the trocar in the right iliac fossa. Arm 2 is placed in the right hypochondrium with bipolar forceps (**Figure 2**).

With the daVinci Si, two alternative approaches can be adopted for the mobilization of the splenic flexure, the first step of the procedure: a supramesocolic and a submesocolic approach. The two approaches are equivalent, and the choice is solely based on surgeon's preference.

In the supramesocolic approach, the patient is firstly positioned with a 5 degrees anti-Trendelenburg and a 15 degrees right tilt.

The procedure starts with the dissection of the gastrocolic ligament in a medial-to-lateral direction, starting from the Bouchet area. The assistant pulls the transverse colon caudally with laparoscopic forceps and the surgeon pulls the omentum in the opposite direction with Arm 2. Starting from the middle transverse colon, the dissection continues laterally, preserving the contralateral gastro-epiploic arcade. This maneuver allows the opening of the omental bursa. Splenocolic and phrenocolic ligaments are sectioned. Previous identification of the inferior pancreatic edge and the root of the mesocolon, dissection reaches the splenic flexure, and the descending colon is mobilized from the left parietocolic gutter. The assistant can now pull the splenic flexure downward and rightward, opening the avascular dissection plane between the Gerota's and the Toldt's fascia. Along this avascular plane the root of the mesocolon is exposed and the origin of the inferior mesenteric vein (IMV) is identified. Mobilization of the splenic flexure is now complete. The robotic system is removed, and patient's position is changed, with 25–30 degrees of Trendelenburg and 15 degrees of right tilt. Robotic docking is performed again adding the third arm. Arm 1 is docked to the trocar in the right iliac fossa mounting the monopolar scissors; Arm 2 is placed in the left hypochondrium/left middle quadrant mounting ProGrasp

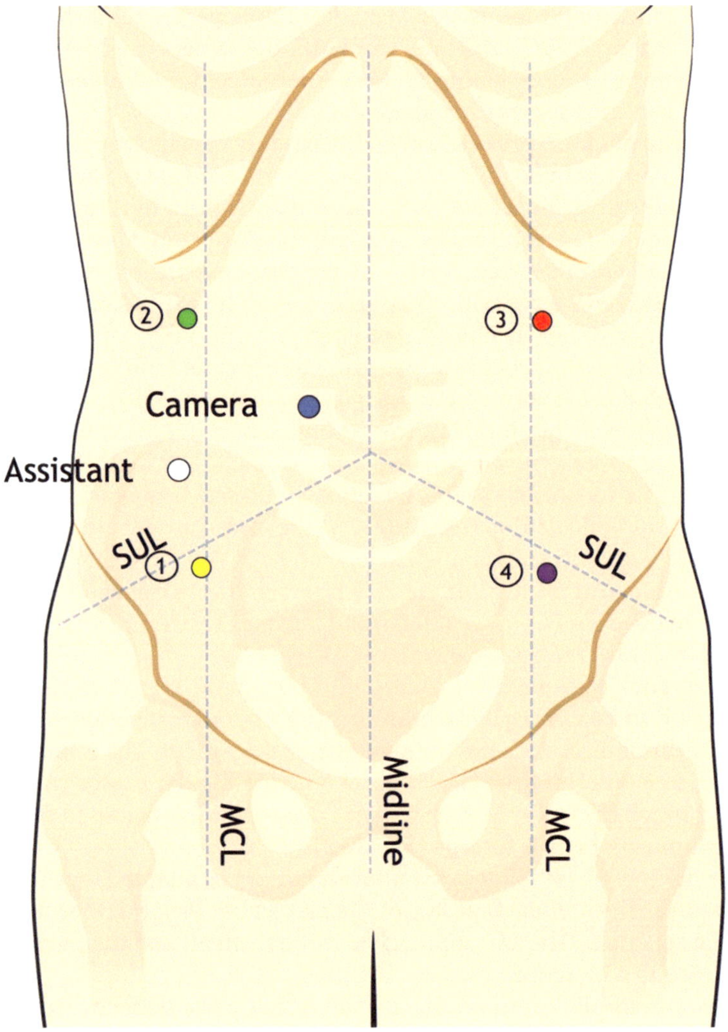

Figure 1.
Position of trocars in LAR with the da Vinci Si surgical platform.

forceps; Arm 3 is placed in the right hypochondrium mounting bipolar forceps. The ProGrasp pulls the mesocolon upward, exposing the IMV and the inferior pancreatic margin. Locoregional perivascular lymphadenectomy is performed, the IMV is isolated, and it is cut between clips. The surgeon proceeds mediolaterally beneath the IMV toward the parietocolic gutter, dissecting the descending mesocolon. During this maneuver, it is important to preserve the left ureter and the gonadic vessels. At the level of the renal artery, the peritoneum is sectioned under the iliac bifurcation, and the inferior mesenteric artery (IMA) is exposed. The ProGrasp in Arm 3 pulls the IMA and locoregional lymphadenectomy is performed between the aorta and the IMA. Periaortic nerves and the mesenteric nervous plexus should be identified and preserved. The IMA is then sectioned between clips, about 2 cm distal its origin from the aorta [26].

The dissection planes of IMA and IMV are now rejoined, and the perivascular lymphadenectomy is completed.

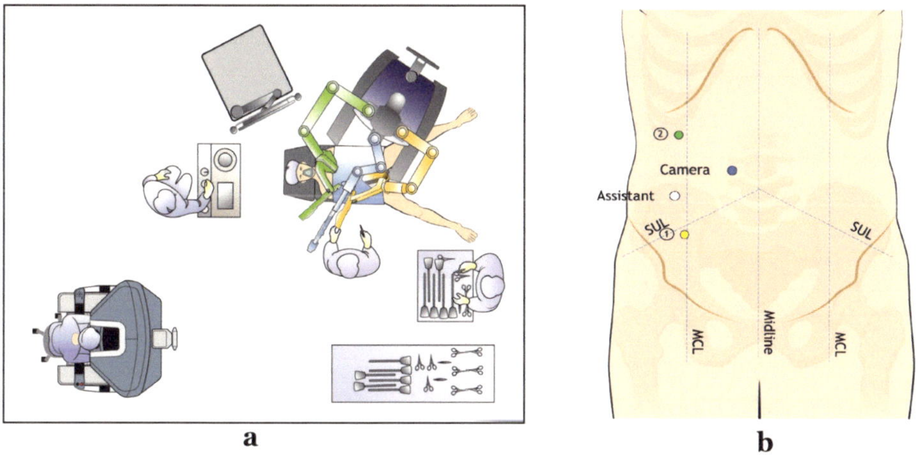

Figure 2.
Operating room setting (a) and trocars used (b) for splenic flexure mobilization.

Mobilization of sigmoid colon from the parietocolic gutter, until the sacral promontory and upper rectum is now performed. During this step, the assistant pulls the descending colon rightward, exposing the left parietocolic gutter and helping the surgeon to identify and preserve the left ureter throughout its course. Once the promontory is reached, the mesorectum starts and TME can be performed. Robotic arms are switched, with Arm 2 positioned in the left iliac fossa mounting the ProGrasp, and Arm 3 in the left hypochondrium mounting the bipolar forceps. Two laparoscopic trocars are available for the assistant, which will use the lateral one for the laparoscopic forceps and the medial one for the laparoscopic aspirator. Initially, the laparoscopic forceps pull the sigmoid colon and proximal rectum cranially and leftward. The ProGrasp pulls the visceral peritoneum of the rectum on the right side and the TME starts. Circumferential mesorectal excision starts from the right posterolateral side, preserving the presacral fascia and the hypogastric nerves underneath. The dissection proceeds until the Waldeyer ligament. Now, the assistant switches the position of the laparoscopic forceps and aspirator, to pull the rectum cranially and rightward. TME continues from right to left side, reaching the anterior compartment. The peritoneum is sectioned at this point reaching the extraperitoneal rectum and the TME continues anteriorly along the plane between the rectum and the bladder-prostate complex in men and along the recto-vaginal septum in female. The laparoscopic forceps pull the rectum cranially and downward, while the ProGrasp pulls upward the peritoneum of the urinary bladder and the prostate to expose the Denonvillier's fascia at this level. During dissection of the Denonvillier's fascia, it is important to preserve the seminal vesicles in men. In female, a vaginal manipulator can be introduced trans-vaginally, for a more efficient separation of the recto-vaginal septum. Mesorectal excision is now completed by sectioning the Waldeyer ligament posteriorly and reaching the levator ani fascia anteriorly and laterally. TME can be considered accurate at this point (**Figure 3**). Indocyanine green (ICG) is administered intravenously to confirm correct vascularization of the rectal stump. The assistant performs the resection of the distal rectum with laparoscopic linear mechanical stapler. Alternatively, the robotic stapler can be positioned on Arm 1.

A suprapubic Pfannenstiel incision is performed, and pneumoperitoneum is deflated. A wound protector is usually inserted at this point to avoid contact

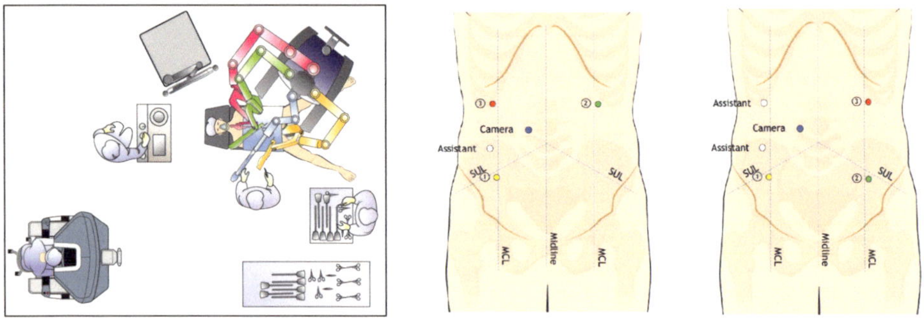

a b c

Figure 3.
Operating room setting (a) during vessel ligation and total mesorectal excision. Trocars used during inferior mesenteric vessels ligation and perivascular lymphadenectomy (b). Trocars used during total mesorectal excision (c).

between the abdominal wall and the colon. The resected colon is extracted. The inferior mesenteric artery peduncle previously cut is identified, and the operator can complete the resection of the sigmoid mesocolon along the artery line to obtain an accurate lymphadenectomy. Once the area of the descending colon is identified for resection, ICG test is performed to confirm the correct vascularization and the colon can be sectioned. Colorectal anastomosis will be performed using a circular stapler. The anvil of the stapler is inserted in the colic lumen, and it is secured by using a purse string suture technique. The colon is reinserted intra-abdominally and pneumoperitoneum is inflated. The operator moves between patient legs and inserts the circular stapler transanally. The mechanical colorectal Knight-Griffen anastomosis is fashioned. The ICG test can be performed up to surgeon's preference. The air leak test is advisable to exclude possible anastomosis leakage. The surgical procedure is now completed (**Figure 4**). Washing of the abdominal cavity is performed, and a drainage is usually placed in the Douglas space. In case of medium-to-low rectal tumors and in case of neoadjuvant chemo-radiotherapy, a temporary loop ileostomy is recommended.

In the submesocolic approach, that is the same for both the two robotic platforms, the patient is positioned in a 25–30 degrees Trendelenburg and 15 degrees right tilt. The robot docking is performed, and the robotic camera is placed in the umbilical trocar. When the Si is used, three Arms are placed from the beginning of the procedure. Arm 1 is introduced through the trocar in the right iliac fossa mounting the monopolar scissors; Arm 2 is placed in the left hypochondrium/left middle quadrant mounting ProGrasp forceps; Arm 3 is placed in the right hypochondrium mounting bipolar forceps.

All the following steps are carried out in a similar manner to the two robotic platforms.

The ProGrasp pulls the mesocolon upward, exposing the IMV and the inferior pancreatic margin. The IMV is isolated, perivascular lymphadenectomy is performed and then the vein is cut between clips. Dissection continues mediolaterally inferiorly to the IMV. The left colon is mobilized from the parietocolic gutter in a caudo-cranial direction and the splenic flexure is reached. Now the assistant can pull medially the descending colon, while the surgeon pulls contralaterally the omentum with the ProGrasp in Arm 3. Latero-medial dissection is performed, completing the mobilization of the splenic flexure.

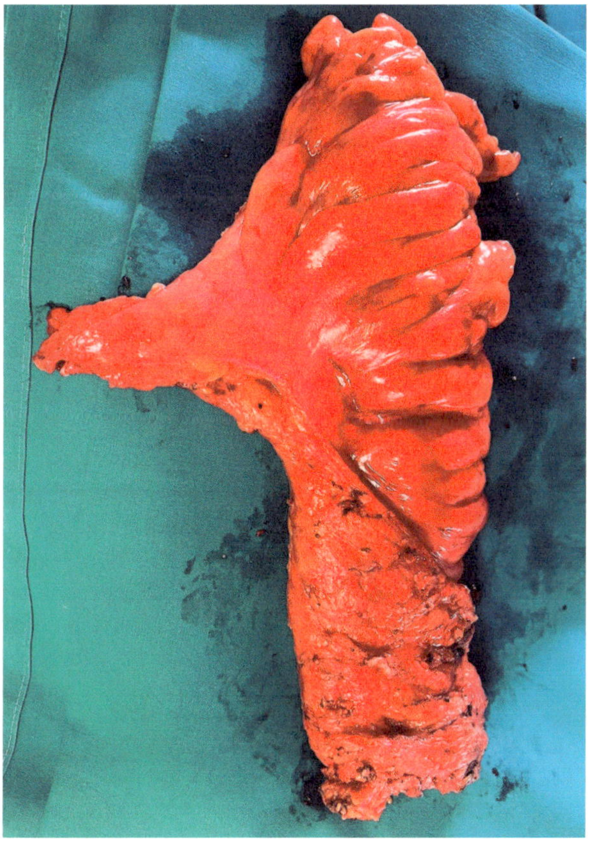

Figure 4.
Rectal specimen after LAR with visible vascular pedicle.

Both supramesocolic and submesocolic approaches lead to the complete mobilization of splenic flexure and left colon. The following steps of the procedure will not be repeated, and they can be found in the section above.

3. Abdomino-perineal resection (miles' operation): surgical procedure

Abdomino-perineal resection was developed by Sir William Miles to reduce the burden of local recurrence in rectal cancer surgery. For decades, Miles' operation was considered the standard of care for all rectal cancer, being the only therapeutic option for these patients. However, the development of perioperative local and systemic therapies, a better understanding of the pathologic tumor dissemination mechanisms [27], and thanks to the development of less mutilating techniques, such as sphincter preservation, TME and LAR, the indication for abdomino-perineal resection have consistently decreased in the decades [28]. First indication of Miles' procedure is ultra-low rectal tumors in which a negative distal margin cannot be obtained. The concept of negative resection margin in rectal surgery has been widely debated among the surgical community. The milestone concept of the "5-cm margin" was challenged by the development of neoadjuvant therapy and the development of TME. To date, a distal resection margin of 1 cm is considered acceptable in case of ultra-low rectal cancer, in the context of a multimodal treatment plan [29]. Moreover, Miles' procedure is indicated in case of involvement of external sphincter or levator ani complex. The abdomino-perineal resection is also the treatment of choice for anal squamous cell carcinoma, when chemoradiation therapy fails [30].

3.1 Surgical steps of miles' operation

The intraperitoneal steps of the abdomino-perineal resection are equivalent to the steps of LAR; hence, you can refer to the appropriate section for it.

Once the dissection reaches the extraperitoneal rectum, TME is performed circumferentially, until the levator ani fascia is reached. It can be recognized because the mesorectum with adipose yellow tissue ends and the white appearance of the levator ani fascia becomes visible. The left colic vein is identified at its confluence in the IMV, and it is sectioned. From this point, the sigmoid mesocolon is sectioned. Now, the proximal section of the colon can be performed with the laparoscopic or robotic mechanical stapler, and the perineal phase can start. The surgeon and the assistant move to the perineal area, which is exposed by lifting patients' legs upward.

A retractor system is positioned, commonly the Lone Star (Lone Star Medical Products Inc., Houston, TX, USA) is used. The perianal region is sectioned circumferentially, 1 cm from the external sphincter margin. It is paramount for the oncological outcome of this procedure to remove the sphincter complex en bloc. The dissection is performed along the pelvic floor and the levator ani fascia. Posteriorly, the surgeon can start form the perineal raphe, from the coccyx along the margin of the sacrum, reaching the plane that was previously dissected in the intra-abdominal phase of the intervention. The dissection proceeds laterally by sectioning the levator ani muscles, and anteriorly, where the vagina or the prostate and urethra are found, in female and male, respectively. At this point, the circumferential perineal dissection is complete, and the surgical specimen can be extracted through the perineum. After accurate washing of the perineal area, the perineum is closed by layers. This is a crucial step, because abdomino-perineal resection often results in perineal wound defects. In addition to risk factors related to wound healing defects, such as smoking, advanced oncologic status and alcohol consumption, the introduction of neoadjuvant radiotherapy significantly increased the rate of wound defects [31] and neoadjuvant chemoradiation and wound complications are predictors of long-term perineal pain [32]. Wound dehiscence in Miles' procedure is the topic of numerous studies, searching for a valid standard closure method of the perineum. However, no ideal solution currently exists, and different approaches have been attempted with more or less success. Primary closure, with levator ani muscles reapproximated with multiple absorbable stitches, remains the most frequent technique. When this closure cannot be obtained, the use of biological or synthetic mesh can be considered [33]. Biological mesh appears to be a valid option, especially in terms of hernia prevention. Its role in preventing wound infections and dehiscence is less clear. Moreover, reconstruction with myocutaneous flap can be considered in selected cases [34]. Regardless the different options, abdomino-perineal resection results often in wound defects that deeply affect patient's quality of life and morbidity, as well as hospitalization and healthcare-associated costs. When the wound fails to heal, a conventional negative pressure wound therapy (NPWT) device can be considered. In a recent systematic review, the use of NPWT represents an encouraging tool in reducing surgical site infection and wound dehiscence in these patients [35].

Once the perineum is sutured, pneumoperitoneum is reinduced. After accurate hemostasis, a surgical drain is placed in the pelvic cavity, the colic stump is brought to the abdominal wall – in the area identified and marked before surgery – and the colonostomy is created.

4. Intersphincteric rectal resection

Sphincter preservation in patients with low rectal cancer is feasible reducing the distance between the tumor and the resection margin. In this way continence can be preserved, but still the oncological radicality of the procedure must be guaranteed.

A conservative procedure can be performed under the following condition:

- Integrity of the sphincter complex: the integrity of the external sphincter (Debray's reflex) and the preservation of the levator ani muscle is essential to maintain normal continence. In particular, the levator ani muscle accentuates the angle of the rectum (Parks mechanism) through the contraction of the puborectal bundles. The rectal resection must therefore fall above the elevator plane and should not damage the external sphincter nerves. The integrity of the mucosal membrane of the anal canal and of the distal end of the rectum are not necessary for a good continence, as the sphincter motor activity is regulated by receptors placed in the external sphincter [36]

- Well vascularized rectal stump [36]

- Transposition of the colon above the pelvic and perineal plane without the risk of traction or lack of perfusion. The impediment to lowering is generally due to the presence of a short Riolano arch or of an accessory middle colic artery [36]

When a free resection margin cannot be obtained without sphincter involvement, an abdomino-perineal resection must be performed.

In ultra-low rectal resections, it is possible to perform a manual coloanal anastomosis or proceed with the intersphincter resection, with partial or total removal of the internal sphincter. This technique aims to obtain appropriate longitudinal and radial margins [37], thanks to the presence of the Debray's reflex and the Parks mechanism, which would guarantee adequate continence [36].

The low rectal cancer can be classified in four groups according to Rullier [38]:

- type I supra-anal (> 1 cm from the anal ring)

- type II juxta-anal (< 1 cm from the anal ring)

- type III intra-anal (internal anal sphincter invasion)

- type IV transanal (external anal sphincter or levator ani invasion)

Type I patients are eligible for ultra-low anterior resection, type 2 for partial intersphinteric resection, type 3 for total intersphinteric resection and type 4 need abdomino-perineal resection. Postoperatively, only 50% of patients presents a good fecal continence; 11% suffers from severe fecal incontinence and 6% of patients requires a definitive colonostomy due to severe postoperative fecal incontinence [38]. Performing a very low colorectal anastomosis can lead to anterior resection syndrome, characterized by involuntary loss of stool, urgency and multiple defecation, due to the loss of the rectal reservoir. Due to these disfunctions, some studies report that patients undergoing an ultra-low anterior resection present a lower quality of life than those undergoing abdominal-perineal amputation, despite the loss of the physiological possibility of defecating and the presence of a definitive ostomy. For these reasons, sphincter preservation procedures must be considered only for those patients who have an adequate sphincter function demonstrated by a manometric examination, and for those who accept a suboptimal functional result [37, 38].

There has been a progressive reduction in Mile's procedures, in favor of LAR which is currently the most used procedure even in cases of ultra-low lesions. Abdominal-perineal amputation is preferred only when disease-free resection margins cannot be guaranteed without resecting the sphincters, or in case of their infiltration [39]. According to Rullier, an intersphinteric rectal resection is performed in two different surgical times: the intraabdominal and the transanal one. The former follows the usual steps of LAR. The transanal time starts with the exposure of the anal canal, using a retractor like Lone Star; for limiting the tumor seeding it is recommended to introduce a gauze into the rectum. The resection starts 1 cm below the tumor with a circular incision that transect the internal anal sphincter by both the mucosa and the muscular layer. Performing a partial or total resection of the internal sphincter depends on the level of the incision (on the dentate line or 1–2 centimeters below). The dissection continues upward between the two sphincters through an avascular plane and can be performed with scissors or an electric scalpel. The resection should start posteriorly and laterally where the external anal sphincter is more visible and proceeds anteriorly. The rectum is closed with a suture as soon as the upper edge of the anal ring is reached in order to avoid intraoperative tumor seeding; then dissection follows the levator ani fibers to reach the previous intrabdominal dissection or a transanal TME (TaTME) is performed [40].

4.1 Transanal total mesorectal excision

In recent years, many efforts have been made to reduce surgical trauma and obtain better operative and postoperative results for patients, but despite the latest technological and surgical advances, rectal cancer surgery is still very complex especially in obese patients, with a narrow pelvis and low tumors. For these reasons, a new surgical approach has recently gained particular attention: the TaTME [41], which according to preliminary results of many centers, has proved to be safe and feasible [42]. The development of this technique resulted from the experience acquired through the different minimally invasive techniques in colorectal surgery: transanal endoscopic microsurgery (TEM) [43], transabdominal transanal (TATA) proctosigmoidectomy [44], transanal minimally invasive surgery (TAMIS) [45] and natural orifice transluminal endoscopic surgery (NOTES) [46, 47]. TaTME is a colorectal resection performed with laparoscopic instruments through a natural orifice: the anal canal [48]. TaTME can facilitate surgery in patients who require anterior resection for low and medium rectal tumors, where intraabdominal insertion of an endoscopic stapler could be limited by the anatomical conformation, such as in obese patients and in males with a narrow pelvis, allowing to achieve complete excision of the mesorectum with clean distal and circumferential resection margins [48, 49]. The TaTME technique developed by Lacie (Cecil Approach) involves the use of a double surgical team, one for the abdominal time and one for the transanal time. Abdominal time coincides with the previously described LAR and involves mobilization of the splenic flexure and of the left colon, identification with section of the inferior mesenteric vein below the inferior margin of the pancreas, identification, and section of the inferior mesenteric artery at its origin. The transanal time begins when the inferior mesenteric artery is sectioned. A transanal surgical device (Buess Rectoscope or Gel Point Platform) is placed and the pneumorectum is performed, with a target pressure of 12–15 mmHg. A purse-string suture of the rectum is performed clockwise distal to the tumor, to prevent tumor spillage, from the anterior wall. The rectal wall is resected by a monopolar hook, with a full-thickness perpendicular transaction, following the holy plane, upwardly. The anterior and posterior planes are dissected at first, because easier to identify than the lateral ones; the lateral resection should be performed following the imaginary line that completes the circumference. Before the communication between transanal and abdominal field, a second purse string suture is performed in the free open edge of the distal stump; this suture will serve to tighten the stapler rod before the anastomosis. When the transanal surgical team is close to the peritoneal reflection, the two teams work together until the rendezvous is completed and the specimen is resected. The specimen can be extracted transanally if the dimension of the pelvis allows it, or transabdominally through a Pfannenstiel incision. The anastomosis could be a handsewn coloanal or a stappled end-to-end one, depending on the resulting stump length. The stapler anvil could be reinserted by the abdominal team if the specimen is extracted transabdominally or by the transanal team if extracted transanally. After tiding the distal purse-string suture around the circular stapler rod, the two parts can be connected, and it is possible to fire the stapler. At this point, the transanal device should be inserted again to verify the anastomosis. The side-to-end hand-sewn anastomosis is performed by pulling the colon wall near the distal rectal margin [50].

5. Conclusions

Surgical resection is a crucial milestone in the multimodal treatment of rectal cancer. A proper and accurate TME represents the most important factor for the post-operative oncological outcome. With the development of minimally invasive techniques in general surgery, the open approach to rectal cancer surgery has been progressively abandoned. More recently, the robotic surgical platform has gained consent in the surgical community. In addition to the well-known advantages of the robotic system over laparoscopy in terms of surgeon's comfort and 3-D visualization, robotic-assisted rectal resection can overcome technical difficulties related to anatomical conditions, such as a narrow pelvis in males and obese patients. Moreover, a learning curve for robotic TME is shorter than for laparoscopic TME. When experienced surgeons perform robotic rectal surgery, the actual operating times do not significantly exceed the laparoscopic ones. Advantages of the robotic technique are counterbalanced by still-elevated costs that hamper its diffusion in surgical centers. No difference in terms of oncological outcomes is reported in the two different minimally invasive approaches.

Different surgical procedures can be offered to the patient affected by rectal cancer, according to its distance from the anal verge and its local extension. The most frequent procedure is low anterior resection. When feasible, a sphincter-preserving procedure should be preferred, and only in case of sphincter involvement or unachievable negative resection margins, abdomino-perineal resection with permanent colonostomy be performed. Different sphincter-preserving techniques have been described, and intersphincteric resection can offer the maintenance of fecal continence. In recent years, transanal TME has been developed, to reduce surgical trauma and improve postoperative results for patients. In this chapter, the currently available options in rectal surgery are reported and the robotic techniques are explained in detail.

Conflict of interest

The authors declare no conflict of interest.

Author details

Francesca De Stefano, Gianfrancesco Intini, Giulia Costantini, Carlo Gennaro, Ali Chahrour and Igor Monsellato*
SS. Antonio and Biagio and Cesare Arrigo Hospital, Alessandria, Italy

*Address all correspondence to: imonsellato@libero.it

References

[1] Wlodarczyk JR, Lee SW. New Frontiers in Management of Early and Advanced Rectal Cancer. 2022. DOI: 10.3390/cancers14040938. Available from: https://www.mdpi.com/journal/cancers

[2] PRM T, Lindblad AS. Adjuvant postoperative radiotherapy and chemotherapy in rectal carcinoma: a review of the gastrointestinal tumor study group experience. Radiotherapy and Oncology. 1988;**13**(4):245-252 [Internet] [cited 2022 May 29] Available from: https://pubmed.ncbi.nlm.nih.gov/3064191/

[3] Sauer R, Becker H, Hohenberger W, Rödel C, Wittekind C, Fietkau R, et al. Preoperative versus postoperative Chemoradiotherapy for rectal cancer. The New England Journal of Medicine. 2004;**17**:1731-1740. DOI: 10.1056/NEJMoa040694. Available from: www.nejm.org

[4] Francois Y, Nemoz CJ, Baulieux J, Vignal J, Grandjean JP, Partensky C, et al. Influence of the interval between preoperative radiation therapy and surgery on downstaging and on the rate of sphincter-sparing surgery for rectal cancer: The Lyon R90-01 randomized trial. Journal of Clinical Oncology. 1999;**17**(8):2396-2402 [Internet] [cited 2022 May 30] Available from: https://pubmed.ncbi.nlm.nih.gov/10561302/

[5] Habr-Gama A, Perez RO, Nadalin W, Sabbaga J, Ribeiro U, Silva E, et al. Operative versus nonoperative treatment for stage 0 distal rectal cancer following chemoradiation therapy: Long-term results. Annals of Surgery. 2004;**240**(4):711-718 [Internet] [cited 2022 May 30] Available from: https://pubmed.ncbi.nlm.nih.gov/15383798/

[6] Wang X, Zheng Z, Zhu H, Yu Q, Huang S, Lu X, et al. Timing to achieve the best recurrence-free survival after neoadjuvant chemoradiotherapy in locally advanced rectal cancer: Experience in a large-volume center in China. International Journal of Colorectal Disease. 2021;**36**(5):1007-1016

[7] Caputo D, Angeletti S, Michele F, Ciccozzi M, Coppola A, Cartillone M, et al. Delayed surgery after radio-chemotherapy for rectal adenocarcinoma is protective for anastomotic dehiscence: a single-center observational retrospective cohort study. Updates in Surgery. 2020;**72**:469-475. [Internet] Available from:. DOI: 10.1007/s13304-020-00770-1

[8] Monsellato I, Alongi F, Bertocchi E, Gori S, Ruffo G, Cassinotti E, et al. Standard (8 weeks) vs long (12 weeks) timing to minimally-invasive surgery after NeoAdjuvant Chemoradiotherapy for rectal cancer: a multicenter randomized controlled parallel group trial (TiMiSNAR). BMC Cancer. 2019;**19**(1):1215

[9] Akgun E, Caliskan C, Bozbiyik O, Yoldas T, Sezak M, Ozkok S, et al. Randomized clinical trial of short or long interval between neoadjuvant chemoradiotherapy and surgery for rectal cancer. The British Journal of Surgery. 2018;**105**(11):1417-1425

[10] Heald RJ, RDH R. Recurrence and survival after total mesorectal excision for rectal cancer. Lancet. 1986;**1**(8496):1479-1482 [Internet] [cited 2022 May 29] Available from: https://pubmed.ncbi.nlm.nih.gov/2425199/

[11] Knol J, Keller DS. Total mesorectal excision technique-past, present, and

future. Clinics in Colon and Rectal Surgery. 2020;**33**(3):134-143. DOI: 10.1055/s-0039-3402776. Epub 2020 Apr 28

[12] van der Pas MHGM, Haglind E, Cuesta MA, Fürst A, Lacy AM, Hop WCJ, et al. Laparoscopic versus open surgery for rectal cancer (COLOR II): Short-term outcomes of a randomised, phase 3 trial. The Lancet Oncology. 2013;**14**(3):210-218

[13] Jayne DG, Guillou PJ, Thorpe H, Quirke P, Copeland J, Smith AMH, et al. Randomized trial of laparoscopic-assisted resection of colorectal carcinoma: 3-year results of the UK MRC CLASICC trial group. Journal of Clinical Oncology. 2007;**25**(21):3061-3068 [Internet] [cited 2022 May 31] Available from: https://pubmed.ncbi.nlm.nih.gov/17634484/

[14] Cui Y, Li C, Xu Z, Wang Y, Sun Y, Xu H, et al. Therapeutics and clinical risk management Dovepress robot-assisted versus conventional laparoscopic operation in anus-preserving rectal cancer: a meta-analysis. Therapeutics and Clinical Risk Management. 2017;**13**:1247. [Internet] Available from:. DOI: 10.2147/TCRM.S142758

[15] Qiu H, Yu D, Ye S, Shan R, Ai J, Shi J. Long-term oncological outcomes in robotic versus laparoscopic approach for rectal cancer: A systematic review and meta-analysis. International Journal of Surgery. 2020;**80**:225-230

[16] Jayne D, Pigazzi A, Marshall H, Croft J, Corrigan N, Copeland J, et al. Effect of robotic-assisted vs conventional laparoscopic surgery on risk of conversion to open laparotomy among patients undergoing resection for rectal cancer. Journal of the American Medical Association. 2017;**318**(16):1569

[17] Pan J, Wang B, Feng Z, Sun Z, Xia C, Zhang Q, et al. Robotic total mesorectal excision versus laparoscopic total mesorectal excision for mid-low rectal cancer with difficult anatomical conditions. Asian Journal of Surgery. 2022;**12**:S1015-584(22)00039-2. DOI: 10.1016/j.asjsur.2022.01.026. Available from: https://pubmed.ncbi.nlm.nih.gov/35168863/ [Online ahead of print]

[18] Baukloh JK, Perez D, Reeh M, Biebl M, Izbicki JR, Pratschke J, et al. Lower gastrointestinal surgery: Robotic surgery versus laparoscopic procedures. Visceral Medicine. 2018;**34**(1):16-22 [Internet] [cited 2022 Jun 1] Available from: https://pubmed.ncbi.nlm.nih.gov/29594165/

[19] Leal Ghezzi T, Campos Corleta O. 30 years of robotic surgery. World Journal of Surgery. 2016;**40**(10):2550-2557. DOI: 10.1007/s00268-016-3543-9

[20] Aliyev V, Arslan NC, Goksoy B, Guven K, Goksel S, Asoglu O. Is robotic da Vinci xi® superior to the da Vinci Si® for sphincter-preserving total mesorectal excision? Outcomes in 150 mid-low rectal cancer patients. Journal of Robotic Surgery. 2022:1-8 [Internet] [cited 2022 May 16] Available from: https://link.springer.com/article/10.1007/s11701-021-01356-8

[21] Felsenreich DM, Gachabayov M, Karas J, Rojas A, Bergamaschi R. A meta-analysis of DaVinci Si versus xi in colorectal surgery. International Journal of Medicine Robotics. 2021;**17**(3):e2222

[22] Huang YM, Huang YJ, Wei PL. Colorectal cancer surgery using the Da Vinci xi and Si systems: Comparison of perioperative outcomes. Surgical Innovation. 2019;**26**(2):192-200

[23] Morelli L, di Franco G, Lorenzoni V, Simone G, Palmeri M, Furbetta N, et al. Structured cost analysis of robotic

TME resection for rectal cancer: A comparison between the da Vinci Si and xi in a single surgeon's experience. Surgical Endoscopy. 2019;**33**:1858-1869. [Internet] DOI: 10.1007/s00464-018-6465-9

[24] Aliyev V, Arslan NC, Goksoy B, Guven K, Goksel S, Asoglu O. Is robotic da Vinci xi® superior to the da Vinci Si® for sphincter-preserving total mesorectal excision? Outcomes in 150 mid-low rectal cancer patients. Journal of Robotic Surgery. 2022. DOI: 10.1007/s11701-021-01356-8. Available from: https://pubmed.ncbi.nlm.nih.gov/35107708/ [Online ahead of print]

[25] Body A, Prenen H, Lam M, Davies A, Tipping-Smith S, Lum C, et al. Neoadjuvant therapy for locally advanced rectal cancer: Recent advances and ongoing challenges. Clinical Colorectal Cancer. 2021;**20**(1):29-41 [Internet] [cited 2022 May 30] Available from: https://pubmed.ncbi.nlm.nih.gov/33531256/

[26] Malakorn S, Sammour T, Bednarski B, You YQN, Chang GJ. Three different approaches to the inferior mesenteric artery during robotic D3 lymphadenectomy for rectal cancer. 2017;**24**(7):1923. DOI: 10.1245/s10434-017-5792-8. Epub 2017 Feb 17

[27] Quirke P, Dixon MF, Durdey P, Williams NS. Local recurrence of rectal adenocarcinoma due to inadequate surgical resection. Histopathological study of lateral tumour spread and surgical excision. Lancet. 1986;**2**(8514):996-999 [Internet] [cited 2022 May 16] Available from: https://pubmed.ncbi.nlm.nih.gov/2430152/

[28] Hawkins AT, Albutt K, Wise PE, Alavi K, Sudan R, Kaiser AM, et al. Abdominoperineal resection for rectal cancer in the twenty-first century: Indications, techniques, and outcomes. Journal of Gastrointestinal Surgery. 2018;**22**(8):1477-1487 [Internet] [cited 2022 May 16] Available from: https://pubmed.ncbi.nlm.nih.gov/29663303/

[29] Yan H, Peng-Yuan W, Wu YC, Liu YC. 4I.s0 a distal resection margin of ≤1 cm safe in patients with intermediate- to low-lying rectal cancer? A systematic review and meta-analysis. Journal of Gastrointestinal Surgery. 2022. DOI: 10.1007/s11605-022-05342-9. [Internet] Available from: DOI: 10.1007/s11605-022-05342-9

[30] Girgis M, Sakai Y, Kim N, Garcia-Henriquez N, Monson JRT, Galante DJ. Selection and outcomes in abdominoperineal resection. Frontiers in Oncology. 2020;**10**:1339 [Internet] Available from: www.frontiersin.org

[31] Musters GD, Buskens CJ, Bemelman WA, Tanis PJ. Perineal wound healing after abdominoperineal resection for rectal cancer: A systematic review and meta-analysis. Diseases of the Colon and Rectum. 2014;**57**(9):1129-1139 [Internet] [cited 2022 May 17] Available from: https://journals.lww.com/dcrjournal/Fulltext/2014/09000/Perineal_Wound_Healing_After_Abdominoperineal.11.aspx

[32] Colov EP, Klein M, Gögenur I. Wound complications and perineal pain after Extralevator versus standard abdominoperineal excision: A Nationwide study. Diseases of the Colon and Rectum. 2016;**59**(9):813-821 [Internet] [cited 2022 May 17] Available from: https://pubmed.ncbi.nlm.nih.gov/27505109/

[33] Schiltz B, Buchs NC, Penna M, Scarpa CR, Liot E, Morel P, et al. Biological mesh reconstruction of the pelvic floor following abdominoperineal excision for cancer: A review. World Journal of Clinical Oncology.

2017;**8**(3):249-254 [Internet] [cited 2022 May 17] Available from: https://pubmed.ncbi.nlm.nih.gov/28638794/

[34] Sheckter CC, Shakir A, Vo H, Tsai J, Nazerali R, Lee GK. Reconstruction following abdominoperineal resection (APR): Indications and complications from a single institution experience. Journal of Plastic, Reconstructive & Aesthetic Surgery. 2016;**69**(11):1506-1512 [Internet] [cited 2022 May 17] Available from: https://pubmed.ncbi.nlm.nih.gov/27538340/

[35] Meyer J, Roos E, Abbassi Z, Toso C, Ris F, Buchs NC. The role of perineal application of prophylactic negative-pressure wound therapy for prevention of wound-related complications after abdomino-perineal resection: a systematic review. International Journal of Colorectal Disease. 2021;**36**(1):19-26 [Internet].[cited 2022 May 17] Available from: https://pubmed.ncbi.nlm.nih.gov/32886194/

[36] Paletto AE, Gaetini A. Nuovo Trattato Di Tecnica Chirurgica. Vol. 4. 2016. EAN: 9788821442193

[37] Saito N, Ito M, Kobayashi A, Nishizawa Y, Sugito M. Sphincter-saving resection for low rectal cancer. Nihon Geka Gakkai Zasshi. 2011;**112**(5):318-324

[38] Rullier E, Denost Q, Vendrely V, Rullier A, Laurent C. Low rectal cancer: Classification and standardization of surgery. Diseases of the Colon and Rectum. 2013;**56**(5):560-567

[39] Mekras A, Michalopoulos A, Papadopoulos VN, Mekras D, Kalles V, Tzeveleki I, et al. Changes in treatment of rectal cancer: Increased use of low anterior resection. Techniques in Coloproctology. 2011;**15**(Suppl 1):S51-S54

[40] Denost Q, Rullier E. Intersphincteric resection pushing the envelope for sphincter preservation. Clinics in Colon and Rectal Surgery. 2017;**30**(5):368-376

[41] Heald RJ. A new solution to some old problems: Transanal TME. Techniques in Coloproctology. 2013;**17**(3):257-258

[42] Simillis C, Hompes R, Penna M, Rasheed S, Tekkis PP. A systematic review of transanal total mesorectal excision: Is this the future of rectal cancer surgery? Colorectal Disease. 2016;**18**:19-36

[43] Buess G, Theiss R, Gunther M, Hutterer F, Pichlmaier H. Endoscopic surgery in the rectum. Endoscopy. 1985;**17**(1):31-35

[44] Bannon JP, Marks GJ, Mohiuddin M, Rakinic J, Nong-Zhou J, Nagle D. Radical and local excisional methods of sphincter-sparing surgery after high-dose radiation for cancer of the distal 3 cm of the rectum. Annals of Surgical Oncology. 1995;**2**(3):221-227

[45] Atallah S, Albert M, Larach S. Transanal minimally invasive surgery: a giant leap forward. Surgical Endoscopy. 2010;**24**(9):2200-2205

[46] Kalloo AN, Singh VK, Jagannath SB, Niiyama H, Hill SL, Vaughn CA, et al. Flexible transgastric peritoneoscopy: A novel approach to diagnostic and therapeutic interventions in the peritoneal cavity. Gastrointestinal Endoscopy. 2004;**60**(1):114-117

[47] Giday S, a, Kantsevoy S V, Kalloo AN. Principle and history of natural orifice Translumenal endoscopic surgery (NOTES). Minimally Invasive Therapy & Allied Technologies. 2006;**15**(6):373-377

[48] Trépanier JS, Fernandez-Hevia M, Lacy AM. Transanal total mesorectal excision: Surgical technique description and outcomes. Minimally Invasive

Therapy and Allied Technologies. 2016;**25**:234-240

[49] de Lacy FB, van Laarhoven JJEM, Pena R, Arroyave MC, Bravo R, Cuatrecasas M, et al. Transanal total mesorectal excision: Pathological results of 186 patients with mid and low rectal cancer. Surgical Endoscopy and Other Interventional Techniques. 2018;**32**(5):2442-2447

[50] Arroyave MC, DeLacy FB, Lacy AM. Transanal total mesorectal excision (TaTME) for rectal cancer: Step by step description of the surgical technique for a two-teams approach. European Journal of Surgical Oncology. 2017;**43**(2):502-505

Section 4

Radiology Based Care

Chapter 6

Magnetic Resonance-Guided Focused Ultrasound in the Treatment of Colorectal Cancer Liver Metastases

Ryan Holman, Orane Lorton, Pauline C. Guillemin, Andrea Peloso, Alexis Ricoeur and Rares Salomir

Abstract

Liver metastases often result secondary to colorectal cancer and curative prognosis is poor. Magnetic resonance high intensity focused ultrasound is a bur-geoning technique with the potential to provide a new image-guidance modality for focused ultrasound ablation of both primary and secondary liver tumors. This is particularly important for colorectal liver metastases cases ineligible for surgical resection, as chemotherapy can often be ineffective at bridging the patient for surgery, and liver transplant has generally been inadequate. At least one system for focused ultrasound ablation of primary and secondary tumors has previously been approved in the European Union, under ultrasound guidance. Magnetic resonance guidance offers many benefits, such as: integration with pre-existing imaging systems, real-time temperature mapping, and ability to assess treatment with MRI during the procedure. This chapter reviews the main aspects in treatment of this disease using this new therapy, including: focused ultrasound physics, magnetic resonance physics, magnetic resonance sequences and protocols in liver imaging, protocols and sequences in magnetic resonance thermometry, standard treatment options and limitations, relevant ongoing clinical trials, previous pilot studies, and outlooks for potential translation of this image-guidance modality as a novel ablative therapy for colorectal liver metastases.

Keywords: interventional radiology, focused ultrasound, liver cancer, thermal ablation, colorectal liver metastases

1. Introduction

Open surgery generally offers the best long-term survival rates for colorectal liver metastases (CRLM); with minimally invasive techniques becoming more common [1]. Magnetic resonance guided high intensity focused ultrasound (MRgHIFU) is noninvasive and non-ionizing, allowing for reduced treatment morbidity. At least one system for ultrasound guided focused ultrasound (USgFUS) ablation has been approved within the European Union for primary and secondary hepatic tumors [2].

 IntechOpen

Although, liver metastases are more common than primary liver tumors, most focused ultrasound studies report outcomes for primary hepatocellular carcinoma (HCC). The use of MRgHIFU for both primary and secondary hepatobiliary tumors is still awaiting certification and has not yet been reported in randomized controlled trials for CRLM or HCC [3]. Discussed here are the focused ultrasound (FUS) physics, the principles of MRI for liver metastases, analysis of the standard treatment approaches for CRLM, and previous studies involving ablation of liver tumors with USgFUS and MRgHIFU.

In 2019, cancer was reported to be the second leading cause of death, globally; amounting to approximately 1 in 6 deaths, worldwide [4]. The primary cause was due to exogenous factors resulting in genetic mutations and amounts to about 90% of reported cases [5]. P53 mutations in tumor suppressor genes are estimated in about 50% of cancers and RAS gene mutations of proto-oncogenes are estimated in about 30% of cancers. Tobacco use is thought to account for the majority of all cancer deaths. This is followed by high body mass index, alcohol use, and malnutrition [5].

HCC is the most common primary liver tumor type. There were approximately 906,000 new primary liver cancer cases in 2020, of which 75–85% were HCC, arriving at approximately 679,500–770,100 new HCC cases [6]. The most prevalent underlying conditions for HCC are Hepatitis-B virus, Hepatitis-C virus, and liver cirrhosis [7, 8]. Primary liver tumor treatment depends on history and staging. If HCC results from decompensated liver cirrhosis, surgical resection is not recommended. These patients do have the option of total liver transplant with 5-year survival rates of about 60–70%. Curative treatment options for late-stage diagnosis or recurrence is rare [8–10]. For HCC, the 10-year survival rate after surgical resection is approximately 25% [11]. However, liver transplant often offers much better outcomes than surgery for HCC. With liver transplant for patients meeting the Milan criteria, 5-year survival rates are near 70%, with less than 10% recurrence rates [11–13]. Liver transplant for HCC constitutes about 25% of liver transplants in the USA and about 40% of liver transplants in Europe [14].

CRLM is the most common form of secondary liver tumor [15]. CRLM occurs in about one-third to one-half of adult CRC cases and the liver metastases is the cause of death in about two-thirds of these patients [16]. In 2020, there were approximately 1.9 million new cases of CRC, of which it might be expected that 633,333–950,000 developed liver metastases [6]. Diagnostic radiologists have listed secondary liver tumor sites at 18–40 times more frequent than primary liver tumors, as the condition often presents with multiple metastases [17]. Historically, CRLM was deemed incurable with untreated 5-year survival rates of less than 2% [18]. Survival rates of patients with distant secondary metastatic tumors can be improved with surgical treatment and systemic chemotherapy [8, 19, 20]. Pediatric liver metastasis is more often secondary to Wilms' tumors or neuroblastomas rather than CRC [21, 22]. About 15% of adult patients exhibit liver metastasis at initial CRC diagnosis [23] and about 70% develop CRLM [2]. Approximately 60% of CRC deaths result from liver metastases [23, 24]. The standard treatment for CRLM is liver resection and is largely considered the best option for long-term curative potential [1, 8, 25, 26], with about a 40% survival rate after 5 years [2, 8, 23, 27], about a 24% survival rate after 10 years [2, 28], about a 20% cure rate [28], and a median survival rate of approximately 30 months [29]. However, for both HCC and CRLM, surgical eligibility is only 20–25% [2]. Liver transplant for CRLM has given good results in recent clinical trials when using tighter inclusion criteria and molecular profiling [30–32], although has historically given dismal survival rates, with high incidence of recurrence, survival rates only marginally better than systemic chemotherapy, and is not a primary option in standard treatment algorithms [1, 33]. Hence, CRLM has an additional treatment difficulty, compared to HCC, because liver transplant does not generally provide long term survival.

2. Focused ultrasound principles

FUS surgery was first reported in 1942 after being applied to cat and dog brain tissue [34, 35] and more elaborate neurological studies later followed [36, 37]. MRgHIFU integrates a FUS transducer into a MRI system with near real-time imaging feedback; capable of temporal resolution less than 1.0 seconds, in-plane resolution less than 1.0 mm, and temperature resolution less than 1.0°C [34]. Thermal tissue ablation results from rapid temperature change of greater than 55°C during heating or −20 to −50°C during cooling [38]. Adequate ablation for coagulative necrosis requires about 10 seconds, with intermittent cooling periods to avoid skin burning [34]. More recent developments enable various feedback methods to regulate temperature, optimize speed, and automate the scanning procedure [39].

FUS works via constructive wave interference. The waves are generated by powering piezoelectric elements with an alternating current [40]. Most modern transducers are phase-array types, composed of hundreds of elements that can be individually controlled, each emitting a low amplitude ultrasonic wave at the focus [40]. Each wave is low enough in amplitude to pass through the tissue without causing significant heating, interfering constructively at the focus. The phase lag of each transducer element is adjusted so the waves are in-phase at the focal region, capable of performing beam steering and refocusing phase aberrations from bone or tissue inhomogeneities. When the waves form a large amplitude oscillation, the heating increases substantially and allows ablation and coagulative necrosis. The wave amplitude and frequency can be controlled by the operator as well as other factors like position, applied power, and pulse modulation. Lower frequencies are better for deep sites like transcranial applications, while high frequencies are used for surface sites [41].

Tissue has an inherent property to absorb ultrasonic energy. The acoustic absorption coefficient measures a tissue's ability to absorb ultrasound. In tissue at 1 MHz, the beam attenuates to about 50% at a depth of about 7 cm [38]. Beam reflection is significant at interfaces with large differences in acoustic absorption coefficient, causing high amounts of reflection at tissue-gas interfaces and tissue-bone interfaces [38]. At large FUS powers, strong rarefactional pressures exist. If this is coupled with lower frequency ultrasound waves, the conditions are favorable to induce tissue nucleation [34, 42]. This results in cavitational heating that can cause detrimental tissue damage or be utilized in techniques like lithotripsy [43, 44] and histotripsy [45, 46]. Low temperature therapies expose cells to about 43–45°C for long time periods. High temperature thermal therapy uses temperature between 50°C and 80°C for short time periods to ablate tissue, cause coagulation, and induce necrosis [47]. The tissue damage is estimated by the equivalent number of thermal doses at 43°C, with necrosis induced after about 240 min at 43°C [48, 49].

3. MRI principles

MRI is based on the concept of nuclear magnetic resonance. Atomic nuclei with an odd number of protons or neutrons exhibit a net spin entailing a charge circulation that forms an individual magnetic field surrounding the atom, giving the protons a magnetic dipole [50–55]. As the hydrogen atoms exhibit ±½ spin, and the nuclear spins exist in two states that are randomly oriented, in absence of a net magnetic field, there is no overall net magnetization. When placed in an external magnetic field, the spins orient parallel and anti-parallel to the direction of the B_0 magnetic field, with a slight propensity for the spins to align in the parallel direction, causing the tissue to express a net equilibrium magnetization [50, 53]. The magnetic moment of the atom rotates like a spinning top, predominately in the direction of the applied magnetic field. This magnetic moment rotates at an angular frequency unique to individual atoms, termed the Larmor frequency.

When a perpendicular radiofrequency field (B_1) is applied at the hydrogen Larmor resonance frequency, only the protons absorb energy, and are tipped from the direction of the main magnetic field, with the flip angle denoting the degree that the spins are displaced from the equilibrium B_0 direction [55]. This excites the protons to precess in a rotational motion around the B_0 field vector. The excited proton magnetization vector then relaxes in the direction of the main B_0 magnetic field, generating a longitudinal and transverse time-varying magnetization signal that is detected by the MRI receiver coils.

The rate at which this magnetization vector relaxes towards the main magnetic field direction is measured in terms of spin-lattice relaxation (T_1) in the direction of the B_0 magnetic field, and the spin-spin relaxation rate (T_2) trans-verse to the B_0 magnetic field direction [50, 53]. The T_1 and T_2 decay rates result from random static magnetic field variations. However, the relaxation rates are also influenced by time varying factors, such as magnetic field inhomogeneities, that combine with tissue static magnetic field to affect the relaxation rate.

The net magnetism applied to each proton results from both the field generated from the MRI system, in addition to the fields generated by the surrounding protons and bulk susceptibility [55, 56]. A chemical shift in the precession frequency results from the magnetic fields generated from these surrounding protons. This can allow identification of specific molecules present in the tissue, that introduce a distinctive chemical shift in the MR signal [55]. The degree of this shift also has a temperature dependence. Using the principle of proton resonance frequency shift (PRFS) thermometry, the individual temperature of each voxel can be quantified from the resulting temperature-dependent phase change due to this chemical shift [56].

4. MRI liver imaging

Radiological imaging is used in a variety of manners in treating CRLM: including, to diagnose a condition, stage the disease, to locate extra-hepatic metastases, for treatment planning, for interventional image-guided procedures, and for post-treatment evaluation [57]. MRgHIFU requires additional MRI sequence protocols, compared to general diagnostic MRI.

4.1 Diagnostic MRI for CRLM

Although CRLM is usually confirmed with computed tomography, MRI is an acceptable and common alternative, and is advantageous at identifying small lesions [1]. Some studies have shown MRI to provide the best results among all diagnostic imaging modalities, though more expensive [58]. The primary objectives for MRI liver tumor diagnosis are to verify the neoplasm presence, staging the lesion, and classifying the type of neoplasm [22]. Accurate assessment of these techniques is crucial to guiding subsequent treatment such as resection, biopsy, and chemotherapy [22]. National Comprehensive Cancer Network (NCCN) guidelines recommend CT be used for initial workup and staging; with MRI recommended for potentially resectable cases, prior to locoregional treatment, and for inadequate imaging with CT [59].

Metastatic liver tumors have been reported as a factor of 18–40 more frequent than primary tumors [17]. The presence of both benign and malignant liver lesions are common. The challenge is often distinguishing the benign liver lesions from malignant lesions, as misdiagnosis can greatly impact staging and treatment planning. CRLM lesions exhibit T_1 signal hypointensity, higher FATSAT-T_2W signal intensity, and higher diffusion-weighted imaging (DWI) signal intensity. On T_2W, the tumor resembles a target; with coagulative necrosis causing a relatively higher signal intensity in the tumor center, followed by a reduced signal exterior due to bulk desmoplasia, and an even lower intensity thin edge from desmoplasia growing at the periphery. This thin edge resembles a ring in the arterial phase when gadolinium is administered. These features can change due to fatty liver infiltration and edema [60].

Standard liver tumor protocols are concerned with imaging the parenchyma, vascular supply, and biliary tract [61]. Basic liver protocols often include: T_2 half acquisition single-shot turbo spin echo (HASTE) localizer, in-op phase T_1 Gradient Recall Echo (GRE), T_2 fast spin echo (FSE) with fat saturation (FATSAT), and gadolinium-enhanced 3D FATSAT T_1 GRE [61, 62]. The HASTE localizer uses a motion insensitive T_2 single-shot spin echo sequence in combination with half-Fourier to acquire a multislice image in about 2 seconds during a single breath hold [63]. The in-op phase Dixon technique, is a spectroscopic technique used to suppress fat signal, quantify the hepatic fat content of the liver, and estimate iron content [63]. The spectroscopic method distinguishes an image at the $-CH_2$ fat chemical shift from an image at the water chemical shift [64]. In-phase and op-phase sequences are often spin-echo or GRE sequences with equal repetition times, but different echo times. It acquires a normal in-phase image containing the water and fat, an opposed-phase image containing the water phase signal lessened by the fat phase contribution. Combining in-phase and op-phase images generates the water only image, and subtraction of the op-phase image from the in-phase image allows isolation of the fat signal [64, 65]. Additionally, the Dixon technique allows the generation of a T_2^* map, from which the local iron content (mg g^{-1}) can be formulated [65, 66].

Of high importance in clinical diagnosis of liver lesions are DWI and hepatocyte-specific magnetic resonance contrast agent imaging, with MRI elastography to a lesser extent [67]. DWI is particularly useful for detection of small metastatic lesions [61]. Liver DWI consists of a T_2 sequence with symmetric diffusion sensitizing gradients centered on the 180° refocusing pulse [67, 68]. Brownian motion of water molecules is more restricted in tumors and provides a noticeable degree of contrast compared to normal tissue [69]. The DWI sequence is generally used without the administration of a contrast agent, making it a completely non-invasive diagnostic sequence. The weighting factor in DWI is adjusted based on the b-value, that is a function of gradient strength and duration. The apparent diffusion coefficient (ADC) maps can be viewed by removing the T_2-weighting from a series of diffusion-weighted images. Hyperintense regions generally correspond to regions of low fluid diffusion [63].

CRLM lesions are a solid liver lesion and a general protocol for identification and characterization can be described as follows. First, a highly T_2-weighted SSTSE to identify benign fluid-filled lesions, such as cysts and hemangiomas. Next, a modestly T_2-weighted FATSAT-TSE or DWI to identify metastatic tumor sites. Then, a Dixon sequence might be used to observe the degree of fat infiltration into the tumor. Lastly, a contrast-enhanced image can be used for T_1-weighted phase imaging to characterize the tumor [70].

Extracellular gadolinium agents are the most common contrast agents for general imaging throughout the body [71]. Two common hepatic specific contrast agents are gadoxetate disodium (Gd-EOB-DTPA, Primovist, Eovist, Bayer Healthcare Pharmaceuticals) and gadobenate dimeglumine (Gd-BOPTA, Bracco Diagnostics) [67]. In some studies, Gd-EOB-DTPA hepatocyte specific MRI contrast agents has shown improved sensitivity and specificity in diagnosis of liver metastasis compared to computed tomography, particularly to the improved ability to detect small metastases [67, 72]. The hepatic-specific contrast agents are specific to tumors originating from hepatocytes, and can help distinguish these lesions from cavernoma or metastatic lesions [71, 73]. Though, these are more expensive than extracellular analogues, have a lower recommended dose and signal, and can exhibit reduced uptake in patients with hepatocyte dysfunction [69]. A comparison of DWI and Gd-EOB-DTPA-T_1W MRI for detecting small lesions from CRLM are shown in **Figure 1** [74].

4.2 MRgHIFU sequence aspects

MRgHIFU requires additional MRI sequences that allow for temperature mapping. MR temperature mapping most commonly utilizes PRFS thermometry [75–77], though other possible techniques allow temperature measurements based on the temperature-dependence of relaxation rates, proton density, water diffusion coefficient, thermo-sensitive contrast agents, and magnetization transfer [78, 79]. Resonance frequency shift results from temperature differences in water molecules and aqueous tissues, due to varying degrees of hydrogen bonding. At increased temperatures, the amount of hydrogen bonding is reduced. This increases nuclear shielding of water protons from the incident magnetic field, generating a lower resonance frequency in the water molecules [78]. This results in a linear-dependence of the phase map values from the chemical shift due to temperature change, at a rate of about -0.01 ppm $°C^{-1}$ [78, 79]. MRgHIFU sequences

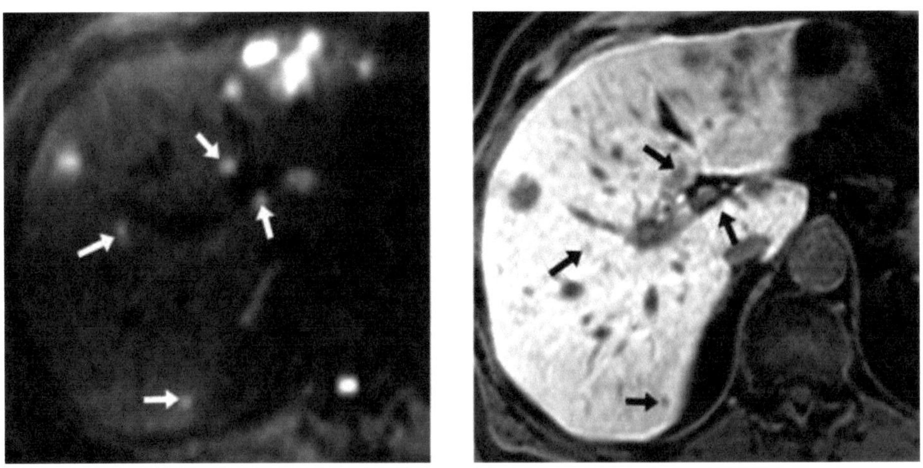

Figure 1.
Comparison of diffusion-weighted MRI with contrast-enhanced T_1W MRI. Left: diffusion-weighted MRI of liver metastases. The arrows indicate small metastatic tumors, less than 1 cm diameter. Right: CE-T_1W image after applying Gd-EOB-DTPA, in the same patient. Reprinted with permission from Koh and Berry [74].

are often based on GRE segmented echo-planar imaging (SEG EPI) sequences. A basic GRE sequence is the fast low-angle shot (FLASH) sequence that utilizes small flip angles to obtain a short echo time (TE) and repetition time (TR) [80]. The sequence further benefits from EPI to accelerate the acquisition rate.

Additional sequences are used to assess tissue peri-ablation and post-ablation. During the peri-ablation period, inflammation in the focal region results from edema, giving more contrast enhancement, and remains for some months. After ablation, T_2 and peripheral T_1 hyperintensity increases significantly due to the presence of hemorrhagic debris at the ablation region. Thickening or nodule formation in the peripheral hyperintense signal can also indicate recurrence or incomplete ablation, during the months following the procedure [67]. Alternative sequences are under study for other aspects of the modality. For example, magnetic resonance acoustic radiation force impulse (MR-ARFI) sequences allow simultaneous displacement and temperature measurements [81, 82], and is implemented in clinical research settings for tracking focal spot and assessing positioning errors [83, 84]. Additionally, MR-ARFI sequences are being studied for phase aberration correction that occurs in transcostal or transcranial procedures [85–87].

Also, thermal ablation needs temperature processing less than about one second. The faster sequences result in reduced signal to noise ratio and increased temperature uncertainty. Echo planar imaging, parallel imaging, alternate trajectories, and undersampling can increase the MRI frame rate [88–90]. In typical rectilinear sampling, the RF pulse frequency and slice-select gradient determine the slice to be imaged, the frequency encoding gradient amplitude controls the k_x-dimension position, and the phase encoding gradient amplitude controls the k_y-dimension position [54]. Alternate trajectories are useful, particularly for fast acquisition times and reducing motion artifacts. Radial trajectories are utilized in some of the fastest real-time MRI sequences [90]. Magnetic field inhomogeneities and magnetic susceptibility are also significant aspects to proper imaging and temperature mapping [91, 92].

5. Surgery for CRLM

Primary colon cancer is classified IV in patients presenting CRLM [2]. Most CRLM patients develop liver metastases after initial CRC treatment, while about 20–34% present liver nodules at initial diagnosis [59]. When CRLM are confined to the liver, the intent should be cure, and surgical resection is actually the standard of care, presenting the best survival rates [59, 93]. Neoadjuvant and adjuvant systemic therapy are recommended in most patients prior to surgical resection, as it can improve instances of recurrence [1, 59]. The response to neoadjuvant chemotherapy has shown to be a strong prognostic factor for outcomes after hepatic resection [94]. The aim of liver resection is to remove all macroscopic disease with clear (negative) margins and leave sufficient functioning liver, with proper vascular and biliary flow [95]. An inadequate future liver remnant volume (FLRV) can lead to post-hepatectomy liver failure, a major cause of morbidity and mortality. Typically, FLRV is intended to be more than 30% of the native tissue and 30% future liver remnant, or more than 350 grams of liver remaining per 70 kg body weight [1]. The anatomic description of functional segments, which is based on the organ's blood supply via the hepatic artery and portal vein, its venous drainage via the hepatic veins, and lastly its biliary drainage, is the foundation of liver surgery. Historically, up to six Couinaud segments can be removed in healthy individuals, returning to original size in about three weeks, with restored liver function in about six weeks [29, 96]. An illustration of the liver segments are given in **Figure 2**.

Typical resection complications occur in 20–50% of patients, although the mortality rate is only 1–3% in high volume centers [29, 97]. Most common complications include pleural effusion or pulmonary atelectasis, venous catheter infection, site-incisional infection, ascites, subphrenic infection, intraperitoneal bleeding, biliary tract hemorrhage, coagulation disorders, and bile leakage [98]. Additionally, inadequate post-operative liver response can result from pre-operative liver dysfunction, prolonged vascular occlusion, and inadequate resid-ual liver volume; leading to hepatic insufficiency that results in ascites, mental impairment, hyperbilirubinaemia, and possible sepsis [98]. Post-operative liver function can be evaluated by dynamic functional testing such as indocyanine green (ICG) clearance rate, or by aminopyrine breath tests for cytochrome P-450 function, and post-treatment monitoring with blood serum tests for analytes including coagulation products and albumin [98].

Surgical resection for synchronous CRLM is an extremely complex scenario and surgery remains one of the major curative treatment options available.

Consideration for surgical resection must be given to: the anatomical distribution of the disease; FRLV; management of the primary disease (in the setting of synchronous CRLM); the timing and role of (neo)adjuvant chemotherapy, and whether all disease can be resected successfully at one sitting. Patients are often administered chemotherapy and chosen to undergo a conventional colon-first procedure, a liver-first procedure, or simultaneous resection [99]. Even for patients presenting multifocal bilateral CRLM, the goal should be a full tumor excision with sufficient remaining functional parenchyma. Though, for multifocal bilateral CRLM, resection and ablation often yield survival rates only faintly superior to chemotherapy alone [99]. The traditional colon-first approach involves complete primary CRC tumor resection, along with systemic chemotherapy, then hepatectomy is performed later if resectable [100]. A “liver-first” approach involves

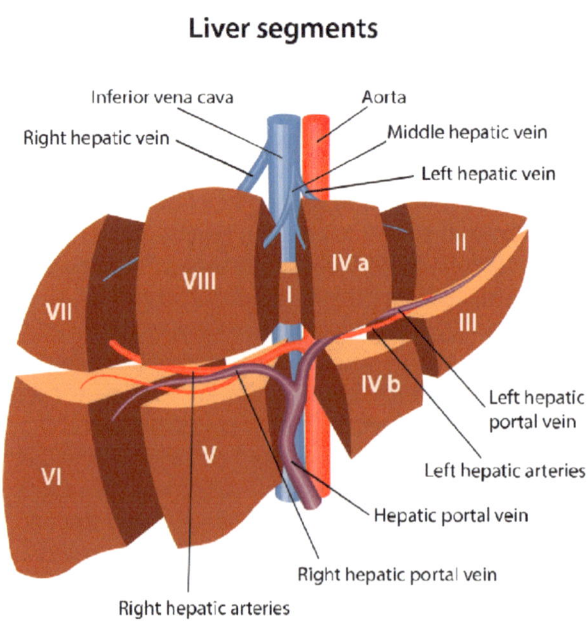

Figure 2.
Illustration identifying locations of individual Couinaud segments. Olga Bolbot/shutterstock.com.

initial systemic chemotherapy, liver tumor removal, then CRC resection [100]. The concept is that the liver tumor is most likely to create further metastasis and the CRC is quite sensitive to systemic chemotherapy [101]. With either approach, approximately only 10–20% of patients are surgical candidates [2, 8, 102]. Reasons include late-stage cancer diagnosis, secondary tumor sites outside the liver, and existing comorbidity ineligibility [2, 8]. Although surgical resections report long-term survival rates, about half of the patients develop widespread metastases within three years [1]. Recurrence after primary liver resection occurs at about a 43% rate in the liver and about a 31% rate in the lungs [8].

Anatomic resections usually involve two or more hepatic segments, while non-anatomic resection involves resection of the metastases with a margin of uninvolved tissue (segmentectomy). Various approaches in liver resection include: right hepatectomy, right lobectomy, left hepatectomy left lobectomy, extended right hepatectomy, and extended left hepatectomy [103]. By performing a segment-based resection, intra-operative hemorrhage and remaining post-treatment ischemic tissue can be avoided, helping to prevent infection and bile duct fistula. Additionally, the segment-based approach allows predetermined calculation of tumor margins and remaining viable parenchyma. Moreover, intrahepatic metastases tend to arise in the same Couinaud segments, allowing better chances to remove small satellite metastatic sites [103, 104].

Modern surgery resection is based on the report of the first successful proce-dure for a right hepatectomy [103, 105]. An illustration of the basic liver anatomy is shown in **Figure 3**. Each Couinaud segment is functionally independent, receiving blood supply from the portal vein and from the hepatic artery; at the same time the outflows is guaranteed by various branches of the hepatic vein. The right hepatic lobe is composed of Couinaud segments 5–8, with the blood supply to the right lobe provided by the right portal vein and right hepatic artery. First, the falciform ligament, coronary ligament, and right triangular ligament are cut to allow increased liver movement. Next, the right hepatic artery, right portal vein, right hepatic duct, and cystic duct are clamped, cut, and ligated. The blood supply to the left lobe is kept intact. This is followed by dissection of the right lobe from the inferior vena cava. Venous outflow from the main and short hepatic veins are divided and ligated. This devascularization creates a line of demarcation due to a color change in the right liver lobe. Then,

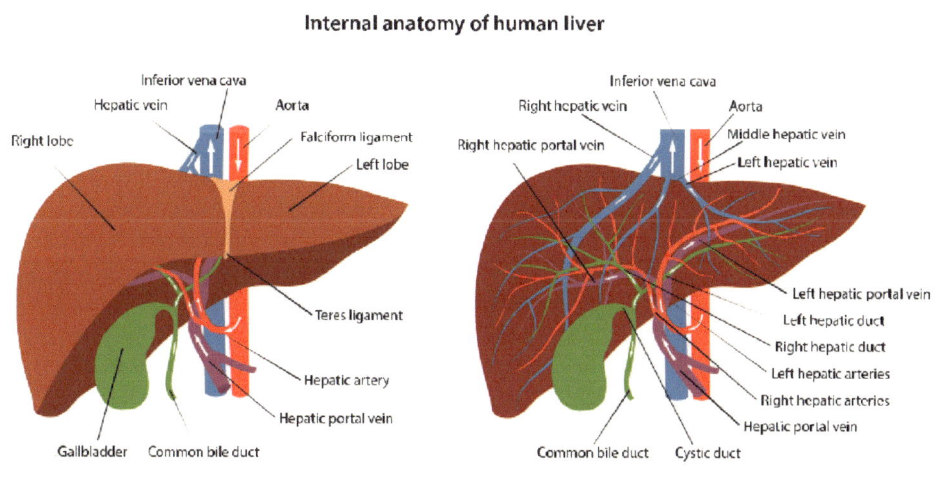

Figure 3.
Overview of the liver anatomy. Olga Bolbot/shutterstock.com.

transection of the liver parenchyma occurs, dividing the right and left lobes along the middle hepatic vein. This is followed by ligation of the middle hepatic vein blood supply. Parenchyma transection can result in large blood loss that can be lessened using a reduced central venous pressure and Pringle's manoeuvre [103, 104, 106]. Three major complications for the procedure include the introduction of an air embolism into the hepatic veins, hemorrhagic bleeding from the hepatic veins, and biliary leakage into the abdominal cavity [107].

The concept of the "two-staged hepatectomy" has been introduced by Adam et al. [108], as a surgical strategy that could be applied to patients with conventionally irresectable metastases to make them eligible for liver resection. This approach involved a combination of systemic chemotherapy to downstage tumors, with or without portal vein embolization (PVE), with subsequent planned staged operations that permitted curative resection of large tumor burden that would otherwise have been considered unresectable. The interval between operations enabled hypertrophy of the remnant liver to theoretically reduce the chance of liver insufficiency and patients would receive chemotherapy during the interval between operations in an effort to control tumor growth.

More recently, the technique known as ALPPS (Associating Liver Partition and Portal Vein Ligation for Staged Hepatectomy) allows removal of extensive tumor load by increasing future liver remnant, allowing increased surgical eligibility, and extended survivability of CRLM patients [109, 110]. Early research included right PVE, which was shown to induce hypertrophy in the left lobe, subsequently allowing increased amounts of liver tissue to be removed in the right lobe [108, 110–112]. This was later applied in two-stage hepatectomies to allow increased amounts of cancerous liver tissue to be removed from both liver lobes, by permitting liver regrowth between procedures [110]. Early two-stage hepatectomies required months for liver regrowth, with tumor progression frequently occurring during this time; however, development of ALPPS allowed the two surgical procedures to be performed within 7–14 days [109, 110]. ALPPS is indicated in case of extensive multifocal CRLM, failure after portal vein embolization, and expected small amounts of FLRV [14].

A generic procedure for two-stage hepatectomy of left lobe wedge resection combined with right lobe hepatectomy includes in situ liver splitting in addition to portal vein ligation [113]. First, the falciform ligament is cut, then tumors locations are confirmed and marked by intraoperative ultrasound. The transection line(s) is identified. Then, the right cystic duct and artery are ligated, followed by dissection and ligation of the right portal vein at the portal bifurcation. The right and middle hepatic veins are isolated, the space between is dissected, and umbilical tape is placed for the hanging maneuver. Then, transection of the parenchyma is performed at the site previously marked with/without Pringle maneuver. The liver is patched, drains placed, abdomen closed, ending the first stage. At this stage the liver is separated but not removed. Then, functional liver testing and weekly volumetry measurements are performed with CT or MRI until the future liver remnant volume surpasses 30%. In the second stage, the incision is reopened, and the hepatic artery and bile duct are ligated on the right lobe that previously underwent portal vein ligation. Then, transection of the right hepatic vein is followed by removal of the right liver lobe and closure of the abdomen.

In the last decade, it has been conceptualized that liver transplantation could offer the theoretical advantage of a real R0 resection, removing also all potentially undetected metastases. Earlier studies in American and European populations showed that transplant after non-neuroendocrine liver metastases from various primary sites yielded one-year survival rates of only 5%, which is compounded by the lack of available donors [33]. More recent studies with tightened inclusion criteria have shown more favorable outcomes and resulted in a large increase in CRLM transplants worldwide [30, 31, 114]. The studies have suggested much longer survival rates after liver transplant for CRLM, when the inclusion criteria included adequate response to chemotherapy, excised primary tumor sites, more than one year between diagnosis and transplant, and liver only metastases [31, 32, 115]. Additional exclusion criteria exist based upon molecular profiling; for instance, exclusion is recommended due to V600 BRAF mutations and MSI from DNA mismatch repair (MMR) mutations [116]. These results have suggested liver transplant possibly provides the best overall survivability compared to other treatment modalities for surgical ineligibility. The drawbacks are smaller study size, the limited availability of liver donors and more specialized training is required across multiple disciplines to conduct the operation [30].

6. Chemotherapy for CRLM

Systemic chemotherapy in CRLM is administered to attain surgical eligibility, for disease control, peri-operatively, or palliatively; since the treatment alone is rarely curative, with 5-year survival rates less than 10%, and historically less than 1% [25, 30, 117]. Polymetastatic liver disease faces treatment limitations with chemotherapy being the primary treatment. The survival rate is poor and a large demand exists for improved treatment options. As surgical resection offers the best long-term survival rates, the aim of systemic chemotherapy is often to downsize tumors to convert ineligible patients to surgical candidates, with systematic review showing a conversion rate for R0 resection in initially ineligible patients at 23% [118]. Chemotherapy regimens are administered neoadjuvantly prior to hepatectomy for cytoreduction, to reduce metastatic tumor size, allowing smaller resection volumes [119]. The regimens are also administered after resection to reduce recurrence [25, 120]. Hepatic intra-arterial infusion is often beneficial because the liver metastasis is supplied by the hepatic artery network, normal tissue is supplied by the portal vein, and locoregional treatment can be performed without exposing much healthy tissue [121–123]. The liver contains a capillary network of sinusoids that filter the blood as shown in **Figure 4**. Approximately 45% of metastatic tumor cells, predominately arriving from the hepatic arterial network [123], become embedded in the sinusoids [89]. Normal liver parenchyma receive about 80% of the blood supply from the portal vein and about 20% from the hepatic artery. In contrast, about 80% of the tumor blood supply arrives from the hepatic artery [116]. This allows locoregional embolization techniques, like radioembolization and chemoembolization, to both embolize the blood supply to specific tumor segments, and deliver locoregional radiotherapy or chemotherapy. These embolization techniques are suggested to be considered for metastatic CRC limited only to the liver, and after unsuccessful chemotherapy [1].

The chemotherapy regimen depends on a number of factors, including: aim of cytoreduction prior to surgery, aim of disease control, aim of palliation, type of somatic gene mutation, and wild-type or mutant phenotype. Somatic mutations of RAS proto-oncogenes have been found in up to 52% of CRLM hepatic resections, with up to 6–12% of resections expressing BRAF mutations, and co-occurring proto-oncogene RAS and TP53 tumor-suppressor mutations as common genetic events [1, 94]. According to ESMO guidelines, first-line chemotherapy for cytoreduction in RAS

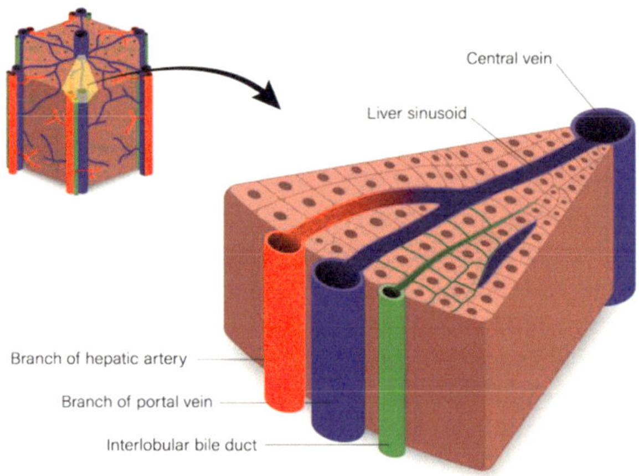

Figure 4.
Histological depiction of liver lobules. These units are microscale components of liver tissue. The liver sinusoids are small capillaries, with blood supplied by small branches of the hepatic artery and portal vein. Dee-sign/shutterstock.com.

tumors should be recommended cytotoxic doublets (FOLFOX/CAPOX/FOLFIRI), in combination with VEGF antibody bevacizumab for RAS mutant-type tumors, and EGFR antibodies for wild-type tumors. FOLFOXIRI with bevacizumab are recommended as a first line treatment for cytoreduction in CRLM BRAF mutant tumors [1].

Chemotherapeutics can also exhibit many adverse side-effects on healthy liver tissue. Side-effects include sinusoidal obstruction syndrome and chemotherapy-associated steatohepatitis, that can lead to liver failure or increased mortality rates [119]. Additionally, the chemotherapy can cause missing metastases, making lesions unidentifiable on radiological imaging, complicating surgical decisions, and increasing the chance of recurrence [119]. Chemotherapy has difficulty supplying tumor cells with adequate drug dose. The maximum dose is limited by systemic toxicity effects and inadequate tumor penetration is common [8, 124]. Intrahepatic arterial delivery can exhibit acute side-effects of hepatocellular atrophy causing cirrhosis and necrosis [123, 125].

Doxorubicin is an anthracycline chemotherapeutic that can be administered during combination therapy. A liposomal form was created relatively early due to the need for better treatment in Kaposi sarcoma from autoimmune deficiency syndrome [126]. Clinical trials of FUS-mediated thermosensitive liposomal doxorubicin drug delivery to liver tumors [127, 128] have shown large increases in intratumoral doxorubicin concentration, and there are ongoing trials with MRgHIFU for pediatric tumors [129]. Similar ongoing trials are studying the enhanced ability for microbubbles to improve chemotherapy delivery to metastatic liver tumors [130].

7. Radiotherapy for CRLM

Radiotherapy emits ionizing radiation at tumors, causing DNA damage, and apoptosis. The technique exhibits some similar drawbacks to focused ultrasound. Cumulative radiation exposure can occur in the beam's near and far field, resulting in unwanted tissue damage [8, 131, 132]. Also, systems require computed tomography guidance and respiratory motion control [8, 133]. Local ablative techniques, including radiotherapy, are generally considered to be limited to patients with unresectable CRLM or oligometastatic disease [1]. CRLM radiotherapy has often been limited by liver parenchyma radio-sensitivity. External beam radiation doses of 70–90 Gy needed for CRLM and HCC tumor treatment exceeds tolerance limits of 35 Gy for radiation-induced liver disease (RILD) [57, 134] that can lead to liver failure and death [25]. The condition occurs two to sixteen weeks after treatment, is identified by ascites, high levels of alkaline phosphatases, and high levels of liver transaminases [135].

Stereotactic body radiation therapy (SBRT) with linear accelerators has recently gained much interest for surgical ineligibility, particularly in oligometastatic disease. With SBRT, fiducial markers are percutaneously placed near the tumor site to allow precise tumor targeting [57]. Though MRI guidance reduces invasiveness, without the need for fiducial markers [116]. SBRT is recommended by ESMO to be considered for patients with oligometastatic disease who are ineligible for surgery and ablative therapy [1]. One major advantage of SBRT compared to ablative therapies is that the treatment is non-thermal, mitigating some of the common side-effects seen in local ablative techniques, such as fluid perfusion effects [116]. Studies have shown that liver failure is infrequent when only a portion of the liver is irradiated [135]. The liver toxicity is mild to moderate, with liver failure in less than 1% of patients [136, 137]. Treatment of oligometastatic CRC in the liver with SBRT, suggests one and two year overall survivability at about 67.1% and 56.5%, respectively [137]. Many early phase clinical trials are recruiting, active, or recently completed, for treatment of primary or secondary hepatic tumors with magnetic resonance guided linear accelerators [138, 139] and magnetic resonance guided SBRT [140–143]. Recent phase I trial results with magnetic resonance guided SBRT, showed improved toxicity, with estimated 2-year overall survival of 51%, and median overall survival of 29 months [144].

8. Focused ultrasound clinical studies for liver cancer

A substantial number of clinical studies, cohorts, and randomized control trials for non-liver MRgHIFU and MRgFUS have been reported, including: treatment with bone osteomas or palliative bone metastasis [145, 146], uterine fibroids [147–151], gynaecological tumor recurrence [152], prostate cancer [153, 154], essential tremor [155, 156], and breast cancer [157]. Many clinical studies have been reported for USgFUS ablation for liver tumors [158–165], with most studies reporting on HCC ablation [166]. Similar to USgFUS, new histotripsy devices using cavitation rather than thermal ablation, are currently being studied for the treatment of primary and secondary tumors, with an active prospective clinical trial [45, 46, 167, 168]. No Phase III trials for USgFUS or MRgHIFU ablation of CRLM have been published [116]. Early USgFUS studies in liver malignancies, not distinguishing between metastatic liver tumors and primary liver tumors, showed a median survival time of 13.4 months, 6-month survival times of 82.6%, and 12-month survival time of 53.4% [159]. More recent systematic reviews of FUS for liver malignancies have given 1 year, 2 year, and 5-year survivability of 81%, 60%, and 39%, respectively [166]. Most studies have been conducted using the Chongqing Haifu JC system, capable of up to 300 W acoustic power and peak intensity up to 20,000 W cm^2 [166]. The system has received the mark Conformite′ Europeenne′ (CE), being the most reported system for clinical liver tumor ablation [2, 3]. The permission is granted to individual commercial models rather than general treatment procedures. The magnetic resonance guided systems that have received regulatory approval for alternative treatments include the ArcBlate (Episonica, Hsinchu, Taiwan), Exablate (Insightec, Tirat Carmel, Israel), and Sonalleve (Profound Medical, Mississauga, Canada) systems.

Local ablative techniques, including focused ultrasound ablation, are generally recommended only in cases of unresectable liver metastases or oligometastatic disease [1]. Most FUS ablation therapy studies for liver tumors are USgFUS for HCC, with less reports of metastatic liver tumor treatment [166]. Particularly advantageous in FUS is the improved side effect profile and reduced morbidity compared to standard treatment options. The treatment can occur multiple times with no cumulative radiation-like side effects. In relation to chemotherapy, it is much more focused, with less toxicity to healthy tissues [8, 169]. Additionally, extracorporeal FUS liver ablation is completely non-invasive and offers very fast recovery times [170]. Benefits of MRgHIFU compared to USgFUS include near real-time temperature mapping, integration into existing imaging systems, less propensity for radiofrequency interference in the imaging system, and capability of assessing treatment response during the procedure. Though ultrasound-guided devices do not provide real-time temperature map-ping, assessment of grey-scale change are indicative of coagulative necrosis [166]. Treatment plans with FUS generally depend on the cancer staging. Curative ablation of early stage tumors often include a 1.5–2.0 cm peripheral tissue margin. The treatment is administered palliatively for late-stage tumors to slow progression or alleviate symptoms [8, 160].

Drawbacks to hepatobiliary focused ultrasound studies have been the need for general anesthesia, long treatment times, scattering by the thoracic cage, high power requirements, respiratory motion, skin burns, osteonecrosis, skin pain, skin edema, rib resection, fever, the need for intrapleural effusion, and reduced thermal dose from fluid perfusion of surrounding vessels [2, 39, 165, 166, 170–177]. A systematic review of USgFUS for the treatment of malignant hepatobiliary tumors indicated the primary complications were skin burns in 15% of cases, followed by localized pain in 5%, then fever at 2% [166]. Major post-treatment complications include fluid and/or air accumulation in the lungs, biliary obstruction, and fistula occurrence [177].

Some studies have reported focused ultrasound ablation in primary and secondary liver tumors in difficult locations, including near major hepatic veins and arteries, and near surrounding organs of the heart, gallbladder, stomach, and intestine [162, 165, 178]. Tumors located near surrounding organs are high-risk. Particularly sensitive are the bowel and gallbladder due to the thin walls and risks of peritonitis [162].

Skin and rib burns have been addressed in a variety of manners. Skin burns have been reported to occur with tumors located near the subcapsular area, resulting from possible rib reflection or reflections from internal gas pockets in the bowel or lung parenchyma [166]. The right lobe is more susceptible as it is predominately located behind the ribs [162]. Intrapleural effusion can distance the tumor site from the subcapsular area, or rib resection can be performed [162, 179]. Particularly troublesome are tumors of the liver dome in Couinaud segments 7 and 8, due to the close proximity to the lungs, the close proximity to the ribs, and that this region tends to remain behind the rib cage under general anesthesia due to reduced respiration [162]. A small cohort for USgFUS reported that proper intraoperative assessment of the soft tissue prevented skin burns in all patients [161].

A variety of techniques have been tested to overcome respiratory motion and rib interaction. Respiratory motion creates complications requiring organ image registration techniques [180] and MRI motion artifact compensation [174, 181]. Numerous preclinical studies have undertaken new technologies to address respiratory motion and rib interactions [39, 172, 174–176, 180, 182–186]. Previous USgFUS human studies have generally been successful at performing ablation through the ribs; though additional measures have included left lung ventilation with endotracheal intubation and general anesthesia to reduce liver movement, intrapleural effusion, and rib resection [160, 162, 179]. MRgHIFU pilot studies used intermittent sonications, and limited to the treatment to the left liver lobe, in tumor sites not blocked by the ribs [170, 187–189].

Handheld intraoperative HIFU devices under ultrasound-guidance are in development, and being tested in early phase clinical trials for CRLM tumor abla-tion. The technique is similar to intraoperative radiofrequency and microwave ablation, but prevents the need for an intraparenchymal probe. Results have been reported using the device for ablating tissue near tumors in segments prior to surgical resection, to assess accuracy and safety. Applications include reduction of hemorrhaging during surgery and potentially bridging more patients for surgical resection [190–193]. The device was shown capable of in vivo hepatic vessel occlusion for diameters of 2 mm [194], and studies have reported diameters of left hepatic arteries and right hepatic veins between 3 and 4 mm [195].

Several small clinical studies have been reported for MRgHIFU ablation for HCC [170, 187–189, 196, 197]. There is currently an ongoing Phase I clinical trial with MRgHIFU for a variety of pediatric solid tumors, in which hepatic tumors are eligible [198].

In the study from Okada et al. [187], MRgHIFU liver tumor ablation was performed on a single patient. The MRI system utilized respiratory gating and ablation was performed on a 15 mm HCC lesion. The procedure required about two hours to ensure complete coagulation by repeated coverage. Gadolinium contrast agent was administered post-treatment and no increased signal intensity was observed at the tumor site, indicating expected ablation contrast. The authors noted the need for better technology for avoiding bowel loops, ribs, and respiratory liver motion. Though, the patient only complained of slight skin heating discomfort during treatment and was released from the hospital the following day.

Anzidei et al. treated a single HCC patient more comprehensively with MR-FUS [188]. The patient refused surgery and percutaneous ablation, then opted for MR-FUS. The individual had no distant metastases, was treated successfully, and later underwent total liver transplant. Excised liver histopathology showed complete coagulative necrosis with only slight recurrence at the ablation periphery. The investigators noted the procedure can be improved with better respiratory motion control and expected that future applications would use automated feedback algorithms.

Gedroyc conducted a series of pilot studies for MRgHIFU liver tumor ablation [170, 189]. It was reported that the absorption from the ribs was problematic and the treatments were limited to patients with exposed tumor sites, such as below the rib line or in the left lobe of the liver. One case was a female with HCC arising from Hepatitis-B infection. She was previously treated with hepatic arterial chemoembolization and laser ablation. Recurrence occurred with a 1.5 cm HCC lesion in the left lobe within Couinaud segment 3, a position that was not covered by the ribs. The site was ablated with MRgHIFU. In another case, the patient was a male with HCC, Hepatitis-C, extensive cirrhosis, and elevated alpha-fetoprotein levels. He was treated for a 3 cm HCC in the anterior portion of the left liver lobe.

9. Conclusions

Optimal treatment strategies for CRLM patients should be made by a multidisciplinary team as part of a tumor board, for establishing diagnostic and treatment strategies [1]. Surgery of CRLM will likely provide the best long-term outcomes and the strategy should focus on complete resection. Although, the majority of patients with CRLM are ineligible for surgery and many surgical cases will experience widespread recurrence. Thermal ablation methods like focused ultrasound are generally only recommended for unresectable CRLM and oligometastatic disease, with at least one system under ultrasound guidance having the CE-mark for CRLM [1, 2]. Due to expected increasing CRLM incidence and high surgical ineligibility, non-invasive technologies like MRgHIFU systems have great potential for clinical translation as an ablative interventional radiology procedure.

Guidelines for FUS pilot studies suggest performing MRgHIFU ablation in CRLM patients prior to the surgical operation, then surgically removing the ablated tumor, and assessing the effectiveness with pathology [2]. Randomized control trials have been suggested to be performed on CRLM patients that are not candidates for surgical resection or RF ablation, and to compare TACE and MRgHIFU to a control group receiving only TACE [2]. In a randomized controlled trial, USgFUS for primary liver tumors in combination with TACE has shown improved treatment over TACE alone, increasing survival times, giving higher remission rates, lower recurrence rates, lower rates of post-operative metastases, and less instances of hemorrhaging in the digestive tract [199, 200].

MRgHIFU has been established in proof-of-concept studies for HCC, limited to the left liver lobe or section not covered by the ribs, requiring intermittent ablation due to respiration, and has not been reported in randomized controlled trials for primary or secondary liver tumors [170, 187–189, 196, 197, 201]. The FUS field has gained much interest in recent years and MRgHIFU ablation of primary and secondary liver tumors appears likely to begin early phase trials in the near future. Previous focused ultrasound studies have developed methods to address many technical complications such as respiratory motion and suppressing prefocal interactions; with focusing through the ribs being one of the major technical difficulties. Long treatment times are another complication and should improve with automated feedback control and faster acquisition times.

Author details

Ryan Holman[1*], Orane Lorton[1], Pauline C. Guillemin[1], Andrea Peloso[2,3], Alexis Ricoeur[4] and Rares Salomir[1,4]

1 Image Guided Interventions Laboratory, Department of Radiology, University of Geneva, Geneva, Switzerland

2 Hepatology and Transplantation Laboratory, Faculty of Medicine, Department of Surgery, Division of Visceral Surgery, University of Geneva, Geneva, Switzerland

3 Department of Surgery, Division of Visceral Surgery, Geneva University Hospitals, Geneva, Switzerland

4 Radiology Department, University Hospitals of Geneva, Geneva, Switzerland

*Address all correspondence to: ryan.holman@unige.ch

References

[1] Van Cutsem E, Cervantes A, Adam R, Sobrero A, Van Krieken JH, Aderka D, et al. ESMO consensus guidelines for the management of patients with metastatic colorectal cancer. Annals of Oncology. 2016;**27**(8):1386-1422

[2] Aubry JF, Pauly KB, Moonen C, Haar G, Ries M, Salomir R, et al. The road to clinical use of high-intensity focused ultrasound for liver cancer: Technical and clinical consensus. Journal of Therapeutic Ultrasound. 2013;**1**(13):1-13

[3] State of the Field Report. Focused Ultrasound Foundation. 2021. Available from: https://www.fusfoundation.org/the-foundation/foundation-reports#SOTF

[4] World Health Organization (WHO). Global Health Estimates 2020: Deaths by Cause, Age, Sex, by Country and by Region, 2000-2019. WHO; 2020. Available from: https://www.who.int/data/gho/data/themes/mortality-and-global-health-estimates/ghe-leading-causes-of-death; [Accessed: December 31, 2021]

[5] Cassidy J, Bissett D, Obe RAS, Payne M, Morris-Stiff G. Oxford Handbook of Oncology. OUP Oxford; 2015

[6] Sung H, Ferlay J, Siegel RL, Laversanne M, Soerjomataram I, Jemal A, et al. Global Cancer Statistics 2020: GLOBOCAN Estimates of Incidence and Mortality Worldwide for 36 Cancers in 185 Countries. CA: A Cancer Journal for Clinicians. 2021;**71**(3):209-249

[7] Shlomai A, de Jong YP, Rice CM. Virus associated malignancies: The role of viral hepatitis in hepatocellular carcinoma. Seminars in Cancer Biology. 2014;**26**:78-88

[8] Lyon PC. Targeted release from lyso-thermosensitive liposomal doxorubicin (ThermoDox®) using focused ultrasound in patients with liver tumours [doctoral dissertation]; 2016

[9] Bruix J, Sherman M. Management of hepatocellular carcinoma. Hepatology. 2005;**42**(5):1208-1236

[10] Bruix J, Sherman M, Llovet JM, Beaugrand M, Lencioni R, Burroughs AK, et al. Clinical management of hepatocellular carcinoma. Conclusions of the Barcelona-2000 EASL conference. European Association for the Study of the Liver. Journal of Hepatology. 2001;**35**(3):421-430

[11] Fan ST. Hepatocellular carcinoma—Resection or transplant? Nature Reviews Gastroenterology & Hepatology. 2012;**9**(12):732-737

[12] Vogel A, Cervantes A, Chau I, Daniele B, Llovet JM, Meyer T, et al. Hepatocellular carcinoma: ESMO Clinical Practice Guidelines for diagnosis, treatment and follow-up. Annals of Oncology. 2018; **29**:iv238-iv255

[13] Clavien PA, Lesurtel M, Bossuyt PM, Gores GJ, Langer B, Perrier A. Recommendations for liver transplantation for hepatocellular carcinoma: An international consensus conference report. The Lancet Oncology. 2012;**13**(1):e11-e22

[14] Petrowsky H, Fritsch R, Guckenberger M, De Oliveira ML, Dutkowski P, Clavien PA. Modern therapeutic approaches for the treatment of malignant liver tumours. Nature Reviews. Gastroenterology & Hepatology. 2020;**17**(12):755-772

[15] Tsilimigras DI, Brodt P, Clavien PA, Muschel RJ, D'Angelica MI, Endo I, et al. Liver metastases. Nature Reviews Disease Primers. 2021;**7**(1):27

[16] Abdalla EK, Adam R, Bilchik AJ, Jaeck D, Vauthey JN, Mahvi D. Improving resectability of hepatic colorectal metastases: Expert consensus statement. Annals of Surgical Oncology. 2006;**13**(10):1271-1280

[17] Hussain SM, Sorrell MF. Colorectal metastases II: MRI findings in a fatty liver. In: Liver MRI Correlation with Other Imaging Modalities and Histopathology. 2nd ed. Berlin, Heidelberg: Springer; 2014. pp. 92-93

[18] Fong Y, Blumgart LH, Cohen AM. Surgical treatment of colorectal metastases to the liver. CA: A Cancer Journal for Clinicians. 1995;**45**(1):50-62

[19] Padman S, Padbury R, Beeke C, Karapetis CS, Bishnoi S, Townsend AR, et al. Liver only metastatic disease in patients with metastatic colorectal cancer: Impact of surgery and chemotherapy. Acta Oncologica. 2013;**52**(8):1699-1706

[20] Ruiterkamp J, Ernst MF, de Munck L, van der Heiden-van der Loo M, Bastiaannet E, van de Poll-Franse LV, et al. Improved survival of patients with primary distant metastatic breast cancer in the period of 1995-2008. A nationwide population-based study in the Netherlands. Breast Cancer Research and Treatment. 2011;**128**(2):495-503

[21] Adeyiga AO, Lee EY, Eisenberg RL. Focal hepatic masses in pediatric patients. American Journal of Roentgenology. 2012;**199**(4): W422-W440

[22] Shelmerdine SC, Roebuck DJ, Towbin AJ, McHugh K. MRI of paediatric liver tumours: How we review and report. Cancer Imaging. 2016;**16**(1):21

[23] Shimada H, Tanaka K, Endou I, Ichikawa Y. Treatment for colorectal liver metastases: A review. Langenbeck's Archives of Surgery. 2009;**394**(6):973-983

[24] Faivre J, Manfredi S, Bouvier AM. Epidemiology of colorectal cancer liver metastases. Bulletin de l'Académie Nationale de Médecine. 2003;**187**(5):815-822; discussion 822-3

[25] Mitchell D, Puckett Y, Nguyen QN. Literature review of current management of colorectal liver metastasis. Cureus. 2019;**11**(1):e3940

[26] Van de Velde CJH. Treatment of liver metastases of colorectal cancer. Annals of Oncology. 2005;**16**:ii144-ii149

[27] Bismuth H, Adam R, Levi F, Farabos C, Waechter F, Castaing D, et al. Resection of nonresectable liver metastases from colorectal cancer after neoadjuvant chemotherapy. Annals of Surgery. 1996;**224**(4):509-520; discussion 520-2

[28] Creasy JM, Sadot E, Koerkamp BG, Chou JF, Gonen M, Kemeny NE, et al. Actual 10-year survival after hepatic resection of colorectal liver metastases: What factors preclude cure? Surgery. 2018;**163**(6):1238-1244

[29] Braccia DP, Heffernan N. Surgical and ablative modalities for the treatment of colorectal cancer metastatic to the liver. Clinical Journal of Oncology Nursing. 2003;**7**(2):178-184

[30] Glinka J, Ardiles V, Pekolj J, Mattera J, Sanchez Claria R, de Santibanes E, et al. Liver transplantation for non-resectable colorectal liver metastasis: Where we are and where we are going.

Langenbeck's Archives of Surgery. 2020;**405**(3):255-264

[31] Hagness M, Foss A, Line PD, Scholz T, Jørgensen PF, Fosby B, et al. Liver transplantation for nonresectable liver metastases from colorectal cancer. Annals of Surgery. 2013;**257**(5):800-806

[32] Dueland S, Grut H, Syversveen T, Hagness M, Line PD. Selection criteria related to long-term survival following liver transplantation for colorectal liver metastasis. American Journal of Transplantation. 2020;**20**(2):530-537

[33] Li K, Yang J, Liu C, Chen P. In: Yan L, editor. Liver Resection of Secondary Liver Cancer. Dordrecht: Springer Netherlands; 2016. pp. 153-157

[34] Hokland SL, Pedersen M, Salomir R, Quesson B, Stodkilde-Jorgensen H, Moonen CT. MRI-guided focused ultrasound: Methodology and applications. IEEE Transactions on Medical Imaging. 2006;**25**(6):723-731

[35] Lynn JG, Zwemer RL, Chick AJ, Miller AE. A new method for the generation and use of focused ultrasound in experimental biology. The Journal of General Physiology. 1942;**26**(2):179-193

[36] Fry WJ, Mosberg JWH, Barnard JW, Fry FJ. Production of focal destructive lesions in the central nervous system with ultrasound. Journal of Neurosurgery. 1954;**11**(5):471-478

[37] Lele PP. Concurrent detection of the production of ultrasonic lesions. Medical & Biological Engineering. 1966;**4**(5):451-456

[38] Tempany CMC, McDannold NJ, Hynynen K, Jolesz FA. Focused ultrasound surgery in oncology: Overview and principles. Radiology. 2011;**259**(1):39-56

[39] Lorton O, Guillemin PC, Mori N, Crowe LA, Boudabbous S, Terraz S, et al. Self-scanned HIFU ablation of moving tissue using real-time hybrid US-MR imaging. IEEE Transactions on Biomedical Engineering. 2018;**66**(8):2182-2191

[40] Mihcin S, Melzer A. Principles of focused ultrasound. Minimally Invasive Therapy & Allied Technologies. 2018;**27**(1):41-50

[41] Izadifar Z, Izadifar Z, Chapman D, Babyn P. An introduction to high intensity focused ultrasound: Systematic review on principles, devices, and clinical applications. Journal of Clinical Medicine. 2020;**9**(2):1-22

[42] Chavrier F, Chapelon JY, Gelet A, Cathignol D. Modeling of high-intensity focused ultrasound-induced lesions in the presence of cavitation bubbles. The Journal of the Acoustical Society of America. 2000;**108**(1):432-440

[43] Harper JD, Metzler I, Hall MK, Chen TT, Maxwell AD, Cunitz BW, et al. First in-human burst wave lithotripsy for kidney stone comminution: Initial two case studies. Journal of Endourology. 2021;**35**(4):506-511

[44] Pishchalnikov YA, Sapozhnikov OA, Bailey MR, Williams JJC, Cleveland RO, Colonius T, et al. Cavitation bubble cluster activity in the breakage of kidney stones by lithotripter shockwaves. Journal of Endourology. 2003;**17**(7):435-446

[45] Xu Z, Hall TL, Vlaisavljevich E Jr, FTL. Histotripsy: The first noninvasive, non-ionizing, non-thermal ablation technique based on ultrasound. International Journal of Hyperthermia. 2021;**38**(1):561-575

[46] Vidal-Jové J, Serres-Creixamś X, Ziemlewicz TJ, Cannata JM. Liver

histotripsy mediated abscopal effect—Case report. IEEE Transactions on Ultrasonics, Ferroelectrics, and Frequency Control. 2021;**68**(9):3001-3005

[47] Kennedy JE. High-intensity focused ultrasound in the treatment of solid tumours. Nature Reviews. Cancer. 2005;**5**(4):321-327

[48] Prakash P, Diederich CJ. Considerations for theoretical modelling of thermal ablation with catheter-based ultrasonic sources: Implications for treatment planning, monitoring and control. International Journal of Hyperthermia. 2012;**28**(1):69-86

[49] Sapareto SA, Dewey WC. Thermal dose determination in cancer therapy. International Journal of Radiation Oncology, Biology, Physics. 1984;**10**(6):787-800

[50] Plewes DB, Kucharczyk W. Physics of MRI: A primer. Journal of Magnetic Resonance Imaging. 2012;**35**(5):1038-1054

[51] Bloch F. Nuclear induction. Physics Review. 1946;**70**:460-474

[52] Purcell EM, Torrey HC, Pound RV. Resonance absorption by nuclear magnetic moments in a solid. Physics Review. 1946;**69**:37-38

[53] Radue EW, Weigel M, Wiest R, Urbach H. Introduction to magnetic resonance imaging for neurologists. Continuum: Lifelong Learning in Neurology. 2016;**22**(5):1379-1398

[54] Westbrook C. MRI at a Glance. 3rd ed. Chichester, England: John Wiley & Sons; 2016

[55] Storey P. In: Prasad PV, editor. Introduction to Magnetic Resonance Imaging and Spectroscopy. Totowa, NJ: Humana Press; 2006. pp. 3-57

[56] de Senneville BD, Quesson B, Moonen CTW. Magnetic resonance temperature imaging. International Journal of Hyperthermia. 2005;**21**(6):515-531

[57] Bajpai S, Kambadakone A, Guimaraes AR, Arellano RS, Gervais DA, Sahani D. Image-guided treatment in the hepatobiliary system: Role of imaging in treatment planning and posttreatment evaluation. Radiographics. 2015;**35**(5):1393-1418

[58] Niekel MC, Bipat S, Stoker J. Diagnostic imaging of colorectal liver metastases with CT, MR imaging, FDG PET, and/or FDG PET/CT: A meta-analysis of prospective studies including patients who have not previously undergone treatment. Radiology. 2010;**257**(3):674-684

[59] National Comprehensive Cancer Network. NCCN Clinical Practice in Oncology: Colon Cancer. NCCN.org 2021, version 3. Available from: https://www.nccn.org/professionals/physiciangls/pdf/colon.pdf

[60] Hussain SM, Sorrell MF. Colorectal metastases I: Typical lesions. In: Liver MRI Correlation with Other Imaging Modalities and Histopathology. 2nd ed. Berlin, Heidelberg: Springer; 2014. pp. 90-91

[61] Donato H, Franca M, Candelaria I, Caseiro-Alves F. Liver MRI: From basic protocol to advanced techniques. European Journal of Radiology. 2017;**93**:30-39

[62] Wile GE, Leyendecker JR. Magnetic resonance imaging of the liver: Sequence optimization and artifacts. Magnetic Resonance Imaging Clinics of North America. 2010;**18**(3):525-547, xi

[63] Runge VM, Nitz WR, Heverhagen JT. The Physics of Clinical MR Taught

Through Images. 4th ed. New York: Thieme; 2018

[64] Dixon WT. Simple proton spectroscopic imaging. Radiology. 1984;**153**(1):189-194

[65] Hussain SM, Sorrell MF. Dixon-based sequence: Assessment of liver fat and iron deposition. In: Liver MRI Correlation with Other Imaging Modalities and Histopathology. 2nd ed. Berlin, Heidelberg: Springer; 2014. pp. 266-267

[66] Wood JC, Enriquez C, Ghugre N, Tyzka JM, Carson S, Nelson MD, et al. MRI R2 and R2* mapping accurately estimates hepatic iron concentration in transfusion-dependent thalassemia and sickle cell disease patients. Blood. 2005;**106**(4):1460-1465

[67] Karaosmanoglu AD, Onur MR, Ozmen MN, Akata D, Karcaaltincaba M. Magnetic resonance imaging of liver metastasis. Seminars in Ultrasound, CT, and MR. 2016;**37**(6):533-548

[68] Liu PS. Liver mass evaluation in patients without cirrhosis: A technique-based method. Radiologic Clinics of North America. 2015;**53**(5):903-918

[69] O'Neill EK, Cogley JR, Miller FH. The ins and outs of liver imaging. Clinics in Liver Disease. 2015;**19**(1):99-121

[70] Hussain SM, Sorrell MF. Solid liver lesions. In: Liver MRI Correlation with Other Imaging Modalities and Histopathology. 2nd ed. Berlin, Heidelberg: Springer; 2014. p. 87

[71] Fidler J, Hough D. Hepatocyte-specific magnetic resonance imaging contrast agents. Hepatology. 2011;**53**(2):678-682

[72] Kim HJ, Lee SS, Byun JH, Kim JC, Yu CS, Park SH, et al. Incremental value of liver MR imaging in patients with potentially curable colorectal hepatic metastasis detected at CT: A prospective comparison of diffusion-weighted imaging, gadoxetic acid-enhanced MR imaging, and a combination of both MR techniques. Radiology. 2015;**274**(3):712-722

[73] Seale MK, Catalano OA, Saini S, Hahn PF, Sahani DV. Hepatobiliary-specific MR contrast agents: Role in imaging the liver and biliary tree. Radiographics. 2009;**29**(6):1725-1748

[74] Koh DM, Berry J. Critical questions in the imaging of colorectal hepatic metastases. Cancer Imaging. 2008;**8** (Spec Iss A):S69-S78

[75] Hindman JC. Proton resonance shift of water in the gas and liquid states. The Journal of Chemical Physics. 1966;**44**(12):4582-4592

[76] Ishihara Y, Calderon A, Watanabe H, Okamoto K, Suzuki Y, Kuroda K, et al. A precise and fast temperature mapping using water proton chemical shift. Magnetic Resonance in Medicine. 1995;**34**(6):814-823

[77] Poorter JD, Wagter CD, Deene YD, Thomsen C, Stahlberg F, Achten E. Noninvasive MRI thermometry with the proton resonance frequency (PRF) method: In vivo results in human muscle. Magnetic Resonance in Medicine. 1995;**33**(1):74-81

[78] Rieke V, Butts PK. MR thermometry. Journal of Magnetic Resonance Imaging. 2008;**27**(2):376-390

[79] Quesson B, de Zwart JA, Moonen CTW. Magnetic resonance temperature imaging for guidance of thermotherapy. Journal of Magnetic Resonance Imaging. 2000;**12**(4):525-533

[80] Haase A, Frahm J, Matthaei D, Hanicke W, Merboldt KD. FLASH imaging: Rapid NMR imaging using low flip-angle pulses. 1986. Journal of Magnetic Resonance. 2011;**213**(2):533-541

[81] Auboiroux V, Viallon M, Roland J, Hyacinthe J, Petrusca L, Morel DR, et al. ARFI-prepared MRgHIFU in liver: Simultaneous mapping of ARFI-displacement and temperature elevation, using a fast GRE-EPI sequence. Magnetic Resonance in Medicine. 2012;**68**(3):932-946

[82] McDannold N, Maier SE. Magnetic resonance acoustic radiation force imaging. Medical Physics. 2008;**35**(8):3748-3758

[83] Payne A, Merrill R, Minalga E, Hadley JR, Odeen H, Hofstetter LW, et al. A breast-specific MR guided focused ultrasound platform and treatment protocol: First-in-human technical evaluation. IEEE Transactions on Biomedical Engineering. 2021;**68**(3):893-904

[84] Bour P, Marquet F, Ozenne V, Toupin S, Dumont E, Aubry JF, et al. Real-time monitoring of tissue displacement and temperature changes during MR-guided high intensity focused ultrasound. Magnetic Resonance in Medicine. 2017;**78**(5):1911-1921

[85] Paquin R, Vignaud A, Marsac L, Younan Y, Lehericy S, Tanter M, et al. Keyhole acceleration for magnetic resonance acoustic radiation force imaging (MR ARFI). Magnetic Resonance Imaging. 2013;**31**(10):1695-1703

[86] Kaye EA, Hertzberg Y, Marx M, Werner B, Navon G, Levoy M, et al. Application of Zernike polynomials towards accelerated adaptive focusing of transcranial high intensity focused ultrasound. Medical Physics. 2012;**39**(10):6254-6263

[87] Hertzberg Y, Volovick A, Zur Y, Medan Y, Vitek S, Navon G. Ultrasound focusing using magnetic resonance acoustic radiation force imaging: Application to ultrasound transcranial therapy. Medical Physics. 2010;**37** (6 Part 1):2934-2942

[88] Mansfield P. Snapshot magnetic resonance imaging (Nobel lecture). Angewandte Chemie (International Ed. in English). 2004;**43**(41):5456-5464

[89] Stehling MK, Turner R, Mansfield P. Echo-planar imaging: Magnetic resonance imaging in a fraction of a second. Science. 1991;**254**(5028):43-50

[90] Zhang S, Block KT, Frahm J. Magnetic resonance imaging in real time: Advances using radial FLASH. Journal of Magnetic Resonance Imaging. 2010;**31**(1):101-109

[91] McIntyrei D, Bowtell R, Commandre M, Hennel F, Mansfield P, Morris P. Overcoming field inhomogeneities in MRI. In: The Bio-Clinical Interface: Bio-Clinical Psychiatry Mapping Brain Function; Edited Proceedings of the Bio-Clinical Interface Conferences, Held in Rouffach, France, between 1992 and 1994. Arcueil, France: John Libbey Eurotext. pp. 349-355

[92] Salomir R, de Senneville BD, Moonen CT. A fast calculation method for magnetic field inhomogeneity due to an arbitrary distribution of bulk susceptibility. Concepts in Magnetic Resonance Part B: Magnetic Resonance Engineering. 2003;**19**(1):26-34

[93] Hayashi M, Inoue Y, Komeda K, Shimizu T, Asakuma M, Hirokawa F,

et al. Clinicopathological analysis of recurrence patterns and prognostic factors for survival after hepatectomy for colorectal liver metastasis. BMC Surgery. 2010;**10**(1):27

[94] Yamashita S, Chun YS, Kopetz SE, Vauthey JN. Biomarkers in colorectal liver metastases. The British Journal of Surgery. 2018;**105**(6):618-627

[95] Adam R, De Gramont A, Figueras J, Guthrie A, Kokudo N, Kunstlinger F, et al. The oncosurgery approach to managing liver metastases from colorectal cancer: A multidisciplinary international consensus. The Oncologist. 2012;**17**(10):1225-1239

[96] Blumgart LH, Leach KG, Karran SJ. Observations on liver regeneration after right hepatic lobectomy. Gut. 1971;**12**(11):922-928

[97] Fang C-H, Liu J, Fang Fan Y, Yang J, Xiang N, Zeng N. Outcomes of hepatectomy for hepatolithiasis based on 3-dimensional reconstruction technique. Journal of the American College of Surgeons. 2013;**217**(2):280-288

[98] Majno P, Azoulay D, Bismuth H. In: Bircher J, Benhamou JP, McIntyre N, Rizzetto M, Rodes J, editors. General Surgical Aspects and the Risks of Liver Surgery in Patients with Hepatic Disease. Oxford Textbook of Clinical Hepatology. Oxford: Oxford University Press; 1999. pp. 1997-2008

[99] Aloia TA, Vauthey JN. Chapter 92—Hepatic metastasis from colorectal cancer. In: Jarnagin WR, editor. Blumgart's Surgery of the Liver, Biliary Tract and Pancreas, 2-Volume Set (Sixth Edition). 6th ed. Philadelphia: Elsevier; 2017. pp. 1339-54.e4

[100] Mentha G, Roth AD, Terraz S, Giostra E, Gervaz P, Andres A, et al. 'Liver first' approach in the treatment of colorectal cancer with synchronous liver metastases. Digestive Surgery. 2008;**25**(6):430-435

[101] Jegatheeswaran S, Mason JM, Hancock HC, Siriwardena AK. The liver-first approach to the management of colorectal cancer with synchronous hepatic metastases: A systematic review. JAMA Surgery. 2013;**148**(4):385-391

[102] Berber E, Pelley R, Siperstein AE. Predictors of survival after radiofrequency thermal ablation of colorectal cancer metastases to the liver: A prospective study. Journal of Clinical Oncology. 2005;**23**(7):1358-1364

[103] Lau WY. Different Approaches to Liver Resection. Singapore: Springer Singapore; 2021. pp. 155-169

[104] Lai ECH, Lau SHY, Lau WY. In: Yan L, editor. Anatomical Liver Resection. Dordrecht: Springer Netherlands; 2016. pp. 111-116

[105] Lortat-Jacob J, Robert H. Well defined technic for right hepatectomy. La Presse Médicale. 1952;**60**(26):549-551

[106] Pack GT, Baker HW. Total right hepatic lobectomy: Report of a case. Annals of Surgery. 1953;**138**(2):253

[107] Woodington GF, Waugh JM. Results of resection of metastatic tumors of the liver. American Journal of Surgery. 1963;**105**(1):24-29

[108] Adam R, Laurent A, Azoulay D, Castaing D, Bismuth H. Two-stage hepatectomy: A planned strategy to treat irresectable liver tumors. Annals of Surgery. 2000;**232**(6):777-785

[109] Alvarez FA, Ardiles V, Sanchez Claria R, Pekolj J, de Santibanes E. Associating liver partition and portal

vein ligation for staged hepatectomy (ALPPS): Tips and tricks. Journal of Gastrointestinal Surgery. 2013;**17**(4): 814-821

[110] de Santibanes E, Clavien PA. Playing play-doh to prevent postoperative liver failure: The "ALPPS" approach. Annals of Surgery. 2012;**255**(3):415-417

[111] Makuuchi M, Thai BL, Takayasu K, Takayama T, Kosuge T, Gunven P, et al. Preoperative portal embolization to increase safety of major hepatectomy for hilar bile duct carcinoma: A preliminary report. Surgery. 1990;**107**(5):521-527

[112] Jaeck D, Oussoultzoglou E, Rosso E, Greget M, Weber JC, Bachellier P. A two-stage hepatectomy procedure combined with portal vein embolization to achieve curative resection for initially unresectable multiple and bilobar colorectal liver metastases. Annals of Surgery. 2004;**240**(6):1037-1049; discussion 1049-51

[113] Schadde E, Clavien PA. In: Clavien PA, Sarr MG, Fong Y, Miyazaki M, editors. ALPPS (Associating Liver Partition with Portal Vein Ligation for Staged Hepatectomy). Berlin, Heidelberg: Springer Berlin Heidelberg; 2016. pp. 447-456

[114] Dueland S, Syversveen T, Solheim JM, Solberg S, Grut H, Bjørnbeth BA, et al. Survival following liver transplantation for patients with nonresectable liver-only colorectal metastases. Annals of Surgery. 2020;**271**(2):212-218

[115] Andres A, Toso C. Liver transplantation for colorectal metastasis: A stepwise approach. Hepatobiliary Surgery and Nutrition. 2020;**9**(3):336

[116] Torres-JimenezJ,Esteban-VillarrubiaJ, Ferreiro-Monteagudo R, Carrato A. Local Treatments in the unresectable patient with colorectal cancer metastasis: A review from the point of view of the medical oncologist. Cancers. 2021;**13**(23)

[117] Gallinger S, Biagi JJ, Fletcher GG, Nhan C, Ruo L, McLeod RS. Liver resection for colorectal cancer metastases. Current Oncology. 2013;**20**(3):e255-e265

[118] Lam VW, Spiro C, Laurence JM, Johnston E, Hollands MJ, Pleass HC, et al. A systematic review of clinical response and survival outcomes of downsizing systemic chemotherapy and rescue liver surgery in patients with initially unresectable colorectal liver metastases. Annals of Surgical Oncology. 2012;**19**(4):1292-1301

[119] Mentha G, Majno P, Terraz S, Rubbia-Brandt L, Gervaz P, Andres A, et al. Treatment strategies for the management of advanced colorectal liver metastases detected synchronously with the primary tumour. European Journal of Surgical Oncology. 2007;**33**(Suppl. 2):S76-S83

[120] Khoo E, O'Neill S, Brown E, Wigmore SJ, Harrison EM. Systematic review of systemic adjuvant, neoadjuvant and perioperative chemotherapy for resectable colorectal-liver metastases. HPB: The Official Journal of the International Hepato Pancreato Biliary Association. 2016;**18**(6):485-493

[121] Bierman HR, Byron JRL, Kelley KH, Grady A. Studies on the blood supply of tumors in man. III. Vascular patterns of the liver by hepatic arteriography in vivo. Journal of the National Cancer Institute. 1951;**12**(1):107-131

[122] Breedis C, Young G. The blood supply of neoplasms in the liver. The American Journal of Pathology. 1954;**30**(5):969-977

[123] Ranieri G, Laforgia M, Nardulli P, Ferraiuolo S, Molinari P, Marech I, et al. Oxaliplatin-based intra-arterial chemotherapy in colo-rectal cancer liver metastases: A review from pharmacology to clinical application. Cancers (Basel). 2019;**11**(2):141-156

[124] Minchinton AI, Tannock IF. Drug penetration in solid tumours. Nature Reviews. Cancer. 2006;**6**(8):583-592

[125] Kemeny MM, Battifora H, Blayney DW, Cecchi G, Goldberg DA, Leong LA, et al. Sclerosing cholangitis after continuous hepatic artery infusion of FUDR. Annals of Surgery. 1985;**202**(2):176-181

[126] Beltrań-Gracia E, Lopeź-Camacho A, Higuera-Ciapara I, Velazqueź-Fernandeź JB, Vallejo-Cardona AA. Nanomedicine review: Clinical developments in liposomal applications. Cancer Nanotechnology. 2019;**10**(1):1-40

[127] Lyon PC, Griffiths LF, Lee J, Chung D, Carlisle R, Wu F, et al. Clinical trial protocol for TARDOX: A phase I study to investigate the feasibility of targeted release of lyso-thermosensitive liposomal doxorubicin (ThermoDox®) using focused ultrasound in patients with liver tumours. Journal of Therapeutic Ultrasound. 2017;**5**(1):1-8

[128] Gray MD, Lyon PC, Mannaris C, Folkes LK, Stratford M, Campo L, et al. Focused ultrasound hyperthermia for targeted drug release from thermosensitive liposomes: Results from a Phase I Trial. Radiology. 2019;**291**(1):232-238

[129] National Library of Medicine (U.S.). A Phase I Study of Lyso-thermosensitive Liposomal Doxorubicin and MR-HIFU for Pediatric Refractory Solid Tumors. Identifier NCT02536183. 2015. Available from: https://clinicaltrials.gov/ct2/show/NCT02536183

[130] National Library of Medicine (U.S.) Ultrasound-enhanced Delivery of Chemotherapy to Patients With Liver Metastasis From Breast- and Colorectal Cancer. Identifier NCT03477019. 2018. Available from: https://clinicaltrials.gov/ct2/show/NCT03477019

[131] Cheng JC, Wu JK, Huang CM, Liu HS, Huang DY, Cheng SH, et al. Radiation-induced liver disease after three-dimensional conformal radiotherapy for patients with hepatocellular carcinoma: Dosimetric analysis and implication. International Journal of Radiation Oncology, Biology, Physics. 2002;**54**(1):156-162

[132] Pan CC, Kavanagh BD, Dawson LA, Li XA, Das SK, Miften M, et al. Radiation-associated liver injury. International Journal of Radiation Oncology, Biology, Physics. 2010;**76**(3 Suppl):S94-S100

[133] Kirichenko A, Gayou O, Parda D, Kudithipudi V, Tom K, Khan A, et al. Stereotactic body radiotherapy (SBRT) with or without surgery for primary and metastatic liver tumors. HPB. 2016;**18**(1):88-97

[134] Ursino S, Greco C, Cartei F, Colosimo C, Stefanelli A, Cacopardo B, et al. Radiotherapy and hepatocellular carcinoma: Update and review of the literature. European Review for Medical and Pharmacological Sciences. 2012;**16**(11):1599-1604

[135] Comito T, Clerici E, Tozzi A, D'Agostino G. Liver metastases and SBRT: A new paradigm? Reports of Practical Oncology and Radiotherapy. 2015;**20**(6):464-471

[136] Aitken KL, Hawkins MA. Stereotactic body radiotherapy for liver metastases. Clinical Oncology (Royal College of Radiologists). 2015;**27**(5):307-315

[137] Petrelli F, Comito T, Barni S, Pancera G, Scorsetti M, Ghidini A. Stereotactic body radiotherapy for colorectal cancer liver metastases: A systematic review. Radiotherapy and Oncology. 2018;**129**(3):427-434

[138] National Library of Medicine (U.S.). The MOMENTUM Study: The Multiple Outcome Evaluation of Radiation Therapy Using the MR-Linac Study (MOMENTUM). Identifier NCT04075305. 2019. Available from: https://clinicaltrials.gov/ct2/show/NCT04075305

[139] National Library of Medicine (U.S.). Feasibility of Online MR-guided Radiotherapy on a 1.5T MR-Linac. Identifier NCT04172753. 2019. Available from: https://clinicaltrials.gov/ct2/show/NCT04172753

[140] National Library of Medicine (U.S.). OAR-Based, Dose Escalated SBRT With Real Time Adaptive MRI Guidance for Liver Metastases. Identifier NCT04020276. 2019. Available from: https://clinicaltrials.gov/ct2/show/NCT04020276

[141] National Library of Medicine (U.S.). Phase II of Adaptative Magnetic Resonance-Guided Stereotactic Body Radiotherapy (SBRT) for Treatment of Primary or Secondary Progressive Liver Tumors. Identifier NCT04242342. 2019. Available from: https://clinicaltrials.gov/ct2/show/NCT04242342

[142] Czito B. Magnetic Resonance Imaging (MRI) Solely For Liver Stereotactic Body Radiation Therapy (SBRT). Identifier NCT02722395. 2016-2017. Available from: https://clinicaltrials.gov/ct2/show/NCT02722395

[143] National Library of Medicine (U.S.). MRI-Guided Stereotactic Body Radiation Therapy in Treating Patients With Liver Metastases or Liver Cancer. Identifier NCT02683200. 2016. Available from: https://clinicaltrials.gov/ct2/show/NCT02683200

[144] van Dams R, Wu TC, Kishan AU, Raldow AC, Chu FI, Hernandez J, et al. Ablative radiotherapy for liver tumors using stereotactic MRI-guidance: A prospective phase I trial. Radiotherapy and Oncology. 2022;**170**:14-20

[145] Giles SL, Brown MRD, Rivens I, Deppe M, Huisman M, Kim YS, et al. Comparison of imaging changes and pain responses in patients with intra-or extraosseous bone metastases treated palliatively with magnetic resonance-guided high-intensity-focused ultrasound. Journal of Vascular and Interventional Radiology. 2019;**30**(9):1351-60 e1

[146] Liberman B, Gianfelice D, Inbar Y, Beck A, Rabin T, Shabshin N, et al. Pain palliation in patients with bone metastases using MR-guided focused ultrasound surgery: A multicenter study. Annals of Surgical Oncology. 2009;**16**(1):140-146

[147] AbdElmagied AM, Vaughan LE, Weaver AL, Laughlin-Tommaso SK, Hesley GK, Woodrum DA, et al. Fibroid interventions: Reducing symptoms today and tomorrow: Extending generalizability by using a comprehensive cohort design with a randomized controlled trial. American Journal of Obstetrics and Gynecology. 2016;**215**(3):338 e1-338 e18

[148] Chen R, Keserci B, Bi H, Han X, Wang X, Bai W, et al. The safety and effectiveness of volumetric magnetic resonance-guided high-intensity focused ultrasound treatment of symptomatic uterine fibroids: Early clinical experience in China. Journal of Therapeutic Ultrasound. 2016;**4**(1):27

[149] Dorenberg EJ, Courivaud F, Ring E, Hald K, Jakobsen JA, Fosse E, et al. Volumetric ablation of uterine fibroids using Sonalleve high-intensity focused ultrasound in a 3 Tesla scanner–first clinical assessment. Minimally Invasive Therapy & Allied Technologies. 2013;**22**(2):73-79

[150] Laughlin-Tommaso S, Barnard EP, AbdElmagied AM, Vaughan LE, Weaver AL, Hesley GK, et al. FIRSTT study: Randomized controlled trial of uterine artery embolization vs focused ultrasound surgery. American Journal of Obstetrics and Gynecology. 2019;**220**(2):174 e1-174 e13

[151] Verpalen IM, de Boer JP, Linstra M, Pol RLI, Nijholt IM, Moonen CTW, et al. The Focused Ultrasound Myoma Outcome Study (FUMOS); a retrospective cohort study on long-term outcomes of MR-HIFU therapy. European Radiology. 2020;**30**(5):2473-2482

[152] Giles SL, Imseeh G, Rivens I, Ter Haar GR, Taylor A, deSouza NM. MR guided high intensity focused ultrasound (MRgHIFU) for treating recurrent gynaecological tumours: A pilot feasibility study. The British Journal of Radiology. 2019;**92**(1098):20181037

[153] Napoli A, Anzidei M, De Nunzio C, Cartocci G, Panebianco V, De Dominicis C, et al. Real-time magnetic resonance-guided high-intensity focused ultrasound focal therapy for localised prostate cancer: Preliminary experience. European Urology. 2013;**63**(2):395-398

[154] Tay KJ, Cheng CWS, Lau WKO, Khoo J, Thng CH, Kwek JW. Focal therapy for prostate cancer with in-BORE MR-guided focused ultrasound: Two-year follow-up of a phase I trial-complications and functional outcomes. Radiology. 2017;**285**(2):620-628

[155] Chang JW, Park CK, Lipsman N, Schwartz ML, Ghanouni P, Henderson JM, et al. A prospective trial of magnetic resonance-guided focused ultrasound thalamotomy for essential tremor: Results at the 2-year follow-up. Annals of Neurology. 2018;**83**(1):107-114

[156] Elias WJ, Lipsman N, Ondo WG, Ghanouni P, Kim YG, Lee W, et al. A randomized trial of focused ultrasound thalamotomy for essential tremor. The New England Journal of Medicine. 2016;**375**(8):730-739

[157] Furusawa H, Namba K, Thomsen S, Akiyama F, Bendet A, Tanaka C, et al. Magnetic resonance-guided focused ultrasound surgery of breast cancer: Reliability and effectiveness. Journal of the American College of Surgeons. 2006;**203**(1):54-63

[158] Wu F, Chen WZ, Bai J, Zou JZ, Wang ZL, Zhu H, et al. Pathological changes in human malignant carcinoma treated with high-intensity focused ultrasound. Ultrasound in Medicine & Biology. 2001;**27**(8):1099-1106

[159] Wu F, Wang ZB, Chen WZ, Wang W, Gui Y, Zhang M, et al. Extracorporeal high intensity focused ultrasound ablation in the treatment of 1038 patients with solid carcinomas in China: An overview. Ultrasonics Sonochemistry. 2004;**11**(3):-149, 54. 4th Conference on the Applications of Power Ultrasound in Physical and Chemical Processing

[160] Wu F, Wang ZB, Chen WZ, Zhu H, Bai J, Zou JZ, et al. Extracorporeal high intensity focused ultrasound ablation in the treatment of patients with large hepatocellular carcinoma. Annals of Surgical Oncology. 2004;**11**(12):1061-1069

[161] Yang T, Ng DM, Du N, He N, Dai X, Chen P, et al. HIFU for the treatment

of difficult colorectal liver metastases with unsuitable indications for resection and radiofrequency ablation: A phase I clinical trial. Surgical Endoscopy. 2021;**35**(5):2306-2315

[162] Tsang SH, Ma KW, She WH, Chu F, Lau V, Lam SW, et al. High-intensity focused ultrasound ablation of liver tumors in difficult locations. International Journal of Hyperthermia. 2021;**38**(2):56-64

[163] Park MY, Jung SE, Cho SH, Piao XH, Hahn ST, Han JY, et al. Preliminary experience using high intensity focused ultrasound for treating liver metastasis from colon and stomach cancer. International Journal of Hyperthermia. 2009;**25**(3):180-188

[164] Illing R, Kennedy J, Wu F, Ter Haar G, Protheroe A, Friend P, et al. The safety and feasibility of extracorporeal high-intensity focused ultrasound (HIFU) for the treatment of liver and kidney tumours in a Western population. British Journal of Cancer. 2005;**93**(8):890-895

[165] Orsi F, Zhang L, Arnone P, Orgera G, Bonomo G, Vigna PD, et al. High-intensity focused ultrasound ablation: Effective and safe therapy for solid tumors in difficult locations. AJR. American Journal of Roentgenology. 2010;**195**(3):W245-W252

[166] Sehmbi AS, Froghi S, Oliveira de Andrade M, Saffari N, Fuller B, Quaglia A, et al. Systematic review of the role of high intensity focused ultrasound (HIFU) in treating malignant lesions of the hepatobiliary system. HPB. 2021;**23**(2):187-196

[167] Schuster TG, Wei JT, Hendlin K, Jahnke R, Roberts WW. Histotripsy treatment of benign prostatic enlargement using the Vortx Rx system: Initial human safety and efficacy outcomes. Urology. 2018;**114**:184-187

[168] Solbiati LA. The HistoSonics System for Treatment of Primary and Metastatic Liver Tumors Using Histotripsy (#HOPE4LIVER). Identifier NCT04573881. 2020. Available from: https://clinicaltrials.gov/ct2/show/NCT04573881

[169] Cranston D. A review of high intensity focused ultrasound in relation to the treatment of renal tumours and other malignancies. Ultrasonics Sonochemistry. 2015;**27**:654-658

[170] Gedroyc WM. New clinical applications of magnetic resonance-guided focused ultrasound. Topics in Magnetic Resonance Imaging. 2006;**17**(3):189-194

[171] Diana M, Schiraldi L, Liu YY, Memeo R, Mutter D, Pessaux P, et al. High intensity focused ultrasound (HIFU) applied to hepato-bilio-pancreatic and the digestive system-current state of the art and future perspectives. Hepatobiliary Surgery and Nutrition. 2016;**5**(4):329-344

[172] Desgranges S, Lorton O, Gui-Levy L, Guillemin P, Celicanin Z, Hyacinthe JN, et al. Micron-sized PFOB liquid core droplets stabilized with tailored-made perfluorinated surfactants as a new class of endovascular sono-sensitizers for focused ultrasound thermotherapy. Journal of Materials Chemistry B. 2019;**7**(6):927-939

[173] Guillemin PC, Gui L, Lorton O, Zilli T, Crowe LA, Desgranges S, et al. Mild hyperthermia by MR-guided focused ultrasound in an ex vivo model of osteolytic bone tumour: Optimization of the spatio-temporal control of the delivered temperature. Journal of Translational Medicine. 2019;**17**(1):350

[174] Mori N, Jud C, Salomir R, Cattin PC. Leveraging respiratory organ motion for non-invasive tumor treatment devices: A feasibility study. Physics in Medicine and Biology. 2016;**61**(11):4247-4267

[175] Muller A, Petrusca L, Auboiroux V, Valette PJ, Salomir R, Cotton F. Management of respiratory motion in extracorporeal high-intensity focused ultrasound treatment in upper abdominal organs: Current status and perspectives. Cardiovascular and Interventional Radiology. 2013;**36**(6):1464-1476

[176] Salomir R, Petrusca L, Auboiroux V, Muller A, Vargas MI, Morel DR, et al. Magnetic resonance-guided shielding of prefocal acoustic obstacles in focused ultrasound therapy: Application to intercostal ablation in liver. Investigative Radiology. 2013;**48**(6):366-380

[177] Jung SE, Cho SH, Jang JH, Han JY. High-intensity focused ultrasound ablation in hepatic and pancreatic cancer: Complications. Abdominal Imaging. 2011;**36**(2):185-195

[178] Zhang L, Zhu H, Jin C, Zhou K, Li K, Su H, et al. High-intensity focused ultrasound (HIFU): Effective and safe therapy for hepatocellular carcinoma adjacent to major hepatic veins. European Radiology. 2009;**19**(2):437-445

[179] Cheung TT, Poon RTP, Yau T, Tsang DSF, Lo CM, Fan ST. High-intensity focused ultrasound as a treatment for colorectal liver metastasis in difficult position. International Journal of Colorectal Disease. 2012;**27**(7):987-988

[180] Preiswerk F, De Luca V, Arnold P, Celicanin Z, Petrusca L, Tanner C, et al. Model-guided respiratory organ motion prediction of the liver from 2D ultrasound. Medical Image Analysis. 2014;**18**(5):740-751

[181] de Zwart JA, Vimeux FC, Palussiere J, Salomir R, Quesson B, Delalande C, et al. On-line correction and visualization of motion during MRI-controlled hyperthermia. Magnetic Resonance in Medicine. 2001;**45**(1):128-137

[182] Lorton O, Guillemin PC, M'Rad Y, Peloso A, Boudabbous S, Charbonnier C, et al. A novel concept of a phased-array HIFU transducer optimized for MR-guided hepatic ablation: Embodiment and first in-vivo studies. Frontiers in Oncology. 2022;**12**

[183] Lorton O, Guillemin PC, Holman R, Desgranges S, Gui L, Crowe LA, et al. Enhancement of HIFU thermal therapy in perfused tissue models using micron-sized FTAC-stabilized PFOB-core endovascular sonosensitizers [Journal Article]. International Journal of Hyperthermia. 2020;**37**(1):1116-1130

[184] Astafyeva K, Somaglino L, Desgranges S, Berti R, Patinote C, Langevin D, et al. Perfluorocarbon nanodroplets stabilized by fluorinated surfactants: Characterization and potentiality as theranostic agents. Journal of Materials Chemistry B. 2015;**3**(14):2892-2907

[185] Lorton O, Guillemin PC, Holman R, Desgranges S, Gui L, Crowe LA, et al. Enhancement of HIFU thermal therapy in perfused tissue models using micron-sized FTAC-stabilized PFOB-core endovascular sonosensitizers. International Journal of Hyperthermia. 2020;**37**(1):1116-1130

[186] Holman R, Gui L, Lorton O, Guillemin P, Desgranges S, Contino-Pépin C, et al. PFOB sonosensitive microdroplets: Determining their interaction radii with focused ultrasound using MR thermometry and a Gaussian convolution kernel computation.

International Journal of Hyperthermia. 2022;**39**(1):108-119

[187] Okada A, Murakami T, Mikami K, Onishi H, Tanigawa N, Marukawa T, et al. A case of hepatocellular carcinoma treated by MR-guided focused ultrasound ablation with respiratory gating. Magnetic Resonance in Medical Sciences. 2006;**5**(3):167-171

[188] Anzidei M, Napoli A, Sandolo F, Marincola BC, Di Martino M, Berloco P, et al. Magnetic resonance-guided focused ultrasound ablation in abdominal moving organs: A feasibility study in selected cases of pancreatic and liver cancer. Cardiovascular and Interventional Radiology. 2014;**37**(6):1611-1617

[189] Gedroyc WM. MR guided focused ultrasound of the liver. In: 2nd International MR-guided Focused Ultrasound Symposium, Focused Ultrasound Foundation. 2010. Available from: https://www.fusfoundation.org

[190] Dupré A, Melodelima D, Perol D, Chen Y, Vincenot J, Chapelon JY, et al. First clinical experience of intra-operative high intensity focused ultrasound in patients with colorectal liver metastases: A phase I-IIa study. PLoS One. 2015;**10**(2):e0118212

[191] Dupré A, Perol D, Blanc E, Peyrat P, Basso V, Chen Y, et al. Efficacy of high-intensity focused ultrasound-assisted hepatic resection (HIFU-AR) on blood loss reduction in patients with liver metastases requiring hepatectomy: Study protocol for a randomized controlled trial. Trials. 2017;**18**(1):1-10

[192] Cambronero S, Rivoire M, Dupré A, Melodelima D. Non-invasive fast, large and selective in vivo HIFU ablation of the liver with a toroidal transducer. In: 2019 IEEE International Ultrasonics Symposium (IUS). 2019. pp. 2126-2128

[193] Dupre A, Melodelima D, Perol D, Chen Y, Vincenot J, Chapelon JY, et al. Evaluation of the feasibility, safety, and accuracy of an intraoperative high-intensity focused ultrasound device for treating liver metastases. Journal of Visualized Experiments. 2019;**143**:e57964

[194] Vaezy S, Zderic V. Hemorrhage control using high intensity focused ultrasound. International Journal of Hyperthermia. 2007;**23**(2):203-211

[195] Silveira LA, Silveira FBC, Fazan VPS. Arterial diameter of the celiac trunk and its branches: Anatomical study. Acta Cirúrgica Brasileira. 2009;**24**(1):43-47

[196] Zaccagna F, Anzidei M, Sandolo F, Cavallo Marincola B, Palla C, Leonardi A, et al. MRgFUS for liver and pancreas cancer treatments: The Umberto I hospital experience. Translational Cancer Research. 2014;**3**(5):430-441

[197] Fischer K, Gedroyc W, Jolesz FA. Focused ultrasound as a local therapy for liver cancer. Cancer Journal. 2010;**16**(2):118-124

[198] National Library of Medicine (U.S.). MR-guided High Intensity Focused Ultrasound (HIFU) on Pediatric Solid Tumors. Identifier NCT02076906. 2014. Available from: https://clinicaltrials.gov/ct2/show/NCT02076906

[199] Zhang Q, Bian S, Lv W, Kou D, Hu H, Guo S, et al. Observation of efficacy of TACE combined with HIFU on patients with middle-advanced liver cancer. European Review for Medical and Pharmacological Sciences. 2019;**23**(3):239-246

[200] Luo Y, Jiang Y. Comparison of efficiency of TACE plus HIFU and TACE alone on patients with primary liver cancer. Journal of the College of

Physicians and Surgeons–Pakistan. 2019;**29**(5):414-417

[201] Wijlemans JW, Bartels LW, Deckers R, Ries M, Mali WP, Moonen CT, et al. Magnetic resonance-guided high-intensity focused ultrasound (MR-HIFU) ablation of liver tumours. Cancer Imaging. 2012;**12**(2):387-394

Section 5

Considering Advanced Therapeutics

Chapter 7

Multidisciplinary Management of Early Rectal Cancer

Sean Ramcharan, Vanessa Cubas, Cortland Linder, Thomas Evans, Julia Merchant and Rakesh Sinha

Abstract

The incidence of colorectal cancers detected at an early stage, that is stage T2 or less, has increased over the last decade, driven primarily by better access to screening and diagnostic pathways. Consequently, timely treatment leads to better outcomes. Early stage rectal cancers (ERC), by virtue of their location, allows for alternative treatment strategies towards organ (rectum) preservation. Local excision techniques have evolved and improved with advances in radiological assessment and minimally invasive surgery. However, decisions on treatment to mitigate local recurrence remain a challenge. This chapter explores the current understanding of the management of ERC and offers insights to the multidisciplinary team to aid treatment strategies.

Keywords: rectal cancer, minimally invasive, multidisciplinary, transanal surgery, TAMIS, TEMS, TEO, radiotherapy, brachytherapy, surveillance, chemotherapy, chemoradiotherapy, intense surveillance

1. Introduction

Since the introduction of bowel cancer screening programs (BCSP) worldwide, the incidence of colorectal cancers (CRC) detected at an early stage, that is T2 or less (TNM Tumour, Node, Metastasis classification) has increased. In fact, 30% of all screen-detected or asymptomatic CRCs are classed as early disease (stage I–II) versus 10% diagnosed at investigation for lower gastrointestinal (LGI) symptoms. Regardless of the diagnostic pathway, the obvious benefit is that early detection leads to timely treatment and better outcomes. This is certainly evident from the improvement in disease-free survival (DFS) and overall survival (OS) outcomes over the last 20 years [1–3].

Early rectal cancers (ERC) are no exception. Fortunately, their location allows for alternative treatment strategies towards organ preservation. Conceptually, local excision began in the 1980s with transanal endoscopic microsurgery (TEMS) and subsequent technological advances in radiological assessment and minimally invasive surgery (MIS) made rectum preservation more feasible.

Overall, the number of patients over 60 years of age with CRC has plateaued. However, the incidence in the younger population (20–39 years) has steadily increased over the last decade, often with advanced disease. This may suggest a change in the biology of CRC amongst this sub-group, the impact of screening for a family history of CRC and better access to diagnostic pathways. Other factors include 'self-diagnosis' of concerning symptoms through internet search engines, cancer awareness campaigns and social media platforms [1].

Increasing public awareness has led to more patients of all ages seeking assessment of lower gastrointestinal (LGI) symptoms sooner and therefore it is likely the incidence of ERCs will continue to rise. Similarly, the incidence detected at BCSPs will improve with the inclusion of patients from 45 years of age (currently 55–60 years), as advocated by some public health policymakers in the US, in the context of the impact of survival benefits to the wider social and healthcare economy [1].

In primary care there has been more uptake of highly sensitive screening tools, such as faecal immunochemical test (FIT), for symptomatic assessment and to better manage the increasing burden of fast-track pathways. Recently, those pathways were challenged by the SARS-COV2 pandemic as more patients with LGI concerns came forward once the restrictions that limited access to primary care and diagnostic pathways were lifted. FIT became a useful tool to screen those needing urgent assessment, though its impact on investigation and treatment delays are yet to be described [2, 3].

The impact of FIT may also include earlier stage diagnosis. As a quantitative screening tool with sensitivities and specificities above 90%, the higher the faecal occult blood level (2–100 μg Hb/g of faeces) the more likely the presence of significant serrated polyps, high risk adenomas or early CRC [3].

2. Early rectal cancer (ERC)

2.1 Definition of ERC

The definition of ERC remains somewhat controversial but is based on the TNM classification. Overall, it is characterised by invasive adenocarcinoma spreading into, but not beyond, the submucosa or muscularis propria, that is, a TNM of T1 or T2, N0 and M0 [4, 5]. Clinically, ERC may present as a polypoid carcinoma, a focus of malignancy within a large pedunculated or sessile adenoma, or a small ulcerating adenocarcinoma [6]. ERCs have a smaller chance of metastasis to local lymph nodes, due to the lack of lymphatics within the mucosa and therefore are potentially treatable without major surgery that excises the mesorectum to mitigate loco-regional spread [5]. However, not all ERCs are the same and treatment strategies must be determined by prognostic factors such as differentiation status and depth of invasion [1, 5].

At publication, there was no international consensus on the definition of ERC, though it is fundamental in discussing treatment options and prognostication with patients. There are several micro- and macroscopic definitions, however these do not capture the overall clinical impact of the disease. As a result, the European Association of Endoscopic Surgery and the European Society of Coloproctology have defined ERC as "a rectal cancer with good prognostic features that might be safely removed while preserving the rectum and have a very limited risk of relapse after local excision" [5].

As with any cancer, the aim of treating ERC is to offer cure while minimising side effects. This is fundamentally achieved by aiming to preserve the rectum. Organ preservation attempts to mitigate the significant risk of total mesorectal excision (TME) surgery which has a 30-day mortality of 3–7%, morbidity of 35% and risk of poor functional outcomes from low anterior resection syndrome (LARS) of up to 20%. While the evidence supports local excision, TME surgery via anterior resection and abdominoperineal excisions (APER) remains the mainstay of treatment with the best prospect of cure. Specifically, it removes the mesorectum to aid histological analysis for loco-regional spread and subsequent decisions on adjuvant treatment [1, 7].

2.2 History of ERC surgery

Abdominoperineal resection (APR), described by Miles et al. in 1901, was the standard operation for much of the twentieth century. In the 1970s, high rates of recurrence were recognised but, more so, the complications of any pelvic surgery led to a re-evaluation of the anatomy and embryology by Crapp and Cuthbertson in 'The Book Shelf—William Waldeyer and the Rectosacral Fascia' [8]. This paved the way to revisiting TME surgery, first described by Abel in 1931, and popularised in 1979 by William (Bill) Heald [9]. TME surgery removes the envelop of the lymphovascular mesorectum by following the 'holy' avascular and embryological mesorectal fascia plane. Heald demonstrated a reduction in recurrence, improved survival, and less bladder and sexual dysfunction. TME remains the gold standard for curative surgery worldwide.

Most would agree that TME surgery for ERCs and high-risk adenomas that have a minimal risk of lymphatic or metastatic spread is 'over-treatment', given the risk of significant morbidity. Until the 1980s, local excision of rectal adenomas and ERCs was performed with trans-anal excision (TAE). This involved open excision of the lesion using an anal retractor, but was restricted by poor visibility, confined operating space and suitable for low rectal lesions only. Technical challenges limited complete oncological resection, resulting in high recurrence rates [1].

In 1984, Buess et al. described the novel technique of transanal endoscopic microsurgery (TEM) [10]. This utilised a stereoscopic viewing system within a rigid rectoscope to give the operator 3D binocular view. A specialised insufflation system created a stable pneumorectum, allowing ample workable space, while dedicated microsurgical instruments provided a high level of precision for oncological resections. Initial results endorsed TEM as an effective technique for rectum-sparing resection of adenomas and malignancy, with low rates of recurrence. However, it was not initially popular. Barriers included a steep learning curve, a lack of other minimally invasive surgical techniques, high equipment costs and staff expertise. With the advent of minimally invasive surgery (MIS) in 1989 from the first laparoscopic cholecystectomy and later extended to colorectal surgery, TEM became more acceptable.

Interest grew as technology progressed, including the development of other natural orifice surgeries and single-incision laparoscopic surgery (SILS). In 2008, the technological advances were combined with the TEM concepts to perform Transanal Minimally Invasive Surgery (TAMIS). A single-incision laparoscopic surgery port is inserted into the rectum through which a pneumorectum is established, and laparoscopic instruments can be passed. This technique allows a platform for precise resection, with low cost and routinely available instruments [1].

Radical surgery carries a significant risk of mortality, morbidity and bowel dysfunction [1, 7]. Before attempting an organ preserving approach it is important to distinguish between malignant and benign lesions. Organ preserving surgery demands a multi-factorial considerations. These include surgical experience, pathological stage, anatomical location of tumour, fitness of patient and patient's wishes. Histologically well differentiated adenocarcinomas with the absence of lymphatic invasion, budding, and submucosal invasion <1 mm are associated with low risk of lymphatic spread [11]. As more treatment options became available, decisions became increasingly complex. Multi-disciplinary team meetings specifically for ERCs and significant polyp and early colorectal cancers (SPECC) are becoming more widely established. In the UK, National Institute of Clinical Excellence (NICE) guidance recommends that all TNM stage 1 rectal cancers are discussed within an ERC/SPECC MDT. This includes all pertinent specialists, i.e. surgeon, radiologist, endoscopist, histopathologist, nurse specialists, and oncologists. MDTs do improve rates of complete resection, operative mortality and patient satisfaction outcomes [4, 11].

2.3 Investigations for ERC

2.3.1 Colonoscopy

ERC may present with rectal bleeding or as an incidental finding during screening. At endoscopic evaluation, macroscopic detection of malignant transformation of any polyp is challenging, and more so the features of spread beyond the muscularis propria. The endoscopist aims to identify the classic changes of cancerous potential by examining mucosal irregularity for pinkness, superficial granularity and nodularity, mucosal fading, depressions, or haemorrhagic spots [6]. Other techniques include magnifying colonoscopy to better examine pit-patterns and air transformation by reducing insufflation pressure to locate depressed areas of invasion. For an ERC, narrow-band imaging and dye techniques, (such as indigo carmine) may reveal the loss of circumferential grooves at the margins of normal mucosa [12, 13].

Tissue biopsy is required unless the tumour can be removed completely via endoscopy. Biopsy and histology are essential for staging and management. However, they frequently under-stage disease due to sampling error from superficial or anatomically challenging locations and inter-observer errors in interpretation of histopathology [12]. Furthermore, biopsies can lead to the "non-lifting sign" from fibrosis, making subsequent local excision more challenging. The authors therefore agree with the recommendation that tissue biopsies should be performed at the most suspicious area of the lesion. Also, where malignancy is unlikely and complete excision is not within the remits of the endoscopist's skill set, biopsy should be avoided to allow subsequent success at excision by a more advanced endoscopist, and unhindered by scarring [4].

2.3.1.1 Kudo classification

Macroscopic classification of adenomas, proposed by the Japanese Society for the Study of Cancer of the Colon and Rectum resembles that of gastric tumours (**Table 1**). Adenomas are subdivided into pedunculated or sessile. Around 42–85% of early colorectal cancers are pedunculated and 15–58% sessile. Adenocarcinomas in pedunculated polyps have less potential to infiltrate the submucosal layer [6, 13].

2.3.1.2 Pit pattern classification

The Pit Pattern Classification (**Table 2**) was first described by Kudo *et al* [6]. Type I and type II lesions have non-neoplastic or benign patterns (*e.g.*, normal, hyperplastic,

Endoscopic features	Type	Description	Example
Protruding Lesions	Ip	Pedunculated	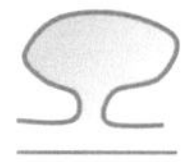
	Isp	Sub/Semi-pedunculated	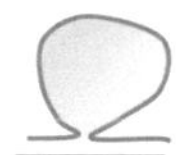
	Is	Sessile	
Flat lesions	IIa	Flat elevation of the mucosa	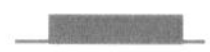
	IIb	Flat mucosal changes	
Depressed lesions	IIc	Mucosal depression	
	IIa + IIc	Flat elevation with central depression	
	IIc + IIa	Mucosal depression with elevated margin	
Laterally spreading lesions	LST	Laterally spreading	

Table 1.
Macroscopic classification for early colorectal cancer [6, 13].

inflammatory polyps); types IIIL, IIIs and IV are adenomatous; and type VI and VN are cancerous. Although Type III is considered to exhibit no invasive characteristics, it is a common pit pattern observed in depressed-types of early cancers [6, 13], and type IV lesions often contain characteristics of advanced neoplasia (e.g. high-grade adenomas or villous components).

2.3.2 Radiological imaging

The most sensitive imaging investigation for differentiating between T1 and T2 lesions is endorectal ultrasonography (ERUS), with an accuracy of 81–92%, however it is very user dependent with considerable inter-observer variability [14, 15]. It is also useful in assessing the presence of residual tumour following polypectomy [16]. ERUS is more specific in assessing invasion when compared to MRI, which is 86% *vs* 69% respectively. Both have similarly high sensitivities (94%) to determine spread beyond the muscularis propria [16].

The precision of ERUS in assessing the depth of invasion appears to vary with the T stage, a lower accuracy for T2 cancers, compared with that of early (T1) and advanced (T3–T4) stages [17]. Additionally, ERUS is less likely to consistently distinguish between inflammation surrounding the tumour and transmural tumour infiltration, which may lead to over-staging from T2 to T3 tumours and, subsequently, overtreatment [18–20]. The staging of bulky, distal and/or stenotic lesions with ERUS is also challenging due to the limited field of view and the inability of rigid probes to traverse the lesion [21, 22].

MRI of the anorectum and pelvis is essential to exclude extension into the muscularis propia, as well as locoregional metastases. Both MRI and ERUS, are equally proficient at evaluating lymph node involvement [15, 23]. Lymph nodes over 8 mm in diameter are generally malignant, however, size alone is not reliable as small nodes

Type	Schematic	Endoscopic	Description	Pathology
I	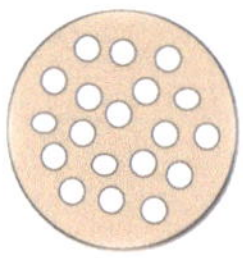	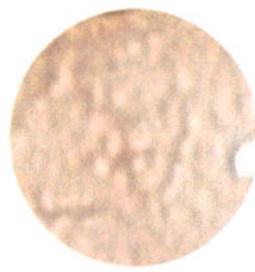	Round pits	Benign/Normal
II	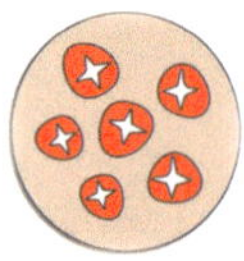	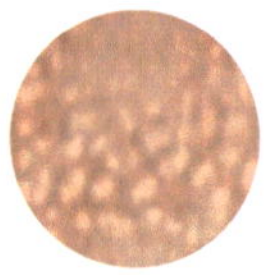	Stellar or papillary pits	Non-neoplastic (e.g. Hyperplastic)
IIIS	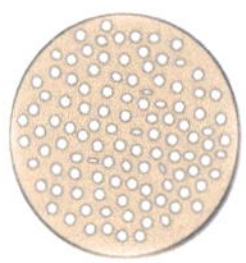	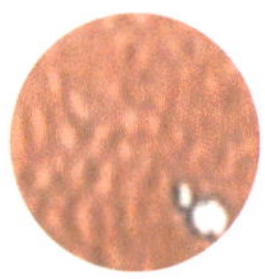	Small tubular or round pits. Smaller than type I pits	Neoplastic
IIIL	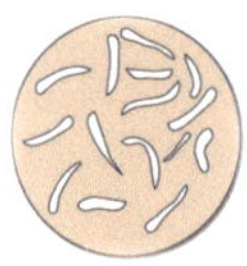	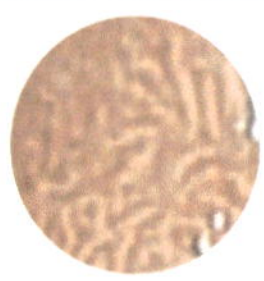	Tubular or roundish pits that are larger than type I pits	Neoplastic
IV	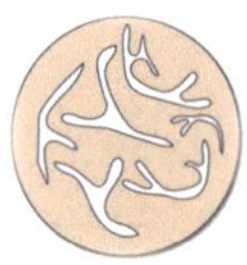	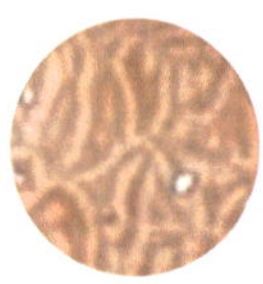	Dendrite-like pits	Neoplastic
VI	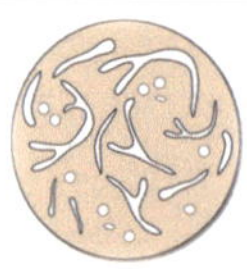	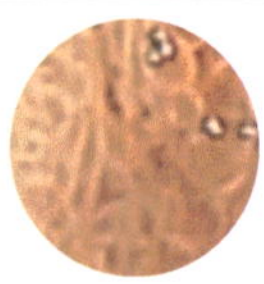	Irregular arrangement and sizes of type IIIs, IIIL, IV type pit patterns.	Neoplastic (invasive)
VN	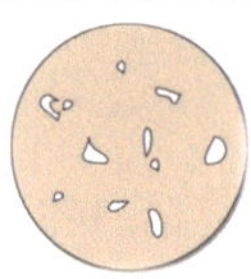	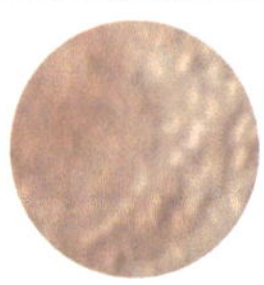	Loss or decrease of pits with an amorphous structure	Neoplastic (submucosal invasion)

Table 2.
Pit pattern classification [6, 13].

may contain metastases while large uninvolved reactive ones adjacent to cancers are common [24–26]. Criteria such as the presence of spiculation, indistinct border and mottled heterogenic pattern are indicative of nodal metastasis [27].

Chest, abdomen and pelvis computerised tomography (CT) must be performed to exclude distant metastasis and the entire colon should be assessed to rule out synchronous adenomas or carcinomas. While it is widely available and provides rapid scanning times, it is of limited value in assessing loco-regional spread in early-stage lesions confined to the rectal wall. Additionally, the lower resolution is unreliable to confidently distinguish the layers of the rectal wall and differentiate desmoplastic or inflammatory changes from tumour infiltration into the mesorectal fat [15]. These limitations often result in a tendency to over-stage early cancers (≤T2) to T3 ones [28].

2.3.3 Lymph node involvement

Lymph node metastasis remains a fundamental prognostic indicator for decisions on adjuvant treatment, specifically chemotherapy, where suitable. It is likely future developments will focus on improving preoperative assessment. Currently, the precision in assessing locoregional spread for T1 tumours suitable for ERC treatment and to differentiate T1 from T2 cancers remain a challenge for the MDT [4, 11].

Immunological localisation and lymph node specific contrast is progressing rapidly, and likely the future for improving staging and management of CRC. Preliminary observations suggest that ultra-small superparamagnetic iron oxide (USPIO) is useful at differentiating normal nodes from ones with metastases [22]. Promising prospects include anti-carcinoembryonic antigen (CEA) antibodies to detect CEA-bearing tumours, recurrent disease, and metastases [27].

Positron emission tomography (PET) is used almost routinely to investigate recurrence and may also detect involved nodes. However, it is not without limitations. The resolution for involved lymph nodes of 1 centimetre or less is inadequate and often indistinguishable to the primary tumour that lies nearby [29].

Endorectal ultrasonography guided needle biopsy of lymph nodes is a minimally invasive and inexpensive technique that may lead to more accurate nodal staging. This technique is not widely used though promising, given the current need to identify local disease and improve decisions for surgery [30, 31].

Unlike breast cancer, the value of sentinel node biopsy in visceral cancers is uncertain. Approximately 20% of patients with node negative disease develop recurrence within 5 years, probably as a consequence of missed micro-metastases by conventional staging [31]. Sentinel node study has the potential to detect micro-metastases and lead to upstaging of the disease and thus reducing tumour related mortality from surgery [32]. Further research of its value in ERC and on the overall effects on survival is needed.

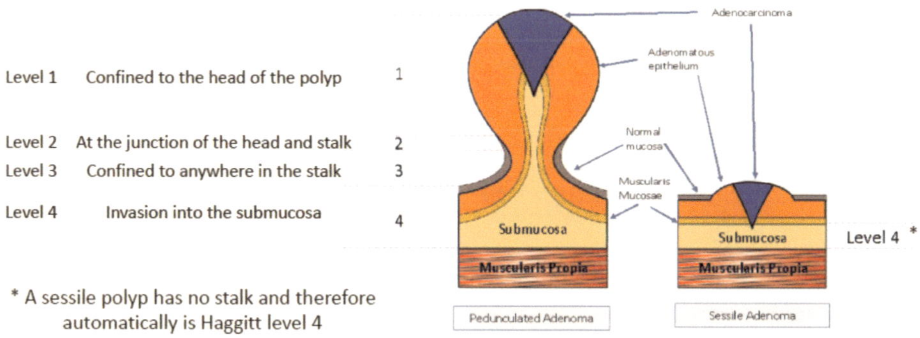

Figure 1.
The Haggitt classification of depth of invasion in malignant pedunculated and sessile polyps [33].

Figure 1 highlights the typical features of a T1 ERC found at colonoscopy and later staged with ERUS and MRI. While the radiology demonstrated a T1 lesion without invasion, the depth into the submucosa is difficult to assess. Unfortunately, this was an SM1 adenocarcinoma with lymphovascular invasion. Overall, In the absence of more accurate staging before resection, we must rely on estimations of the likelihood of undetectable loco-regional spread primarily based on histology.

2.3.4 Histology of ERC

2.3.4.1 Features of malignant transformation of adenomas

Risk factors associated with malignancy include grade of epithelial dysplasia, location and histological type [33]. However, the most significant factor is size. Adenomas of less than 5 mm have almost 0% risk of transformation whereas risk to those >2 cm is around 40% [34, 35]. Adenomas are classified as tubular, tubulovillous and villous. Villous adenomas have the highest risk at 29.8% and tubular the lowest at 3.9%. Epithelial dysplasia is defined as low grade versus high grade. Low grade dysplasia is typically neoplastic change seen only in the epithelial glands. High grade dysplasia shows glandular irregularity, crowding with a cribriform architecture and prominent glandular budding. High grade dysplasia is usually, though not exclusively associated with malignancy. Rectal adenomas have the highest risk of transformation at 23% when compared to the right (6.4%) and left colon (8%) [36].

2.3.4.2 Haggitt classification

Haggitt's submucosal invasion classification within a polyp is widely used. Levels 1, 2 and 3 apply to pedunculated lesions only. An invasive carcinoma in a sessile polyp is an automatic level 4 lesion (**Figure 2**) [37].

2.3.4.3 Kikuchi classification

The limitation of the Haggitt classification is that it is not as suitable for sessile tumours. The Kikuchi classification aims at depicting the extent of submucosal invasion and therefore more practical for these lesions (**Figure 3**) [38].

This classification can be correlated to the Haggitt level: levels 1, 2, and 3 are Sm1. Level 4 can be Sm1, Sm2 or Sm3.

Overall there are 3 histopathology features that inform the risk of local recurrence: SM level, tumour diameter and lympho-vascular (LV) invasion (**Table 3**).

Sm1	Invasion into the upper 1/3 of submucosa	
	Sm1a	Less than a quarter invading upper 1/3 of submucosa
	Sm1b	Quarter to half invading upper 1/3 of submucosa
	Sm1c	More than half invading upper 1/3 of submucosa
Sm2	Invasion into the upper 2/3 of submucosa	
Sm3	Invasion into the lower 1/3 of submucosa	

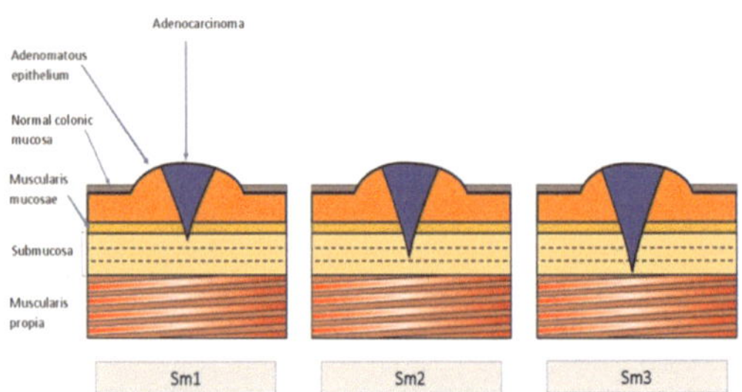

Figure 2.
Kikuchi Classification [38].

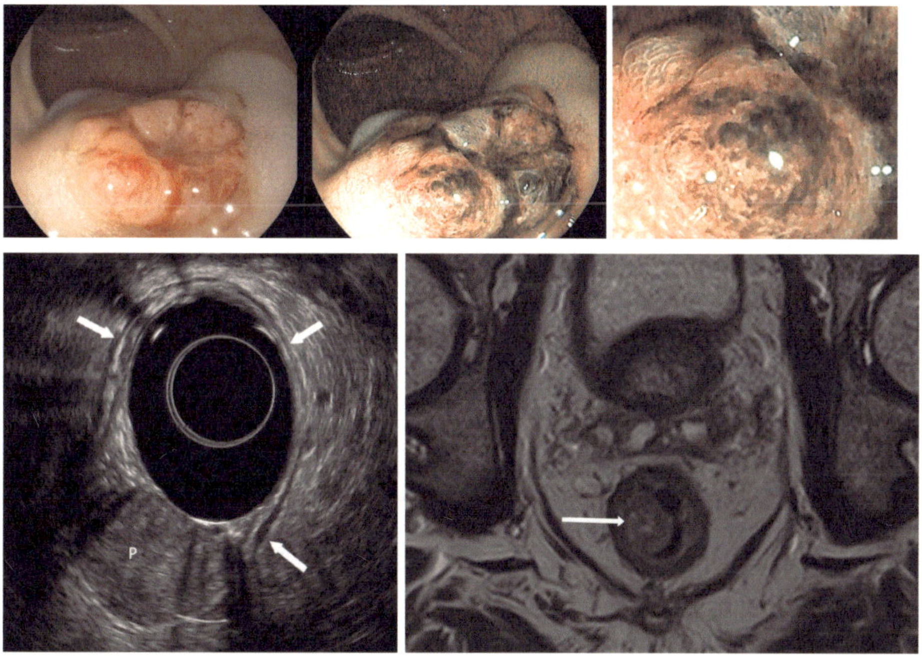

Figure 3.
Upper pictures of an early rectal cancer at colonoscopy, with the middle image showing narrow-band filters (Pentax i-scan) to display type V Kudo pit pattern and magnified in the upper right image. ERUS of the same polyp suggests a T1 cancer, with the arrows identifying the intact muscularis propria, which are also demonstrated on the MRI (lower right image). After TAMIS excision, histology revealed accurate preoperative staging but the presence of lymphovascular invasion.

SM level	LV invasion	Maximum tumour diameter (cm)					
		≤1	1·1–2	2·1–3	3·1–4	4·1–5	≥ 5·1
SM1	No	3·0	3·6	4·4	5·4	6·6	8·1
SM1	Yes	5·2	6·4	7·7	9·4	11·4	13·7
SM2–3	No	10·5	12·7	15·3	18·5	22·1	26·4
SM2–3	Yes	17·8	21·4	25·5	30·3	35·7	41·8

Table 3.
the risk of local recurrence from the histopathology of SM level, tumour diameter and lympho-vascular (LV) invasions [39].

3. Management of ERC

3.1 The multidisciplinary team (MDT)

There are significant challenges for the MDT in treating ERC. As the early stage incidence becomes more common, newer treatments and strategies will emerge to address the complexities in balancing outcomes against morbidity. While this may further complicate decisions, fundamentally the MDT relies heavily on macroscopic and radiological features of the ERC. Once a lesion has been determined as malignant, or at least has suspicious morphology at endoscopy, despite limited histological evidence, the decision on how best to remove it safely must be made. In recognition of these challenges there has been an increase in polyp-focused MDTs, though significant variations in those treatment decisions exist [5].

Any decision relies on accurate delivery of information to the patients to facilitate their own decisions in their shared care. Discussions must include the tumour characteristics, grade and location, as well as patient factors such as age, sex, comorbidities, and performance status. Patients must then be informed of the MDTs discussion as well and address their concerns on stoma rates, recurrence risks and the incidence of post-operative complications.

With the increasing complexity of those decision and number of patients coming through MDTs, protocol tools have attempted to unify standards, but remain far from perfect [8]. A recent Cochrane review in 2017 demonstrated that the use of these tools can improve a patient's knowledge of risk and, interestingly, seems to increase the likelihood of patients choosing less radical surgery [6].

Therefore, decisions require experienced specialists in MDT meetings aided by accurate staging as possible and formal assessment of patient risk. For individual risk assessment for treatment, prediction models are quite common such as p-possum scoring, performance status and ASA scores. More surgery specific models, such as the American College of Surgeons (ACS) surgical risk calculator, are also available, however the evidence for their use to inform patients of outcomes in ERC is limited. Decisions are made avoiding the methodological limitations of these models and once again rely on the experience of the MDT [9, 10].

3.2 Options for treating ERC

As for any rectal cancer, options for ERC treatment must be patient-centred. The initial workup determines tumour stage, location, circumferential resection margins (CRM) margins, and presence or absence of metastatic disease. Patient fitness and preference, alongside the availability of treatment, including available research trials should also be considered by the MDT.

3.2.1 Traditional TME surgery

For many years TME surgery was the only acceptable curative treatment of any rectal cancer, involving either an anterior resection or abdominoperineal resection. This facilitates full staging of local disease postoperatively as lymphadenectomy will guide the need for adjuvant treatment. However, the significant risk, particularly in frail patients, and that of a stoma when fitted to avoid the risks of anastomotic leak, must be considered and discussed with the patient.

Disease recurrence is very much related to tumour grade, accepted as less than 5% with well to moderately differentiated and node negative cancers [11]. Anastomotic leak and significant complication rates vary depending on pelvic factors, patient health, intraoperative findings, tumour height, previous surgery and neoadjuvant treatment but are typically quoted between 4 and 10%.

3.2.2 Organ preservation techniques

Transanal Endoscopic Microsurgery (TEM), Transanal Endoscopic Operations (TEO) & Transanal minimally invasive surgery (TAMIS).

Historically, local excision was only possible under direct vision, using an anal retractor and towards organ preservation. The TEM platform later emerged as forerunner to definitive treatment for ERCs by MIS with no adverse features [39–41]. This approach should only be considered in patients with cT1 disease with no evidence of lymph node involvement [40]. TEM allows for complete local disease control with accurate, local excision. It allows a full-thickness excision of the affected bowel wall and primary closure. For pT1, SM1, node negative ERCs, it offers comparable oncological results as TME surgery, with significantly less morbidity [42]. The recurrence rates of T1 lesions without adverse features vary but are largely agreed to be in the region of 10–15% (see **Table 3**). However, in T2 lesions, also without adverse features, this jumps to 25% [43]. The same study shows little difference in R1 (involved margin) resection rates, around 5%, when compared to traditional TME surgery. Alternative platforms include TEO and, gaining wider popularity, TAMIS (see **Figure 4**). While there is a steep learning curve for all transanal techniques, TAMIS allows transferable skills gained at laparoscopic resections and the outcomes are similar to TEMS [1].

The ongoing advancement of minimally invasive technology is likely to improve the accessibility of ERC surgery. The transference of robotic skills to TAMIS, known as R-TAMIS, promises to aid accurate dissection and better intraluminal control of suturing to close the rectal wall defect. It may allow repair of perforations that breach the peritoneal reflection which occur on resecting anterior lesions and would otherwise have required abdominal (open or laparoscopic) access [1].

3.2.3 Contact radiotherapy/Brachytherapy

Local radiotherapy (brachytherapy or Papillon, CXB) is effective in some instances [44], and as standalone treatment. It was first popularised by Jean Papillon in France in

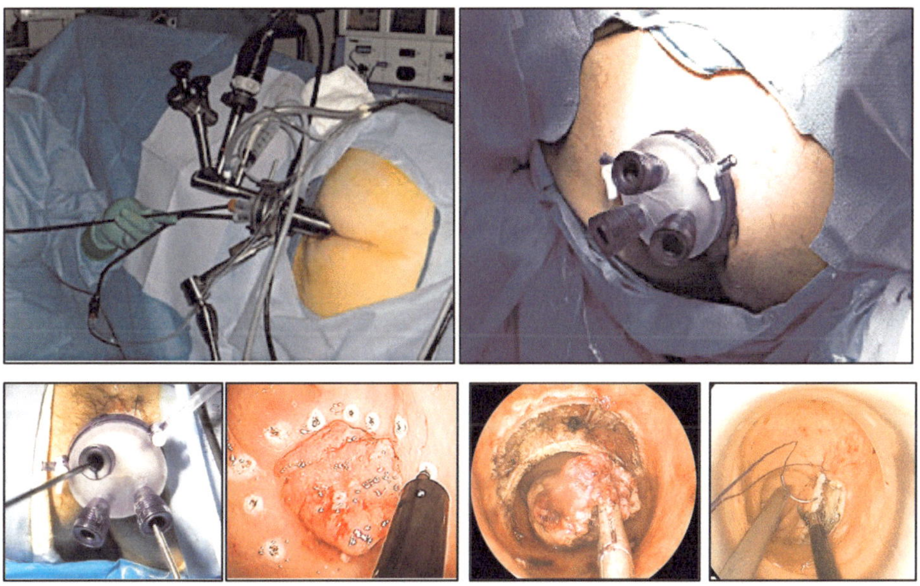

Figure 4.
TEMs (upper left) versus TAMIS (upper right) setup at the anus. While TEMs offers binocular and near 3D views, TAMIS via a less rigid platform allows greater freedom of movement and transferability of minimally invasive skills and tools. Using standard laparoscopic instruments via the GelPOINT Path™ platform (lower left image), a full thickness resection of the ERC is achieved (lower images second and third from left) and the rectal wall defect is sutured with a continuous absorbable, such as a 3–0 PDS suture (lower right).

the 1950s and has gained recent popularity. This strategy can be considered in patients with exophytic, mobile cancers under 3 cm. It is a curative, non-operative approach for some T1 cancers, however primarily suitable for elderly or frail patients unfit for major resections. Its main disadvantage is the lack of histological specimen and failure to treat the mesorectum, unless combined with external beam radiotherapy (EBR). Overall, the complete clinical response rate ranges between 10 and 30% when combined with chemotherapy. Professor Sun Myint et al. outline the criteria for ERCs suitable for CXB that may successfully result in a complete response as follows [45]:

- Inclusion criteria for CXB alone for ERCs with curative intent.

    1. mobile exophytic ERC (cT1).

    2. well to moderately differentiated adenocarcinoma.

    3. tumour size <3 cm.

    4. no evidence of suspicious lymph nodes.

    5. no evidence of distant metastases.

    6. tumour within 12 cm of the anal verge.

    7. patient suitable for long-term follow-up.

- Exclusion criteria.

    1. poorly differentiated adenocarcinoma.

    2. presence of lymphatic or vascular invasion.

    3. bulky rectal cancer involving more than half the circumference (> 3 cm).

    4. fixed rectal adenocarcinoma with deep ulceration (cT3, cT4).

The described regimen involves two weekly outpatient treatments, in which 30 Grey of 50KV is delivered to the target area through a rigid applicator. Standard dosage is 60 Grey in 2 fractions over 2 weeks.

3.2.4 Total neoadjuvant therapy (TNT)

There has been increasing use of the non-operative approach to rectal cancer treatment since Habr-Gama et al. of Brazil published their outcomes. It removes the need for major surgery by aiming to achieve complete clinical response with neoadjuvant chemoradiotherapy and 'watch and wait' monitoring for recurrence by intensive follow-up. It not currently known whether induction chemotherapy followed by chemoradiotherapy or vice versa is the superior regimen, but the inclusion of radiotherapy significantly improves complete pathological response rates. Surgery is only undertaken for recurrent disease [46]. Until recently there were concerns most of the data came from a single centre, though it continues to gain wider acceptance and currently the subject of RCTs worldwide. As a more focused treatment, there is likely to be greater numbers of patients considering and undergoing TNT [1]. The NCCN recommends FOLFOX or CAPEOX (12–16 weeks) then long course chemoradiotherapy with capecitabine or infusional 5-FU, followed by restaging. MDTs and patients must be aware however, that local recurrence rates are around 30–35% and distant metastases of 15% occur within a year of treatment.

3.2.5 The malignant polyp- endoscopic approach

The endoscopic mucosal resection (EMR) technique involves injecting a solution, traditionally saline, under the lesion to expand the submucosal space and elevate the lesion away from the muscle layer below. If the lesion does not 'lift' then this can be an important feature indicating local invasion. It may also not lift with background colitis and scarring from previous excisions or biopsies. Injections improve resections as flat lesions become more bulbous and easier to grip. EMR for lesions less the 25 mm in the rectum are usually suitable for en bloc resection [47].

Endoscopic submucosal dissection (ESD) is a relatively new technique that offers en bloc mucosal excision. This has the benefit of a high-quality pathological specimen to facilitate accurate assessment of deep and lateral margins and the depth of submucosal invasion. If R0 resection is obtained with no high risk features then recurrence rates are very low. However, ESD has a higher risk of perforation, but manageable non-surgically with endoclips. It is therefore reserved for higher risk lesions and requires a steep learning curve. It involves lifting the lesion, mucosal incision, making a 'groove' down to the muscle layer, submucosal dissection, elevation of a mucosal flap, and completing the resection en bloc [47].

3.3 The Conundrums: Minimising recurrence after organ-preserving treatment

In principle, locoregional treatment is appropriate for the least invasive tumours as they are less likely to have occult lymph node metastases (1–2% for Kikuchi SM1 invasion versus 2–8% for ≥SM2). The gamble with preservation surgery is that estimation of recurrence is only assessable at histopathology.

The best outcome that will not require further treatment is a well to moderately differentiated adenocarcinoma, ≤ SM1, and R0 margins only (see **Table 3**). Therefore, the main challenges for the MDT are non-assessable excision margins (typically from cautery damage), poor differentiation, >SM1 invasion, presence of vascular invasion or R1 margins. These factors are associated with 5–18% local recurrences. If any of these features are present, the MDT ought to consider more radical treatment, specifically adjuvant therapy (such as chemotherapy with EBR and/or brachytherapy) and/or TME excision. If TME surgery is decided, the patient must be aware that scarring from local excision may increase the risk of collateral damage to pelvic nerves, levator muscle, prostate or vagina, and increase the incidence of bleeding and low anterior resection syndrome (LARS).

One of the more challenging discussions is the possibility of residual locoregional disease after excision of a SM2 or SM3 cancer without other adverse risk factors. The patient must be aware of a 5–12% incidence of locoregional recurrence. Decisions are made to in effect halve that risk with either TME surgery or adjuvant brachytherapy +/− EBR +/− chemotherapy. The patients must be aware that TME surgery has significant morbidity of up to 10% and potentially functional concerns, such as LARS. From current literature, it is difficult to estimate the risk of recurrence by brachytherapy+/− EBR, though suggested to be less than 5%. It remains an area in need of high quality RCTs.

For tumours staged T2, lymph-node negative and less 4cm in diameter, local excision after neoadjuvant chemoradiotherapy has been shown in clinical trials to be a safe alternative to TME surgery [48, 49] with minimal adverse impact on anorectal function 1year after surgery. Longer term data suggests some compromise to function [50]. This strategy is not routinely recommended outside of clinical trials, but may be explored at the MDT for elderly, frail patients with significant perioperative risks [51].

There is currently little evidence that healthy young patients with proven ERC should undergo organ preserving excision. TME surgery remains the 'gold standard' [52, 53]. Expert staging and treatment demand a thorough understanding of the anatomy of the rectum and the variability of characteristics in relation to gender and body habitus. Ultimately variations in presentation, patient features, and surgical factors, including the availability of therapeutic options prevents defining borders of ERC management to a viable and universal protocol. The MDT discussions must reflect that complexity and rely on up-to-date evidence of new treatments or consider enrolment into trials.

Differing treatment strategies may be appropriate depending on site of the ERC. Organ-preserving approaches are less relevant for a young patient with no comorbidities and a mid or upper ERC. However, the MDT should explore neoadjuvant therapy for a similar patient with a very low ERC, given the potential risks and impact on quality of life for a low anastomosis or abdominoperineal resection. Once the risks are discussed, an early, localised adenocarcinoma adjacent to the anal sphincter muscle may be appropriately treated with primary chemo-radiotherapy only and intense follow-up towards preserving anal sphincter function. The difference of just a few centimetres in location or millimetres in invasion can have an enormous impact on treatment options and decision-making. What remains unanswered is the longer-term impact of avoiding radical surgery.

If adverse pathology is diagnosed after local excision, proceeding to completion resection via TME surgery may be required. This may necessitate stomas, exenteration surgery for very advanced disease or adjuvant treatments. Nevertheless, those risks must be made clear to the patient before embarking on any treatment for ERC towards shared clinical decision-making and against potential litigation. Strategies to manage this particular question are quickly evolving, though likely to become a common problem with no simple answer, which mandates the MDT to be up to date with the options available.

3.4 Surveillance

To date there is much variation in surveillance protocols after definitive ERC treatment. Overall, follow-up, intense or otherwise, is unlikely to significantly reduce OS. Furthermore, they are costly and cause significant patient anxiety. However, they may improve DFS and therefore quality of life while living with recurrent cancer. The recognised variations in ERC treatment will support differing approaches by MDTs on follow-up regimes. The authors recommend regular review of protocol updates and changes to patient circumstances and health condition.

The authors support an intense regime for ERCs locally treated with surgery +/− chemoradiotherapy+/− brachytherapy, in line with the Brazilian protocol proposed by Habr-Gama et al. [46]. Those with recurrent disease after local excision and subsequently treated with curative intent will require modifications to their protocol, often based on MDT preferences.

Recommended 5-year surveillance, 'intense' protocol for ERC:

• Physical examination & serum CEA	Every 3 to 6 months for 5 years
• Rectosigmoidoscopy	Every 3 to 6 months for first 3 years
• Colonoscopy	First and third to fourth year
• MRI	3–6 months for first 3 years
• CT scan	Yearly for 5 years

If there are other high-risk polyps in the large bowel, colonoscopy may be required yearly until no further concerning polyps are identified followed by then standard bowel surveillance as per hospital guidance.

4. Conclusion

Organ-preservation strategies to treat ERC are effective and, when carefully considered, have acceptable outcomes comparable to TME surgery. Technological advances have improved accessibility of MIS and interest in non-operative treatment continues to grow. However, there are important gaps in the evidence on surgical versus non-surgical treatment. Also, there is a lack of understanding of how patients weigh and prioritise their perceptions of potential benefits over that of morbidity and the risk of local recurrence. Decisions on ERCs other than a 'good' T1 (that is an SM1, R0, no lympho-vascular invasion) treated by local excision remain a challenge, specifically when balancing the likelihood of over- versus under-treatment. It is therefore imperative on well-informed specialists of the MDT to offer the best estimates on outcomes towards shared decision-making with patients.

Overall, the prospects for ERC treatment are very promising. As the current trend to organ-preservation continues, along with current and future research, so too will our understanding of therapeutic strategies improve towards standardising management.

Acknowledgements

We acknowledge the contributions from Drs. Scott Sanders and Farah Sandhu of the Histopathology Department, South Warwickshire NHS Foundation Trust and University of Warwick, UK. This chapter was supported by the Departments of Gastrointestinal Surgery, Histopathology and Radiology of the National Health Service, South Warwickshire NHS Foundation Trust, UK. We also acknowledge support of the School of Medicine, University of Warwick, UK, and the Institute of Cancer and Genomics, University of Birmingham, UK. We would also like to thank Dr. N Pargass for her help in verifying the references in finalising this chapter.

Conflict of interest

The authors declare no conflict of interest.

Author details

Sean Ramcharan[1,2,3*], Vanessa Cubas[1], Cortland Linder[1], Thomas Evans[1], Julia Merchant[1] and Rakesh Sinha[1,2]

1 Department of Gastrointestinal Surgery, Warwick Hospital, South Warwickshire NHS Foundation Trust, Warwick, Warwickshire, UK

2 School of Medicine, University of Warwick, Warwick, Warwickshire, UK

3 Institute of Cancer and Genomics, University of Birmingham, Birmingham, West Midlands, UK

*Address all correspondence to: sean.ramcharan@swft.nhs.uk

References

[1] Merchant J, McArthur D, Ferguson H, Ramcharan S. Concepts and prospects of minimally invasive colorectal cancer surgery. Clinical Radiology. 2021;**76**(12): 889-895. DOI: 10.1016/j.crad.2021.09.013

[2] Kanth P, Inadomi JM. Screening and prevention of colorectal cancer. BMJ. 2021;**374**:1855. DOI: 10.1136/bmj.n1855

[3] Balamou C, Koïvogui A, Rodrigue CM, Clerc A, Piccotti C, Deloraine A, et al. Prediction of the severity of colorectal lesion by fecal hemoglobin concentration observed during previous test in the French screening program. World Journal of Gastroenterology. 2021 Aug 21;**27**(31): 5272-5287. DOI: 10.3748/wjg.v27.i31.5272

[4] Geh I, Gollins S, Renehan A, Scholefield J, Goh V, Prezzi D, et al. Association of coloproctology of great britain & Ireland (ACPGBI): Guidelines for the management of cancer of the colon, Rectum and Anus (2017)—Anal Cancer. Colorectal Disease. 2017;**19** (Suppl 1):82-97. DOI: 10.1111/codi.13709

[5] Morino M, Risio M, Bach S, Beets-Tan R, Bujko K, Panis Y, et al. European association for endoscopic surgery; european society of coloproctology. Early rectal cancer: The European Association for Endoscopic Surgery (EAES) clinical consensus conference. Surgical Endoscopy. 2015;**29**(4): 755-773. DOI: 10.1007/s00464-015-4067-3

[6] Kudo S, Tamura S, Nakajima T, Yamano H, Kusaka H, Watanabe H. Diagnosis of colorectal tumorous lesions by magnifying endoscopy. Gastrointestinal Endoscopy. 1996; **44**:8-14

[7] REACCT Collaborative. Characteristics of early-onset vs late-onset colorectal cancer: A review. JAMA Surgery. 2021;**156**(9):865-874. DOI: 10.1001/jamasurg.2021.2380 Erratum in: JAMA Surg. 2021 Sep 1;156 (9):894. PMID: 34190968

[8] Crapp AR, Cuthbertson AM. William Waldeyer and the rectosacral fascia. Surgery, Gynecology & Obstetrics. 1974; **138**(02):252-256

[9] Heald RJ. A new approach to rectal cancer. British Journal of Hospital Medicine. 1979;**22**(03):277-281

[10] Saclarides TJ, Smith L, Ko ST, Orkin B, Buess G. Transanal endoscopic microsurgery. Diseases of the Colon and Rectum. 1992; **35**(12):1183-1191. DOI: 10.1007/BF02251975

[11] Available from: https://www.nice.org.uk/guidance/ng151 [Accessed: July 16, 2022]

[12] Day DW, Jass JR, Price AB, Shepherd NA, Sloan JM, Talbot IC, et al. Epithelial tumours of the large intestine. In: Morson and Dawson's Gastrointestinal Pathology. 4th ed. Blackwell Science: Oxford; 2003. pp. 551-609

[13] Kudo S, Kashida H, Nakajima T, Tamura S, Nakajo K. Endoscopic diagnosis and treatment of early colorectal cancer. World Journal of Surgery. 1997;**21**:694-701

[14] Starck M, Bohe M, Simanaitis M, Valentin L. Rectal endosonography can distinguish benign rectal lesions from invasive early rectal cancers. Colorectal Disease. 2003;**5**:246-250

[15] Bipat S, Glas AS, Slors FJ, Zwinderman AH, Bossuyt PM, Stoker J. Rectal cancer: Local staging and assessment of lymph node involvement with endoluminal US, CT, and MR imaging—A meta-analysis. Radiology. 2004;**232**:773-783

[16] Kruskal JB, Sentovich SM, Kane RA. Staging of rectal cancer after polypectomy: Usefulness of endorectal US. Radiology. 1999;**211**:31-35

[17] Puli SR, Bechtold ML, Reddy JB, Choudhary A, Antillon MR, Brugge WR. How good is endoscopic ultrasound in differentiating various T stages of rectal cancer? Meta-analysis and systematic review. Annals of Surgical Oncology. 2009;**16**:254-265

[18] Garcia-Aguilar J, Pollack J, Lee SH, Hernandez de Anda E, Mellgren A, Wong WD, et al. Accuracy of endorectal ultrasonography in preoperative staging of rectal tumors. Diseases of the Colon and Rectum. 2002;**45**:10-15

[19] Hulsmans FJ, Tio TL, Fockens P, Bosma A, Tytgat GN. Assessment of tumor infiltration depth in rectal cancer with transrectal sonography: Caution is necessary. Radiology. 1994;**190**:715-720

[20] Maier AG, Barton PP, Neuhold NR, Herbst F, Teleky BK, Lechner GL. Peritumoral tissue reaction at transrectal US as a possible cause of overstaging in rectal cancer: Histopathologic correlation. Radiology. 1997;**203**:785-789

[21] Krajewski KM, Kane RA. Ultrasound staging of rectal cancer. Seminars in Ultrasound, CT, and MR. 2008;**29**: 427-432

[22] Lin S, Luo G, Gao X, Shan H, Li Y, Zhang R, et al. Application of endoscopic sonography in preoperative staging of rectal cancer: Six-year experience. Journal of Ultrasound in Medicine. 2011; **30**:1051-1057

[23] Kim JH, Beets GL, Kim MJ, Kessels AG, Beets-Tan RG. High-resolution MR imaging for nodal staging in rectal cancer: Are there any criteria in addition to the size? European Journal of Radiology. 2004;**52**:78-83

[24] Akasu T, Sugihara K, Moriya Y, Fujita S. Limitations and pitfalls of transrectal ultrasonography for staging of rectal cancer. Diseases of the Colon and Rectum. 1997;**40**(Suppl):S10-S15

[25] Dworak O. Morphology of lymph nodes in the resected rectum of patients with rectal carcinoma. Pathology, Research and Practice. 1991;**187**: 1020-1024

[26] Kotanagi H, Fukuoka T, Shibata Y, Yoshioka T, Aizawa O, Saito Y, et al. The size of regional lymph nodes does not correlate with the presence or absence of metastasis in lymph nodes in rectal cancer. Journal of Surgical Oncology. 1993;**54**:252-254

[27] Hardman N, Murray B, Zwickl M, Kolbinger F, Pluschke G. Application of genetically-engineered anti-CEA antibodies for potential immunotherapy of colorectal cancer. The International Journal of Biological Markers. 1992;7(3): 203-209

[28] Heo SH, Kim JW, Shin SS, Jeong YY, Kang HK. Multimodal imaging evaluation in staging of rectal cancer. World Journal of Gastroenterology. 2014 Apr 21;**20**(15):4244-4255

[29] Llamas-Elvira JM, Rodríguez-Fernández A, Gutiérrez-Sáinz J, et al. Fluorine-18 fluorodeoxyglucose PET in the preoperative staging of colorectal

cancer. European Journal of Nuclear Medicine and Molecular Imaging. 2007; **34**:859-867. DOI: 10.1007/s00259-006-0274-4

[30] Shami VM, Parmar KS, Waxman I. Clinical impact of endoscopic ultrasound and endoscopic ultrasound-guided fine-needle aspiration in the management of rectal carcinoma. Diseases of the Colon and Rectum. 2004; **47**(1):59-65. DOI: 10.1007/s10350-003-0001-1

[31] Hunerbein M, Totkas S, Moesta KT, Ulmer C, Handke T, Schlag PM. The role of transrectal ultrasound-guided biopsy in the postoperative follow-up of patients with rectal cancer. Surgery. 2001;**129**:164-169

[32] Saha S, Elgamal M, Cherry M, et al. Challenging the conventional treatment of colon cancer by sentinel lymph node mapping and its role of detecting micrometastases for adjuvant chemotherapy. Clinical & Experimental Metastasis. 2018;**35**:463-469

[33] Salmo E, Haboubi N. Adenoma and malignant colorectal polyp: Pathological considerations and clinical applications. EMJ Gastroenterol. 2018;**7**:92-102

[34] Gschwantler M, Kriwanek S, Langner E, Goritzer B, Schrutka-Kolbl C, Brownstone E, et al. High-grade dysplasia and invasive carcinoma in colorectal adenomas: A multivariate analysis of the impact of adenoma and patient characteristics. European Journal of Gastroenterology & Hepatology. 2002;**14**:183-188

[35] Nusko G, Mansmann U, Altendorf-Hofmann A, Groitl H, Wittekind C, Hahn EG. Risk of invasive carcinoma in colorectal adenomas assessed by size and site. International Journal of Colorectal Disease. 1997;**12**:267-271

[36] Dixon MF. Gastrointestinal epithelial neoplasia: Vienna revisited. Gut. 2002; **51**:130-131

[37] Haggitt RC, Glotzbach RE, Soffer EE, Wruble LD. Prognostic factors in colorectal carcinomas arising in adenomas: Implications for lesions removed by endoscopic polypectomy. Gastroenterology. 1985;**89**:328-336

[38] Kikuchi R, Takano M, Takagi K, Fujimoto N, Nozaki R, Fujiyoshi T, et al. Management of early invasive colorectal cancer. Risk of recurrence and clinical guidelines. Diseases of the Colon and Rectum. 1995;**38**:1286-1295

[39] Morino M, Risio M, Bach S, et al. Early rectal cancer: The European Association for Endoscopic Surgery (EAES) clinical consensus conference. Surgical Endoscopy. 2015;**29**:755-773

[40] Bach SP, Hill J, Monson JR, et al. A predictive model for local recurrence after transanal endoscopic microsurgery for rectal cancer. The British Journal of Surgery. 2009;**96**:280-290

[41] Junginger T, Goenner U, Hitzler M, et al. Long-term oncologic outcome after transanal endoscopic microsurgery for rectal carcinoma. Diseases of the Colon and Rectum. 2016;**59**:8-15

[42] Goldwag J, Marsicovetere P, Scalia P, et al. The impact of decision aids in patients with colorectal cancer: A systematic review. BMJ Open. 2019;**9**: e028379. DOI: 10.1136/bmjopen-2018-028379

[43] Tsai Ben M, Finne Charles O, Nordenstam Johan F, Dimitrios C, Madoff Robert D, Mellgren Anders MD. Transanal endoscopic microsurgery resection of rectal tumors: Outcomes and recommendations. Diseases of the Colon

& Rectum. 2010;**53**(1):16-23. DOI: 10.1007/DCR.0b013e3181bbd6ee

[44] Gérard JP, Ortholan C, Benezery K, et al. Contact X-ray therapy for rectal cancer: Experience in Centre Antoine-Lacassagne, Nice, 2002–2006. International Journal of Radiation Oncology, Biology, Physics. 2008;**72**: 665-670

[45] Myint AS. Jean Pierre Gerard Minimally invasive contact X-ray brachytherapy as an alternative option in patients with rectal cancer not suitable for bespoke surgical resection. Minimally invasive surgery. 2018;**2**:34. DOI: 10.20517/2574-1225.2018.52

[46] Habr-Gama A, Gama-Rodrigues J, Sro Juliro GP, Proscurshim I, Sabbagh C, Lynn PB, et al. Local recurrence after complete clinical response and watch and wait in rectal cancer after neoadjuvant chemoradiation: Impact of salvage therapy on local disease control. International Journal of Radiation Oncology, Biology, Physics. 2014;**88**: 822-828

[47] Mihir W, Sachin W. Gastrointestinal Interventional Endoscopy Advanced Techniques: Advanced Techniques. 1st ed. Springer International; 2020. pp. 153-162. DOI: 10.1007/978-3-030-21695-5

[48] Lezoche E, Baldarelli M, Lezoche G, et al. Randomized clinical trial of endoluminal locoregional resection versus laparoscopic total mesorectal excision for T2 rectal cancer after neoadjuvant therapy. The British Journal of Surgery. 2012;**99**:1211-1218

[49] Garcia-Aguilar J, Renfro LA, Chow OS, et al. Organ preservation for clinical T2N0 distal rectal cancer using neoadjuvant chemoradiotherapy and local excision (ACOSOG Z6041): Results of an open-label, single-arm, multi-institutional, phase 2 trial. The Lancet Oncology. 2015;**16**:1537-1546

[50] Gornicki A, Richter P, Polkowski W, et al. Anorectal and sexual functions after preoperative radiotherapy and full-thickness local excision of rectal cancer. European Journal of Surgical Oncology. 2014;**40**:723-730

[51] Smith FM, Rao C, Oliva PR, et al. Avoiding radical surgery improves early survival in elderly patients with rectal cancer, demonstrating complete clinical response after neoadjuvant therapy: Results of a decision-analytic model. Diseases of the Colon and Rectum. 2015; **58**:159-171

[52] Hallam S, Messenger DE, Thomas MG. A systematic review of local excision after neoadjuvant therapy for rectal cancer: Are ypT0 tumors the limit? Diseases of the Colon and Rectum. 2016;**59**:984-997

[53] Bach S, Gilbert A, Brock K, Korsegen S, Geh I, Hill J. Radicle surgery versus organ preservation via short-course radiotherapy followed by transanal endoscopic microsurgery for early stage rectal cancer (TREC): A randomised, open- label feasibility study. The Lancet Gastroenterology & Hepatology. 2020;**6**:92-105

Chapter 8

Immunotherapy for Colorectal Cancer in the Era of Precision Medicine

Daniel Sur, Alecsandra Gorzo and Claudia Burz

Abstract

Colorectal cancer (CRC) is considered the third most common cancer type and the second cause of cancer-related death worldwide, representing a significant global public health issue. Approximately 20% of patients present with metastatic disease, while up to 50% of those with early stages will eventually develop metastasis. During the last two decades, sustained efforts have been made to discover the molecular landscape of CRC and identify novel therapeutic targets. These efforts changed the treatment paradigm for CRC and improved survival significantly in metastatic disease. Immunotherapy represents a novel and exciting treatment option with promising results in gastrointestinal malignancies. The application of immunotherapy in CRC showed impressive results in a subset of patients with high microsatellite instability/deficient mismatch repair (MSI-H/dMMR) phenotype. An in-depth analysis of these particular MSI-H/dMMR tumors revealed that they are characterized by a high mutational load resulting in an increased number of neoantigens and a highly infiltrated tumor microenvironment. The Food and Drug Association (FDA) has recently approved immune checkpoint inhibitors (ICIs) pembrolizumab and nivolumab +/− ipilimumab for first-line and non-first-line therapy of MSI-H/dMMR metastatic CRC, contributing to the continuum of care in these patients. This chapter aims to overview the immune landscape and immunotherapeutic strategies in CRC.

Keywords: colorectal cancer, immunotherapy, pembrolizumab, nivolumab, ipilimumab, MSI-H/dMMR

1. Introduction

According to the GLOBOCAN database, colorectal cancer (CRC) represents the second most frequent cancer type diagnosed in women and the third in men. Globally, the highest incidence rates of CRC are seen in New Zeeland, Australia, North America, and Europe [1]. In contrast, the lowest incidence is found in South-Centre Asia and Africa. The existing discrepancies among geographic regions are mainly attributed to lower screening rates in undeveloped countries, socioeconomic status, lifestyle, and dietary disparities [2]. Age is considered a risk factor for CRC. However, recent epidemiologic studies reported an increased incidence in people under 50 years old due to lifestyle changes and genetic implications [3].

Despite the sustained efforts focused on developing new treatment options for CRC, metastatic CRC (mCRC) patients still have a very poor prognosis [4]. For advanced and metastatic CRC treatment, the breakthrough was the addition of oxaliplatin and irinotecan to the original 5-fluorouracil (5-FU) regimen. The combination almost doubled the survival rates and has been the standard of care for more than 20 years. The addition of targeted agents, such as bevacizumab (anti-VEGF), panitumumab, and cetuximab (anti-EGFR), further increased the efficacy of the treatment [5]. In recent times, treatment strategies focused on altering the immune system, like immune checkpoint inhibitors (ICIs), have made their way into oncology practice after showing promising results in solid tumors like melanoma and lung cancer. These approaches have been demonstrated to be less effective in CRC patients [6]. However, a better understanding of the tumor immune contexture and CRCs' molecular subtypes demonstrated that a specific subset of patients having a hypermutated phenotype might benefit from ICIs [7]. Mainly, these tumors are distinguished by a robust immune activation and high microsatellite instability (MSI-H) due to dysfunctions of the mismatch repair (MMR) genes-dMMR. By contrast, in tumors with low microsatellite instability (MSI-L) and proficient mismatch repair (pMMR) function, ICIs are ineffective [8]. To date, many novel combinatorial approaches have been researched in order to overcome the relative resistance seen in CRCs.

This chapter aims to overview the immune landscape and immunotherapeutic strategies in CRC.

2. Immune landscape of colorectal cancer

The pathogenesis of CRC is a very complex multistep event linked to the accumulations of both the epigenetic and genetic alterations [9]. Other exogenous factors, including lifestyle, diet, and microbiota, contribute to this process [10]. Moreover, another essential aspect correlated with CRC development is the host immune dysfunction, primarily relying on escape mechanisms and immune evasion, which create a favorable environment for tumor growth [11]. The immune system can distinguish tumor antigens after their presentation via major histocompatibility complex (MHC) proteins present on antigen-presenting cells adenomatous polyposis coli to T cell receptors (TCR) found on the surface of T cells. The interaction between MHC proteins and TCR is insufficient for T cell activation. These pathways are further modulated by co-inhibitory and co-stimulatory signals, which tumor cells exploit to evade recognition and destruction [12, 13]. Among the co-stimulatory molecules that positively influence T cell activation and expansion after interaction with their ligands, we mention CD80 and CD86, found on cancer cells or APC. Other co-stimulatory molecules recently described include 4-1BB, GITR, and X40 [14].

On the other hand, co-inhibitory molecules, including cytotoxic T lymphocyte antigen 4 (CTLA4), programmed cell death protein-1 (PD-1), LAG-3, and TIM-3, antagonize the effects mentioned above upon interaction with their ligands. These signaling pathways prevent excessive immune responses and autoimmune phenomena [15]. Tumor cells often hijack these mechanisms, overexpress co-inhibitory molecules, which promote the activation of immunosuppressive regulatory T cells (Treg) instead of effector T cells (Teff), and, therefore, evade immune surveillance [16].

ICIs using anti-PD1, anti-PD-L1 (programmed cell death protein-ligand 1), and anti-CTLA4 molecules have been successfully used in various cancer types to promote an effective antitumor immune response and overcome immune evasion mechanisms (**Figure 1**).

It was initially assumed that CRC is not an immunogenic cancer type, and therefore, immunotherapy would not be successful in this setting. Further studies identified a subset of patients harboring MSI-H/dMMR phenotype that could benefit from these therapeutic strategies [17]. Mutations in MMR genes are associated with microsatellite instability (MSI) and, therefore, a high tumor mutational burden. Consequently, these tumors contain an increased number of neoantigen, which will be recognized as foreign and will generate a robust immune response by the host. Moreover, MSI-H/dMMR tumors are characterized by the upregulation of immune checkpoints (PD-1 and PD-L1), which further enhances immune evasion [18].

2.1 Colorectal cancer molecular subtypes

Furthermore, CRC has been classified into four consensus molecular subtypes (CMS) to correlate the tumor phenotype with the clinical behavior and guide treatment. CMS1 (MSI immune subtype, 14%) tumors are frequently located in the proximal colon and are characterized by an increased immune infiltration in the tumor microenvironment (TME) (particularly CD8+, CD4+, and NK). In addition, these tumors have a high BRAFV600E mutation rate, are hypermethylated, and are associated with an impaired MMR system [19]. Owing to their particular phenotype, the immune-activated CMS1 subgroup has a clinical benefit from treatment with ICIs.

The CMS2 subtype (canonical, 37%) result from the canonical adenoma-to-carcinoma sequence. This cell phenotype is typically characterized by loss of tumor suppressor gene adenomatosis polyposis coli, followed by Kirsten rat sarcoma virus (KRAS) mutation and TP53 loss [20]. Moreover, these tumors present with low levels of hypermethylation and microsatellite stability (MSS). The CMS2 subtype is also characterized by the activation of WNT and MYC pathways, high expression of oncogenes epidermal growth factor receptor (EGFR), human epidermal growth factor receptor 2 (HER2), and a significant risk of distant relapse. However, CMS2 tumors have the highest 5-year overall survival (OS), at 77% among all the subtypes [21].

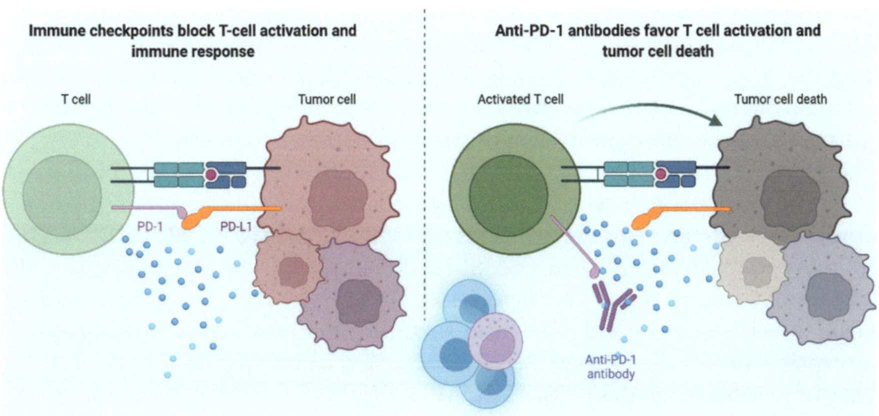

Figure 1.
Mechanism of anti-PD-1 antibodies.

CMS3 tumors (metabolic, 13%) have a chromosomal instability (CIN) genomic phenotype but with fewer copy number alterations. 30% of these tumors have microsatellite instability and an intermediate gene hypermethylation level. Moreover, CMS3 tumors are enriched with Kirsten rat sarcoma virus (KRAS) mutations [19, 20].

CMS4 (mesenchymal, 23%) has a phenotype distinguished by the activation of pathways associated with epidermal-mesenchymal transition (EMT) and by the overexpression of proteins involved in complement signaling and extracellular matrix remodeling [22]. The tumor microenvironment of CMS4 tumors is pro-inflammatory, with high levels of Treg, T helper, and myeloid derivated suppressor cells. CMS4 tumors are often diagnosed in advanced stages, have a poor prognosis, and show no benefit from adjuvant chemotherapy. Regarding the metastatic setting, CMS4 tumors are resistant to anti-EGFR, independently of KRAS status [23].

In a recent translational study of over 1700 tumor samples, 55% of them had ≥2 CMS subgroups, suggesting that intratumoral heterogenicity is a common finding [24]. However, intratumoral heterogenicity was associated with worse OS and reduced disease-free survival (DFS) [25].

3. Clinical evidence of immune checkpoint inhibitors in colorectal cancer

Immunotherapy based on ICIs has changed the treatment paradigm in various tumor types, including lung cancer, melanoma, renal cell carcinoma, etc. These strategies showed minimal clinical activity in nonselected CRC patients [26]. The first glimpse of hope came from a phase I clinical trial investigating the efficacy of the anti-PD-1, nivolumab, in advanced solid tumors, including CRC. Of 14 CRC patients, only one with an MSI-H/dMMR phenotype had a durable complete response (CR) [27]. Further, extensive research has been developed to understand the immune contexture of MSI-H/dMMR tumors, their response to ICIs, and possible combinatorial strategies (**Tables 1** and **2**).

3.1 Metastatic setting

3.1.1 Pembrolizumab

Pembrolizumab is an anti-PD-1 humanized IgG4 Kappa monoclonal antibody (mAb). Its role is to target PD-1 molecules from the T cell's surface and, therefore, to prevent the interaction with its ligands, PD-L1 and PD-L2. By blocking this interaction, pembrolizumab can resuscitate the cytotoxic activity of T cells and promote the recruitment of other immune cells in the tumor microenvironment [28].

The phase Ib KEYNOTE-028 trial (NCT02054806) investigated pembrolizumab's clinical efficacy in patients with PD-L1-positive advanced solid tumors. Only one accomplished a partial response among the 23 PD-L1-positive mCRC patients. Once again, this patient reportedly had an MSI-H/dMMR phenotype, suggesting that this feature could further predict the response to ICIs [29]. Starting from the hypothesis that tumors with an increased number of somatic mutations due to dMMR might be susceptible to ICIs, the phase II KEYNOTE-016 trial investigated the clinical efficacy of pembrolizumab in MSI-H/dMMR CRC, MSS/pMMR CRC, and MSI-H/dMMR non-CRC. Among the MSI-H/dMMR CRC patients, the progression-free survival (PFS) rate and overall response rate (ORR) were 79% (seven out of nine patients) and 40% (four out of 10 patients), respectively. Similar positive results

Study name	Phase	Trial population	Treatment	ORR	PFS	OS
NCT01876511 (KEYNOTE-016)	2	Refractory dMMR mCRC refractory pMMR mCRC refractory dMMR non-CRC	Pembrolizumab	Refractory dMMR mCRC: 40% refractory pMMR mCRC: 0% refractory dMMR non-CRC: 71%	At 20 weeks refractory dMMR mCRC: 78% refractory pMMR mCRC: 11% refractory dMMR non-CRC: 67%	For dMMR mCRC and dMMR non-CRC mediat OS was not reached For pMMR mCRC median OS 5 months
NCT02460198 KEYNOTE-164	2	Refractory MSI-H/dMMR mCRC Cohort A ≥ 2 previous treatment lines Cohort B ≥ previous treatment lines	Pembrolizumab	Cohort A: 33% Cohort B: 33%	Estimated PFS at 12 mo Cohort A: 34% Cohort B: 41%	Estimated OS at 12 mo Cohort A: 72% Cohort B: 76%
NCT02563002 KEYNOTE-177	3	Treatment naïve MSI-H/dMMR mCRC Arm A- pembrolizumab Arm B investigator's choice chemotherapy	Pembrolizumab vs. standard chemotherapy as 1st line treatment	Arm A: 43.8% Arm B: 33.1%	Median follow-up of 32.4 mo Arm A- 16.5 mo Arm B- 8.2 mo	Median survival not reached
NCT02060188 CheckMate 142	2	Refractory MSI-H/dMMR mCRC	Nivolumab	31%	At 12 mo: 50%	At 12 mo: 73%
	2	Refractory MSI-H/dMMR mCRC	Nivolumab + ipilimumab	55%	At 12 mo- 71% PFS rate	At 12 mo: 85% OS rate
	2	Treatment naïve MSI-H/dMMR mCRC	Nivolumab + ipilimumab	Median follow-up of 29 mo: 69%	at 24 mo: 74% PFS rate	At 24 mo: 79% OS rate

Table 1.
Key clinical trials of ICIs in MSI-H/dMMR mCRC.

Study name	Phase	Trial population	Treatment	Primary endpoint	Study purpose
NCT04014530 ATAPEMBRO	I/II	MSI-H/dMMR mCRC pMMR mCRC dMMR endometrial carcinoma	Ataluren (premature stop codon suppressor) + pembrolizumab	AEs MTD (maximum tolerated dose) of Ataluren ORR	• To determine the safety and efficacy of the combination ataluren + pembrolizumab
NCT04008030 CheckMate 8HW	III	dMMR/MSI-H mCRC	Nivolumab Nivolumab + ipilimumab Investigator's choice chemotherapy	PFS	• To compare the clinical benefit of nivolumab monotherapy or nivolumab + ipilimumab • To compare the clinical benefit of nivolumab + ipilimumab versus investigator's choice chemotherapy
NCT03104439	II	MSI-H/dMMR mCRC MSS mCRC Pancreatic cancer	Nicolumab + ipilimumab + radiation therapy	DCR (disease control rate)	• To establish the clinical efficacy of combining nivolumab + ipilimumab + radiation therapy
NCT02997228 COMMIT SWOG1610	III	Treatment naïve dMMR/ MSI-H mCRC	mFOLFOX6 + bevacizumab + atezolizumab mFOLFOX6 + bevacizumab + atezolizumab	PFS	• To determine the clinical efficacy of mFOLFOX6/bevacizumab and atezolizumab compared to atezolizumab monotherapy
NCT02912559 ATOMIC Alliance A021502	III	Stage III MSI-H/dMMR CRC	mFOLFOX6 + atezolizumab mFOLFOX6	DFS	• To compare the association of standard chemothereapy+atezolizumab versus standard chemotherapy in the adjuvant setting
NCT03186326 SAMCO	II	Previously treated MSI-H/ dMMR mCRC	Standard chemotherapy (FOLFOX/ FOLFIRI +/– targeted therapy) Avelumab	PFS	• To compare the efficacy of avelumab versus second line standard chemotherapy
NCT03475953 REGOMUNE	I/II	Metastatic solid tumors (MSI-H/dMMR mCRC)	Avelumab + regorafenib	RP2D (recommended phase 2 dose)	• To determine the safety and efficacy of low dose regorafenib in combination with avelumab
NCT03435107	II	Previously treated MSI-H/ dMMR mCRC and POLE mu- tated mCRC	Durvalumab	ORR	• To evaluate the efficacy of durvalumab in later lines of therapy

Table 2.
Selected ongoing clinical trials of ICIs in MSI-H/dMMR CRC.

were observed in MSI-H/dMMR non-CRC cohort, with 71% ORR (five out of seven patients). Contrarily, in the MSS/pMMR cohort, the ORR was 0% and the PFS rate was 11%. In the MSI-H/dMMR CRC cohort, the median OS and PFS were not reached. Moreover, a high somatic mutational load was significantly associated with a longer PFS ($p = 0.02$) [30]. These preliminary results inspired the initiation of the KEYNOTE-164 trial. This phase II study investigated the efficacy of pembrolizumab in two cohorts of previously treated MSI-H/dMMR advanced CRC patients. Cohort A included the patients previously treated with ≥2 lines of standard therapy, while cohort B included the patients treated with ≥1 line of therapy. With a median follow-up of 31.3 months (mo) for cohort A and 24.2 mo for cohort B, the results showed an ORR of 33% (95% CI; 21–46%). The median OS was 31.4 mo (95% CI; 21.4 mo to not reached) in cohort A, and it was not reached in cohort B [31]. Furthermore, another phase II trial, KEYNOTE-158, investigated the antitumor activity of pembrolizumab in previously treated MSI-H/dMMR non-CRC patients. The ORR was 34.3%, the median PFS was 4.1 mo, and the media OS was 34.5 mo [32]. Considering these results, in May 2017, the Food and Drug Association (FDA) approved pembrolizumab to treat unresectable or metastatic MSI-H/dMMR CRC patients who progressed after conventional chemotherapy with oxaliplatin, fluorouracil, and irinotecan, and for previously treated metastatic or unresectable MSI-H/dMMR solid tumors that have no other satisfactory treatment option [33].

Based on the robust and sustained results seen in refractory mCRC, the phase III KEYNOTE-177 trial investigated the clinical efficacy of pembrolizumab as first-line treatment compared to standard chemotherapy in MSI-H/dMMR mCRC patients. At a median follow-up of 32 mo, pembrolizumab doubled the PFS compared to chemotherapy (8.2 mo versus 16.5 mo; $p = 0.0002$). The ORR was significantly higher with pembrolizumab than with standard chemotherapy (44% versus 33%). Moreover, the grade 3–5 AEs (adverse events) rate was 66% for standard chemotherapy and only 22% for pembrolizumab [34]. Even if the OS data are not mature yet, a high crossover rate to the immunotherapy arm has been reported. Based on these results, which demonstrate the superiority of pembrolizumab over standard chemotherapy, in June 2020, the FDA approved the treatment with pembrolizumab as first-line treatment in MSI-H/dMMR mCRC patients [35].

3.1.2 Nivolumab +/− Ipilimumab

Nivolumab is an anti-PD-1 humanized IgG4 mAb that, similar to pembrolizumab, disrupts the interaction between the PD-1 receptor and its ligands (PD-L1 and PDL2). The clinical benefit of nivolumab has been documented in many tumor types as melanoma, lung cancer, and renal cell carcinoma [28].

Ipilimumab is a mAb directed against the surface protein CTLA-4, expressed on activated and regulatory T cells. The CTLA-4 molecule negatively regulates T-cell function by inducing T cell anergy and tolerance [36]. Therefore, CTLA-4 blockade intends to counteract the immune tolerance to cancer cells. To support this idea, James Allison and colleagues showed that antibodies against CTLA-4 enhance the antitumor activity of immune cells in mice transplanted with fibrosarcoma and colon cancer [37].

The phase II CheckMate-142 trial was a large initiative to evaluate the clinical benefit of nivolumab alone or associated with other anticancer therapies in mCRC patients with or without MSI-H/dMMR phenotype. The study has an atypical design which initially included six cohorts: 1—nivolumab monotherapy; 2—nivolumab + ipilimumab (every 3 weeks, for four doses, followed by nivolumab monotherapy every

2 weeks); 3—nivolumab + ipilimumab (every 6 weeks, for four doses, followed by nivolumab monotherapy every 2 weeks); 4—nivolumab + ipilimumab + cobimetinib; 5—nivolumab + BMS-986016; and 6—nivolumab + daratumumab.

Out of 74 MSI-H/dMMR mCRC patients from cohort 1, 31.1% (23 out of 74) achieved an OR, while 69% (51 out of 74) had disease control for ≥12 weeks. Moreover, responses have been obtained in patients with or without KRAR, BRAF mutations, or a history of Lynch syndrome. Additionally, this study reported an OR of 25% in BRAF-mutated patients. These results outperform the ones obtained using standard chemotherapy (<10%) and combination strategies with EGFR, BRAF, or MEK inhibitors (10–16%) [38].

The results from cohort 3, including MSI-H/dMMR mCRC patients treated with nivolumab and ipilimumab, have also been released. At a median follow-up of 13.4 mo, the ORR was 55% (65 out of 119 patients), the median PFS was not reached, and a durable response (≥6 weeks) was seen in 83% of patients. Nonetheless, it is important to note that this trial was not randomized, and the direct comparison could be, at some point, misleading. The phase II CheckMate-142 trial results guided the FDA approval of nivolumab +/− ipilimumab in previously treated MSI-H/dMMR mCRC patients [39].

The CheckMate-142 trial further investigated the clinical benefit of nivolumab + ipilimumab as first-line treatment in MSI-H/dMMR mCRC patients. The trial's primary endpoint was ORR. With a median follow-up of 29 mo, the ORR was 69% and CR 13%. The median PFS and OS were not yet reached. Based on these results, nivolumab is recommended as front-line treatment in MSI-H/dMMR mCRC patients as monotherapy or with ipilimumab [40].

In recent years, other ICIs have made their way into oncological practice and are under clinical investigation, including atezolizumab (anti-PD-L1), avelumab (anti-PD-L1), and durvalumab (anti-PD-L1).

3.2 Neoadjuvant and adjuvant setting

Preclinical studies hypothesized that ICIs might be more effective in neoadjuvant and adjuvant settings. In this regard, the phase II NICHE trial included 40 stages I–III CRC cancer patients with or without MSI-H/dMMR phenotype. All the patients were treated with two doses of nivolumab and one of ipilimumab. All the patients obtained pathological responses in the MSI-H/dMMR group, suggesting that immunotherapy warrants further investigations in the neoadjuvant setting [41]. The ATOMIC study, a phase III randomized controlled trial, is currently investigating Atezolizumab + FOLFOX regimen compared to FOLFOX alone in 700 patients with MSI-H/dMMR stage III CRC. The study's primary endpoint is disease-free survival (DFS), and the results are highly expected [42]. Currently, two sizeable ongoing phase III clinical trials are investigating the addition of anti-PD-L1 avelumab (NCT03827044) or anti-PD-1 pembrolizumab (NCT02912559) to standard adjuvant chemotherapy regimes in stage III MSI-H/dMMR CRC patients.

4. Strategies beyond ICI

4.1 Adoptive cell transfer (ACT)

Another revolutionary treatment option aiming to augment the host's immune system is represented by ATCs. The approach consists of transferring the patient's immune cells, which were previously genetically engineered, and expanded to destroy cancer cells. ACT can include tumor-infiltrating lymphocytes (TILs), natural killer (NK), chimeric antigen receptor T-cell therapy (CAR-T), or engineered T cell receptors (TCR).

ACTs have achieved impressive success in several tumor types in the last two decades, especially in hematologic malignancies, like B cell lymphoma and leukemia [43].

ACT usage for cancer treatment originates from the observation of TILs, representing a population of lymphocytes infiltrating the tumor or located at its' margins. TILs represent the host's natural antitumor immune response and can recognize tumor-specific antigens presented by MHC 1 [44].

In 2016, a group of researchers identified in the TILs from CRC metastatic lesions a polyclonal population of CD8+ cells directed against KRAS G12D. After expansion, this TILs population was further reinfused into the patient and eradicated six out of seven lung metastases. So far, harvesting TILs from colorectal tumors has faced many difficulties [45]. One of the concerning issues is the contamination with intestinal flora, which can be overcome by acquiring tumor-specific T cells from tumor-draining lymph nodes [46]. Another ideal source for aseptically harvesting TILs in CRC might be liver metastasis. However, further research is needed to overcome all the impediments to the usage of TILs in CRC and other solid tumors.

CAR-T cell therapies have been extensively studied in hematologic malignancies, with less evidence in solid tumors at the moment. This kind of personalized medicine combines genetic therapy with immunotherapy. It involves T cells harvesting from the patient, which are genetically modified to express a chimeric antigen receptor (CAR) that can recognize a tumor-associated antigen (TAA) [47, 48]. The clinical trials investigating CAR-T cells in CRC treatment targeted various TAAs, including carcinoembryonic antigen (CEA), mesothelin (MSLN), EGFR, HER2, and natural killer group 2 member D (NKG2D) [49]. A phase I clinical trial investigated CAR-T cell therapy targeting CEA in previously treated CEA-positive mCRC patients. Out of the 10 patients included in the study, seven experienced stable disease for longer than 30 months. Moreover, the study reported a sustained decline in CEA serum levels [50]. Apical surfaces of the intestinal epithelium express the membrane-bound receptor guanylyl cyclase C (GUCY2C). Magee et al. tested the efficacy of a GUCY2C-specific CAR-T cell molecule in an mCRC mice model. The result showed that GUCY2C CAR-T cells reduced the number of lung metastasis in mice, lowering morbidity and improving survival [51].

Although ACTs have shown therapeutic potential in many cancer types, there are still many obstacles to their effectiveness in solid tumors, including CRC.

4.2 Cancer vaccines

Cancer vaccines are a form of active immunotherapy thought to enhance the antitumor immune response by evoking TAA in order to be targeted by the immune system. In mCRC, several vaccine types have been studied, including peptides, dendritic cells, autologous tumor cells, and recombinant viral vectors [52]. The vaccine must supply enough tumor antigens to induce a robust immune response and, therefore, to obtain a substantial clinical benefit [53]. Unfortunately, these requests are challenging to be acquired; thus, the clinical trials investigating cancer vaccines reported mixed results.

A benefit of peptide-based vaccines is that they are affordable in terms of production and storage. A recently developed peptide vaccine, PolyPEPI1018 consisting of

12 epitopes derived from seven antigens frequently expressed in mCRC, demonstrated increased CD8+ T cell and CD4+ T cell responses against three antigens after only one dose [54].

Since plasmid DNA encoding influenza nucleoprotein A was discovered to trigger a specific T cell response, DNA vaccines have received much attention. These types of vaccines consist of bacterial plasmids created to provide tumor antigens that will be further presented via MHC proteins and stimulate an immune response [55]. MYB is an oncoprotein abnormally expressed in many tumor types, including CRC. In CRC transgenic mice, MYB-based vaccines showed good therapeutic efficacy. However, several corners about DNA vaccines include poor immunogenicity and potential interactions with the host's genome [56].

RNA-based vaccines, another widely investigated therapeutic and prophylactic form of immunotherapy, consist of a platform that encodes tumor-specific antigens. After the internalization of mRNA transcript by the target cell, the translation takes place in the cytoplasm and is followed by tumor antigen presentation via MHC proteins, triggering a robust immune response. mRNA vaccines offer several benefits, making them appealing therapeutic options. They are nonintegrating molecules, affordable, relatively fast to produce, and easy to modify [57]. A phase I/II trial is currently investigating an mRNA-based vaccine (mRNA 4650) for treating various tumor types, including gastrointestinal, melanoma, genitourinary, and CRC [58]. There are only two anticancer vaccines approved in oncological practice: Provenge (sipuleucel-T) for prostate cancer treatment and Oncophage for kidney cancer [59, 60]. At the moment, cancer vaccines are extensively studied in clinical trials and will hopefully improve treatment strategies for CRC.

5. Correct treatment sequence after the implementation of ICI in CRC armamentarium

Nowadays, most CRC patients (75%) are diagnosed with an early stage (I–III) due to performant screening programs providing a chance for cure. However, 25% of them have metastatic disease at presentation and, therefore, poor prognosis [61].

For early-stage CRC, the standard of care consists of upfront surgery of the primary tumor and regional lymph nodes, followed by adjuvant chemotherapy in selected patients [62]. Following surgical resection, the 5-year DFS is 95% for stage I, 82–88% for stage II, and 45–50% for stage III CRC [63]. The primary role of adjuvant chemotherapy is to eradicate the micrometastatic residual disease after surgery. Identifying micrometastatic residual disease is unreliable; therefore, the gold standard used to confirm the clinical benefit of adjuvant chemotherapy is the 5-year OS [64]. Since the most challenging issue of the existing treatment parading in early-stage CRC is the incapacity to detect micrometastatic disease, the available guidelines recommend adjuvant chemotherapy for all stage III CRC patients. For stage II CRC, the benefit of adjuvant chemotherapy is still debatable. To date, it is recommended only for patients with high-risk clinicopathologic features (positive resection margins, <12 examined lymph nodes, T4, perineural invasion, lymphovascular emboli, perforation, and obstruction). The preferred chemotherapy regimens for this setting are a combination of fluoropyrimidine and oxaliplatin (FOLFOX or CAPOX) [65]. The addition of oxaliplatin led to OS improvement, and the risk of death was further reduced by 16%, 17%, and 12% in the MOSAIC, XELODA, and NSABP C-07 trials [66–68].

In the last 20 years, the prognosis of mCRC patients has significantly improved due to remarkable progress made in precision medicine. The currently available guidelines recommend resectioning metastasis performed either upfront or after previous downsizing treatment in selected patients [69]. In a recent meta-analysis, the 5-year survival rate was approximately 38% in patients who underwent resection of the liver metastasis [70]. If, however, this goal is not realistic, systemic therapy has shown significant survival benefits for mCRC patients. The fundamental development in mCRC treatment was the addition of oxaliplatin (a platinum derivate) and irinotecan (a topoisomerase I inhibitor) to 5-FU-based chemotherapy. Therefore, FOLFOX (5-FU, folinic acid, and oxaliplatin) and FOLFIRI (5-FU, folinic acid, and irinotecan) demonstrated better response rates and DFS compared to 5-FU alone, representing the mainstay of first-line chemotherapy [71, 72].

Further, after decades of clinical and translational research, an important step toward precision medicine was discovering treatment options based on the tumor's molecular characteristics. The first biologic therapy included in the mCRC treatment strategy was bevacizumab, a mAb targeting vascular endothelial growth factor-A (VEGF-A) [73]. Bevacizumab is recommended for RAS-mutated mCRC either as first-line or second-line in combination with chemotherapy [74]. Similarly, cetuximab and panitumumab are anti-EGFR mAbs associated with chemotherapy in the first and second lines of treatment but for restricted patients harboring RAS/BRAF-WT (wild-type) tumors [75]. Moreover, aflibercept (a synthetic receptor for VEGF-B, VEGF-A, and PIGF) and ramucirumab (anti-VEGFR-2) demonstrated clinical benefit in the second-line therapy while combined with chemotherapy [76, 77]. In further line, regorafenib (a multikinase inhibitor) also showed clinical efficacy [78]. Owing to improved surgical procedures and expanded therapeutic options, most mCRC patients experience an improved survival between 24 and 36 months, allowing a continuum of care [79].

Even if MSI-H/dMMR tumors represent a small subset of mCRC (5% or all cases), the discovery and introduction of ICIs into the continuum of care has been a significant step forward in precision medicine. Based on the clinical benefit observed in clinical trials, the current guidelines recommend nivolumab ± ipilimumab and pembrolizumab as first-line and non-first-line therapy for MSI-H/dMMR mCRC patients [33, 34, 40, 80]. Surprisingly, the phase III KEYNOTE-177 trial, which compared pembrolizumab with standard first-line therapy in MSI-H/dMMR mCRC, demonstrated a doubling PFS in pembrolizumab-treated patients (16.5 months). This outcome is the longest PFS ever reported by phase III trials for any first-line therapeutic options in mCRC [34]. Additionally, pembrolizumab and nivolumab ± ipilimumab are also recommended in the neoadjuvant setting for resectable MSI-H/dMMR mCRC patients [81].

According to the CMS classification, mCRCs with MSI-H/dMMR phenotype are considered immune-activated and belong to the CMS1 subgroup. Conversely, MSS/pMMR tumors, representing 95% of all mCRCs, display a low immune infiltrate, do not respond to ICIs, and are a serious challenge for clinical management [19]. It has been revealed that radiotherapy, chemotherapy, and targeted agents can induce immunogenic cell death (ICD), releasing tumor neoantigens and increasing the immune infiltrate in the tumor microenvironment (TME). Based on this hypothesis, many clinical trials are currently investigating the combination of ICIs with other anticancer therapies in MSS/pMMR mCRC to overcome the primary resistance to immunotherapy [82, 83].

6. Biomarkers

6.1 Microsatellite instability (MSI)

"Short tandem repeats" or microsatellites are repeated noncoding DNA sequences with a length from one to six base pairs. DNA polymerases are more predisposed to make errors either by removing or by inserting additional bases in these particular regions, leading to mismatched DNA strands [84]. Therefore, the MSI molecular phenotype is a consequence of deficient MMR proteins. The most directed genes from the MMR family associated with genome instability are MLH1, MLH2, PMS2, and MSH6. It is estimated that only 15% of CRCs are microsatellite unstable (MSI-H) [85]. Germline MMR gene mutation is the hallmark of Lynch syndrome, an autosomal dominant condition associated with an increased risk of colorectal (80%), endometrial (60%), stomach, small intestine, kidney, bladder, and brain tumors [86]. However, the MSI phenotype appears due to somatic mutations in most cases, usually caused by epigenetic silencing of the MLH1 promoter. Less commonly, the inactivation of MMR proteins can occur due to somatic biallelic MMR gene mutations. It is worth mentioning that a subset of MSI-H tumors has no detected alterations in the MMR genes [87]. These tumors were shown to overexpress various micro-RNAs (miRNAs), like miRNA-21 and 122, that might silence MMR genes [88].

Considering that the human genome comprises hundreds of thousands of microsatellites, the MSI assay evaluates only five of them via polymerase chain reaction (PRC) for practical reasons. Therefore, a tumor is defined as MSI-H if at least two microsatellites have a shift in size, and a size shift in only one locus represents an MSI-L tumor. By contrast, tumors with no unstable microsatellites are defined as microsatellite stable (MSS). The immunohistochemistry (IHC) assay of key MMR proteins has a high concordance rate and similar performance characteristics to the MSI assay via PRC. Hence, loss of protein expression defines a tumor as dMMR, while the presence of all MMR proteins labels the tumors as pMMR (MMR proficient) [89]. Besides IHC and PCR, next-generation sequencing (NGS) is a novel approach for detecting MSI status with high sensitivity (95%) and specificity (98%) [90]. To further clarify the notions, MSI-H and dMMR are considered the same types of tumor, and MSS and pMMR tumors are also mostly overlapping.

Regardless of the origin (sporadic or hereditary), all the MSI-H/dMMR CRCs have some characteristic histologic features. The high mutational load resulting from the deficiency of MMR proteins leads to the accumulation of a robust number of tumors neoantigens with great immunological potential [91]. MSI-H/dMMR tumors are frequently located in the right colon, have mucinous histology, are poorly differentiated, and, more importantly, have increased TILs. Moreover, MSI-H/dMMR tumors were reported to highly express immune checkpoints (CTLA4, PD-1, and PD-L1) [92].

6.2 PD-L1 expression

The detection of PD-L1 using immunohistochemical staining is one of the most explored predictive biomarkers for the response to ICIs. Studies reported that upregulation of PD-L1 is correlated with high infiltration of effector T cells. Moreover, these tumors have a high likelihood of responding to ICI. In contrast to other tumor types like non-small-cell lung cancer (NSCLC), melanoma, and gastric cancer, the PD-L1 expression predicted no response to ICIs in mCRC patients [93]. An update from the CheckMate-142 trial investigating nivolumab +/− ipilimumab in MSI-H/dMMR CRC demonstrated that the ORR was irrespective of PD-L1 expression [39]. Moreover, the KEYNOTE-016 trial investigating the clinical benefit of pembrolizumab in mCRC with both MSS and MSI-H phenotypes showed no statistically significant correlation between PD-L1 expression and OR or PFS [31].

The reported disparities among tumors could be explained by the dynamic nature of this surface protein, which is influenced by the TME and treatment options. Furthermore, the lack of standardization for PD-L1 expression assay limits its clinical significance [94].

6.3 POLE/POLD1

POLE (DNA polymerase epsilon) and POLD1 (DNA polymerase delta) are two enzymes responsible for the correct genome replication during the cell cycle. Somatic mutation of either POLE or POLD genes affects their proofreading function, increasing the predisposition to numerous cancer types, including CRC [95]. Similar to the MSI-H/dMMR, these tumors have an ultramutated phenotype [96]. POLE-mutated CRCs express an upregulation of immune checkpoint molecules and also have a high level of TILs. Moreover, these tumors seem to be a rare finding (1% of CRCs), appear more frequently in young male patients, and have an early stage at presentation [97].

To date, limited evidence is available regarding the clinical benefit of ICIs in POLE/POLD1-mutated tumors. An excellent response to pembrolizumab was seen in a patient suffering from endometrial cancer who had a POLE mutation seen at genomic profiling. Since MSI-H/dMMR CRCs have similar characteristics (hypermutated phenotype, upregulated immune checkpoints, and inflamed TME), it was supposed that POLE/POLD1-mutated CRCs might be better suited for ICIs [98]. Further data are, however, needed to support this hypothesis.

6.4 Immunoscore

The immunoscore represents an immunohistochemical and digital pathology-based assay derived from the immune contexture. It quantifies two lymphocyte populations, CD8+ and CD3+, both in the tumor core (TC) and invasive margins (IM). The purpose of immunoscore was to translate the immune contexture into a viable biomarker for CRC [99]. The immunoscore ranks from I0 (immunoscore 0), characterized by a low density of CD8+ and CD3+ in both TC and IM, to I4 (immunoscore 4), with a high density of both lymphocyte populations in both regions. The advantage of immunoscore appears to be dual. First, this score is reported to be a prognostic factor for DFS and OS in early CRC. Moreover, it also seems to be an important tool for novel therapeutic approaches, including immunotherapy [100].

The prognostic value of immunoscore is supported by several studies. According to the phase III NCCTG N0147 trial, a high immunoscore was statistically significantly associated with a longer 3-year DFS than a low immunoscore in stage III CRC patients [101]. An international consortium including 14 centers from 13 countries assessed the prognostic value of immunoscore in stage I–III CRC patients (samples from 2681 patients). Patients with high immunoscore had a statistically significant lower risk of recurrence at 5 years compared to low immunoscore (HR = 0.20, 95%

CI 0.10–0.38; $p < 0.0001$). In the multivariant analysis, the association between immunoscore and the time to recurrence (TTR) was independent of T stage, N stage, patient's age, sex, microsatellite instability, or other existing prognostic factors ($p < 0.0001$) [102]. Besides its prognostic value, immunoscore holds great potential as a predictive biomarker. An international study conducted by the Society for Immunotherapy of Cancer analyzed the association of immunoscore with the effect of adjuvant chemotherapy in time to recurrence (TTR) in stage III CRC patients. A high immunoscore was associated with the lowest risk of recurrence, and it showed a significant correlation with prolonged TTR, DFS, and OS in this subset of patients (all $p < 0.001$) [103]. The immune context might also predict the clinical response to ICIs. CD8+ T cells were reportedly a good predictor of response to CTLA4 blockade in melanoma patients. Moreover, CD8+ lymphocytes were associated with response to anti-PD-1 molecules [100, 104].

To date, immunoscore was introduced among the "Essential and Desirable Diagnostic Criteria" for CRC in the fifth edition of the World Health Organization (WHO) classification of digestive tumors. This detail brings us closer to the notion of TNM-I classification ("I" from "immune") [105].

7. Conclusions and future perspectives

Immunotherapy evolved into a desirable treatment option for CRC because of the success seen in various solid tumors and the reliable side effects. However, the role of immunotherapy is still restricted to a very small subset of patients with an MSI-H/dMMR phenotype. At the moment, many clinical trials are exploring combinatorial strategies of conventional therapy and ICIs to overcome primary resistance to ICIs in CRC. To extend the clinical benefit of cancer immunotherapies, novel delivery platforms are currently under investigation, including nanoparticles, implants, biomaterials, and scaffolds. Using these delivery systems may help reduce toxicities and ensure localized and controlled drug delivery [106]. Moreover, metagenomic studies underline the critical role of microbiota in CRC pathogenesis and response to treatment, including ICIs. Nonetheless, the implementation of radiomic analyses could further identify the antitumor activity of targeted therapies or immunotherapy [107].

Future technological progress is expected to provide a more profound knowledge of the immune system and the tumor and microenvironment gene expression to ensure a continuum of care based on precision medicine.

Acknowledgements

This section of your manuscript may also include funding information.

List of abbreviations

AEs	adverse events
APC	antigen-presenting cells

CAR	chimeric antigen receptor
CAR	T-chimeric antigen receptor T-cell therapy
CEA	carcinoembryonic antigen
CMS	consensus molecular subtypes
CRC	colorectal cancer
CTLA4	cytotoxic T lymphocyte antigen 4
DCR	disease control rate
dMMR	mismatch repair deficient
EMT	epidermal-mesenchymal transition
FDA	Food and Drug Association
GUCY2C	membrane-bound receptor guanylyl cyclase C
ICIs	immune checkpoint inhibitors
IHC	immunohistochemistry
IM	invasive margins
KRAS	Kirsten rat sarcoma virus
mAb	monoclonal antibody
mCRC	metastatic colorectal cancer
MHC	major histocompatibility complex
miRNAs	micro-RNA
Mo	months
MSI-H	microsatellite instability-high
MSLN	mesothelin
MSS	microsatellite stable
NGS	next-generation sequencing
NK	natural killer
NKG2D	natural killer group 2 member D
NSCLC	non-small cell lung cancer
ORR	overall response rate
OS	overall survival
PD-1	programmed cell death protein-1
PD-L1	programmed cell death protein- ligand 1
PFS	progression-free survival
POLD1	DNA polymerase delta
POLE	DNA polymerase epsilon
PRC	polymerase chain reaction
PR2D	recommended phase 2 dose
TAA	tumor-associated antigen
TC	tumor core
TCR	engineered T cell receptors
TCR	T cell receptors
Teff	effector T cells
TILs	tumor-infiltrating lymphocytes
TME	tumor microenvironment
Treg	immunosuppressive regulatory T cells
TTR	time to recurrence
VEGF-A	vascular endothelial growth factor-A
WHO	World Health Organization

Author details

Daniel Sur[1,2]*, Alecsandra Gorzo[2] and Claudia Burz[2,3]

1 Department of Medical Oncology, University of Medicine and Pharmacy "Iuliu Hatieganu", Cluj-Napoca, Romania

2 Department of Medical Oncology, The Oncology Institute "Prof.dr.Ion Chiricuta", Cluj-Napoca, Romania

3 Department of Allergology and Immunology, The Oncology Institute "Prof.dr.Ion Chiricuta", Cluj-Napoca, Romania

*Address all correspondence to: dr.geni@yahoo.co.uk

References

[1] Xi Y, Xu P. Global colorectal cancer burden in 2020 and projections to 2040. Translational Oncology. 2021;**14**:101174

[2] Marley AR, Nan H. Epidemiology of colorectal cancer. International Journal of Molecular Epidemiology and Genetics. 2016;7:105-114

[3] Siegel RL, Jakubowski CD, Fedewa SA, Davis A, Azad NS. Colorectal Cancer in the Young: Epidemiology, Prevention, Management. American Society of Clinical Oncology Educational Book. 2020 May;**40**:e75-88. DOI: 10.1200/EDBK_279901

[4] Carlomagno C, De Stefano A, Rosanova M, De Falco S, Attademo L, Fiore G, et al. Multiple treatment lines and prognosis in metastatic colorectal cancer patients. Cancer Metastasis Reviews. 2019;**38**:307-313. DOI: 10.1007/s10555-018-9748-7

[5] Stintzing S. Management of colorectal cancer. F1000Prime Reports. 2014;**6**:108

[6] Bever KM, Le DT. An expanding role for immunotherapy in colorectal cancer. Journal of the National Comprehensive Cancer Network. 2017;**15**:401-410. DOI: 10.6004/jnccn.2017.0037

[7] Sur D, Lungulescu C, Puscariu I-I, Volovat SR, Preda M, Mateianu EA, et al. Immunotherapy-related publications in colorectal cancer: A bibliometric analysis. Healthcare. 2022;**10**:75. DOI: 10.3390/healthcare10010075

[8] Lichtenstern CR, Ngu RK, Shalapour S, Karin M. Immunotherapy, inflammation and colorectal cancer. Cells. 2020;**9**:618

[9] Grady WM, Markowitz SD. The molecular pathogenesis of colorectal cancer and its potential application to colorectal cancer screening. Digestive Diseases and Sciences. 2015;**60**:762-772. DOI: 10.1007/s10620-014-3444-4

[10] Øines M, Helsingen LM, Bretthauer M, Emilsson L. Epidemiology and risk factors of colorectal polyps. Best Practice & Research Clinical Gastroenterology. 2017;**31**:419-424. DOI: 10.1016/j.bpg.2017.06.004

[11] Schmitt M, Greten FR. The inflammatory pathogenesis of colorectal cancer. Nature Reviews. Immunology. 2021;**21**:653-667. DOI: 10.1038/s41577-021-00534-x

[12] Jhunjhunwala S, Hammer C, Delamarre L. Antigen presentation in cancer: Insights into tumour immunogenicity and immune evasion. Nature Reviews. Cancer. 2021;**21**:298-312. DOI: 10.1038/s41568-021-00339-z

[13] Gorzo A, Galos D, Volovat SR, Lungulescu CV, Burz C, Sur D. Landscape of immunotherapy options for colorectal cancer: Current knowledge and future perspectives beyond immune checkpoint blockade. Life. 2022;**12**:229. DOI: 10.3390/life12020229

[14] Liu W, Zang X. Structures of immune checkpoints: An overview on the CD28-B7 family. In: Jin T, Yin Q, editors. Structural Immunology. Springer; 2019. pp. 63-78

[15] Huang C, Zhu H-X, Yao Y, Bian Z-H, Zheng Y-J, Li L, et al. Immune checkpoint molecules. Possible future therapeutic implications in autoimmune diseases. Journal of Autoimmunity. 2019;**104**:102333. DOI: 10.1016/j.jaut.2019.102333

[16] Li X, Shao C, Shi Y, Han W. Lessons learned from the blockade of immune checkpoints in cancer immunotherapy. Journal of Hematology & Oncology. 2018;**11**:31. DOI: 10.1186/s13045-018-0578-4

[17] Golshani G, Zhang Y. Advances in immunotherapy for colorectal cancer: A review. Therapeutic Advances in Gastroenterology. 2020;**13**:1756284820917527. DOI: 10.1177/1756284820917527

[18] Llosa NJ, Cruise M, Tam A, Wicks EC, Hechenbleikner EM, Taube JM, et al. The vigorous immune microenvironment of microsatellite instable colon cancer is balanced by multiple counter-inhibitory checkpoints. Cancer Discovery. 2015;**5**:43-51. DOI: 10.1158/2159-8290.CD-14-0863

[19] Thanki K, Nicholls ME, Gajjar A, Senagore AJ, Qiu S, Szabo C, et al. Consensus molecular subtypes of colorectal cancer and their clinical implications. International Biological and Biomedical Journal. 2017;**3**:105-111

[20] Dienstmann R, Vermeulen L, Guinney J, Kopetz S, Tejpar S, Tabernero J. Consensus molecular subtypes and the evolution of precision medicine in colorectal cancer. Nature Reviews. Cancer. 2017;**17**:79-92. DOI: 10.1038/nrc.2016.126

[21] Cancer Genome Atlas Network. Comprehensive molecular characterization of human colon and rectal cancer. Nature. 2012;**487**:330-337. DOI: 10.1038/nature11252

[22] Martini G, Dienstmann R, Ros J, Baraibar I, Cuadra-Urteaga JL, Salva F, et al. Molecular subtypes and the evolution of treatment management in metastatic colorectal cancer. Therapeutic Advances in Medical Oncology. 2020;**12**:1758835920936089. DOI: 10.1177/1758835920936089

[23] De Sousa E, Melo F, Wang X, Jansen M, Fessler E, Trinh A, et al. Poor-prognosis colon cancer is defined by a molecularly distinct subtype and develops from serrated precursor lesions. Nature Medicine. 2013;**19**:614-618. DOI: 10.1038/nm.3174

[24] Marisa L, Blum Y, Taieb J, Ayadi M, Pilati C, Le Malicot K, et al. Intratumor CMS heterogeneity impacts patient prognosis in localized colon cancer. Clinical Cancer Research. 2021;**27**:4768-4780. DOI: 10.1158/1078-0432.CCR-21-0529

[25] Eide PW, Moosavi SH, Eilertsen IA, Brunsell TH, Langerud J, Berg KCG, et al. Metastatic heterogeneity of the consensus molecular subtypes of colorectal cancer. NPJ Genomic Medicine. 2021;**6**:1-9. DOI: 10.1038/s41525-021-00223-7

[26] Esfahani K, Roudaia L, Buhlaiga N, Del Rincon SV, Papneja N, Miller WH. A review of cancer immunotherapy: From the past, to the present, to the future. Current Oncology. 2020;**27**:87-97. DOI: 10.3747/co.27.5223

[27] Kalyan A, Kircher S, Shah H, Mulcahy M, Benson A. Updates on immunotherapy for colorectal cancer. Journal of Gastrointestinal Oncology. 2018;**9**:160-169. DOI: 10.21037/jgo.2018.01.17

[28] Sahin IH, Akce M, Alese O, Shaib W, Lesinski GB, El-Rayes B, et al. Immune checkpoint inhibitors for the treatment of MSI-H/MMR-D colorectal cancer and a perspective on resistance mechanisms. British Journal of Cancer. 2019;**121**:809-818. DOI: 10.1038/s41416-019-0599-y

[29] O'Neil BH, Wallmark JM, Lorente D, Elez E, Raimbourg J, Gomez-Roca C, et al. Safety and antitumor activity of the anti-PD-1 antibody pembrolizumab in patients with advanced colorectal carcinoma. PLoS One. 2017;**12**:e0189848. DOI: 10.1371/journal.pone.0189848

[30] Le DT, Durham JN, Smith KN, Wang H, Bartlett BR, Aulakh LK, et al. Mismatch repair deficiency predicts response of solid tumors to PD-1 blockade. Science. 2017;**357**:409-413. DOI: 10.1126/science.aan6733

[31] Le DT, Kim TW, Van Cutsem E, Geva R, Jäger D, Hara H, et al. Phase II open-label study of pembrolizumab in treatment-refractory, microsatellite instability-high/mismatch repair-deficient metastatic colorectal cancer: KEYNOTE-164. Journal of Clinical Oncology. 2020;**38**:11-19. DOI: 10.1200/JCO.19.02107

[32] Marabelle A, Le DT, Ascierto PA, Di Giacomo AM, De Jesus-Acosta A, Delord J-P, et al. Efficacy of pembrolizumab in patients with noncolorectal high microsatellite instability/mismatch repair-deficient cancer: Results from the phase II KEYNOTE-158 study. Journal of Clinical Oncology. 2020;**38**:1-10. DOI: 10.1200/JCO.19.02105

[33] Research C for DE and. FDA grants accelerated approval to pembrolizumab for first tissue/site agnostic indication [Internet]. FDA. FDA; 2019 [cited 24 Apr 2022]. Available from: https://www.fda.gov/drugs/resources-information-approved-drugs/fda-grants-accelerated-approval-pembrolizumab-first-tissuesite-agnostic-indication

[34] Shiu K-K, Andre T, Kim TW, Jensen BV, Jensen LH, Punt CJA, et al. KEYNOTE-177: Phase III randomized study of pembrolizumab versus chemotherapy for microsatellite instability-high advanced colorectal cancer. JCO. 2021;**39**:6-6. DOI: 10.1200/JCO.2021.39.3_suppl.6

[35] Research C for DE and. FDA approves pembrolizumab for first-line treatment of MSI-H/dMMR colorectal cancer [Internet]. FDA. FDA; 2020 [cited 24 Apr 2022]. Available from: https://www.fda.gov/drugs/drug-approvals-and-databases/fda-approves-pembrolizumab-first-line-treatment-msi-hdmmr-colorectal-cancer

[36] Letendre P, Monga V, Milhem M, Zakharia Y. Ipilimumab: From preclinical development to future clinical perspectives in melanoma. Future Oncology. 2017;**13**:625-636. DOI: 10.2217/fon-2016-0385

[37] Leach DR, Krummel MF, Allison JP. Enhancement of antitumor immunity by CTLA-4 blockade. Science. 1996;**271**:1734-1736. DOI: 10.1126/science.271.5256.1734

[38] Overman MJ, McDermott R, Leach JL, Lonardi S, Lenz H-J, Morse MA, et al. Nivolumab in patients with metastatic DNA mismatch repair-deficient or microsatellite instability-high colorectal cancer (CheckMate 142): An open-label, multicentre, phase 2 study. The Lancet Oncology. 2017;**18**:1182-1191. DOI: 10.1016/S1470-2045(17)30422-9

[39] Morse MA, Overman MJ, Hartman L, Khoukaz T, Brutcher E, Lenz H, et al. Safety of nivolumab plus low-dose ipilimumab in previously treated microsatellite instability-high/mismatch repair-deficient metastatic colorectal cancer. The Oncologist. 2019;**24**:1453-1461. DOI: 10.1634/theoncologist.2019-0129

[40] Lenz H-J, Van Cutsem E, Luisa Limon M, Wong KYM, Hendlisz A,

Aglietta M, et al. First-line nivolumab plus low-dose ipilimumab for microsatellite instability-high/mismatch repair-deficient metastatic colorectal cancer: The phase II CheckMate 142 Study. Journal of Clinical Oncology. 2022;**40**:161-170. DOI: 10.1200/JCO.21.01015

[41] Chalabi M, Fanchi LF, Dijkstra KK, Van den Berg JG, Aalbers AG, Sikorska K, et al. Neoadjuvant immunotherapy leads to pathological responses in MMR-proficient and MMR-deficient early-stage colon cancers. Nature Medicine. 2020;**26**:566-576. DOI: 10.1038/s41591-020-0805-8

[42] Sinicrope FA, Ou F-S, Shi Q, Nixon AB, Mody K, Levasseur A, et al. Randomized trial of FOLFOX alone or combined with atezolizumab as adjuvant therapy for patients with stage III colon cancer and deficient DNA mismatch repair or microsatellite instability (ATOMIC, Alliance A021502). JCO. 2017;**35**:TPS3630-TPS3630. DOI: 10.1200/JCO.2017.35.15_suppl.TPS3630

[43] Fan J, Shang D, Han B, Song J, Chen H, Yang J-M. Adoptive cell transfer: Is it a promising immunotherapy for colorectal cancer? Theranostics. 2018;**8**:5784-5800. DOI: 10.7150/thno.29035

[44] Paijens ST, Vledder A, de Bruyn M, Nijman HW. Tumor-infiltrating lymphocytes in the immunotherapy era. Cellular & Molecular Immunology. 2021;**18**:842-859. DOI: 10.1038/s41423-020-00565-9

[45] Tran E, Robbins PF, Lu Y-C, Prickett TD, Gartner JJ, Jia L, et al. T-cell transfer therapy targeting mutant KRAS in cancer. The New England Journal of Medicine. 2016;**375**:2255-2262. DOI: 10.1056/NEJMoa1609279

[46] Karlsson M, Marits P, Dahl K, Dagöö T, Enerbäck S, Thörn M, et al. Pilot study of sentinel-node-based adoptive immunotherapy in advanced colorectal cancer. Annals of Surgical Oncology. 2010;**17**:1747-1757. DOI: 10.1245/s10434-010-0920-8

[47] Jin K-T, Chen B, Liu Y-Y, Huan-Rong L, Yan J-P. Monoclonal antibodies and chimeric antigen receptor (CAR) T cells in the treatment of colorectal cancer. Cancer Cell International. 2021;**21**:83. DOI: 10.1186/s12935-021-01763-9

[48] Sur D, Havasi A, Cainap C, Samasca G, Burz C, Balacescu O, et al. Chimeric antigen receptor T-cell therapy for colorectal cancer. Journal of Clinical Medicine. 2020;**9**:182. DOI: 10.3390/jcm9010182

[49] Li H, Yang C, Cheng H, Huang S, Zheng Y. CAR-T cells for colorectal cancer: Target-selection and strategies for improved activity and safety. Journal of Cancer. 2021;**12**:1804-1814. DOI: 10.7150/jca.50509

[50] Zhang C, Wang Z, Yang Z, Wang M, Li S, Li Y, et al. Phase I escalating-dose trial of CAR-T therapy targeting CEA+ metastatic colorectal cancers. Molecular Therapy. 2017;**25**:1248-1258. DOI: 10.1016/j.ymthe.2017.03.010

[51] Magee MS, Kraft CL, Abraham TS, Baybutt TR, Marszalowicz GP, Li P, et al. GUCY2C-directed CAR-T cells oppose colorectal cancer metastases without autoimmunity. Oncoimmunology. 2016;**5**:e1227897. DOI: 10.1080/2162402X.2016.1227897

[52] Butterfield LH. Cancer vaccines. BMJ. 2015;**350**:h988

[53] Saxena M, van der Burg SH, Melief CJM, Bhardwaj N. Therapeutic cancer vaccines. Nature Reviews. Cancer. 2021;**21**:360-378. DOI: 10.1038/s41568-021-00346-0

[54] Hubbard JM, Cremolini C, Graham RP, Moretto R, Mitchelll JL, Wessling J, et al. A phase I study of PolyPEPI1018 vaccine plus maintenance therapy in patients with metastatic colorectal cancer with a predictive biomarker (OBERTO). JCO. 2019;**37**:3557-3557. DOI: 10.1200/JCO.2019.37.15_suppl.3557

[55] Ferraro B, Morrow MP, Hutnick NA, Shin TH, Lucke CE, Weiner DB. Clinical applications of DNA vaccines: Current progress. Clinical Infectious Diseases. 2011;**53**:296-302. DOI: 10.1093/cid/cir334

[56] Cross RS, Malaterre J, Davenport AJ, Carpinteri S, Anderson RL, Darcy PK, et al. Therapeutic DNA vaccination against colorectal cancer by targeting the MYB oncoprotein. Clinical & Translational Immunology. 2015;**4**:e30. DOI: 10.1038/cti.2014.29

[57] Kowalzik F, Schreiner D, Jensen C, Teschner D, Gehring S, Zepp F. mRNA-Based Vaccines. Vaccines. 2021;**9**:390. DOI: 10.3390/vaccines9040390

[58] Cafri G, Gartner JJ, Hopson K, Meehan RS, Zaks TZ, Robbins P, et al. Immunogenicity and tolerability of personalized mRNA vaccine mRNA-4650 encoding defined neoantigens expressed by the autologous cancer. JCO. 2019;**37**:2643-2643. DOI: 10.1200/JCO.2019.37.15_suppl.2643

[59] Keshavarz-Fathi M, Rezaei N. Chapter 14 - Concluding Remarks and Future Perspectives on Therapeutic Cancer Vaccines. In: Rezaei N, Keshavarz-Fathi M, editors. Vaccines for Cancer Immunotherapy. Tehran, Iran: Academic Press; 2019. p. 171-176. DOI:10.1016/B978-0-12-814039-0.00014-X

[60] Ogi C, Aruga A. Clinical evaluation of therapeutic cancer vaccines. Human Vaccines & Immunotherapeutics. 2013;**9**:1049-1057. DOI: 10.4161/hv.23917

[61] Chakrabarti S, Peterson CY, Sriram D, Mahipal A. Early stage colon cancer: Current treatment standards, evolving paradigms, and future directions. World Journal of Gastrointestinal Oncology. 2020;**12**:808-832. DOI: 10.4251/wjgo.v12.i8.808

[62] Costas-Chavarri A, Nandakumar G, Temin S, Lopes G, Cervantes A, Cruz Correa M, et al. Treatment of patients with early-stage colorectal cancer: ASCO resource-stratified guideline. JCO Global Oncology. 2019;**5**:1-19. DOI: 10.1200/JGO.18.00214

[63] Böckelman C, Engelmann BE, Kaprio T, Hansen TF, Glimelius B. Risk of recurrence in patients with colon cancer stage II and III: A systematic review and meta-analysis of recent literature. Acta Oncologica. 2015;**54**:5-16. DOI: 10.3109/0284186X.2014.975839

[64] Sargent D, Sobrero A, Grothey A, O'Connell MJ, Buyse M, Andre T, et al. Evidence for cure by adjuvant therapy in colon cancer: Observations based on individual patient data from 20,898 patients on 18 randomized trials. Journal of Clinical Oncology. 2009;**27**:872-877. DOI: 10.1200/JCO.2008.19.5362

[65] Argilés G, Tabernero J, Labianca R, Hochhauser D, Salazar R, Iveson T, et al. Localised colon cancer: ESMO clinical practice guidelines for diagnosis, treatment and follow-up. Annals of Oncology. 2020;**31**:1291-1305. DOI: 10.1016/j.annonc.2020.06.022

[66] Twelves CJ. Xeloda in adjuvant colon cancer therapy (X-ACT) trial: Overview of efficacy, safety, and cost-effectiveness. Clinical Colorectal Cancer. 2006;**6**:278-287. DOI: 10.3816/CCC.2006.n.046

[67] Yothers G, O'Connell MJ, Allegra CJ, Kuebler JP, Colangelo LH, Petrelli NJ, et al. Oxaliplatin as adjuvant therapy for colon cancer: Updated results of NSABP C-07 trial, including survival and subset analyses. Journal of Clinical Oncology. 2011;**29**:3768-3774. DOI: 10.1200/JCO.2011.36.4539

[68] André T, Boni C, Mounedji-Boudiaf L, Navarro M, Tabernero J, Hickish T, et al. Oxaliplatin, fluorouracil, and leucovorin as adjuvant treatment for colon cancer. New England Journal of Medicine. 2004;**350**:2343-2351. DOI: 10.1056/NEJMoa032709

[69] Modest DP, Pant S, Sartore-Bianchi A. Treatment sequencing in metastatic colorectal cancer. European Journal of Cancer. 2019;**109**:70-83. DOI: 10.1016/j.ejca.2018.12.019

[70] Kanas GP, Taylor A, Primrose JN, Langeberg WJ, Kelsh MA, Mowat FS, et al. Survival after liver resection in metastatic colorectal cancer: Review and meta-analysis of prognostic factors. Clinical Epidemiology. 2012;**4**:283-301. DOI: 10.2147/CLEP.S34285

[71] Goldberg RM, Sargent DJ, Morton RF, Fuchs CS, Ramanathan RK, Williamson SK, et al. A randomized controlled trial of fluorouracil plus leucovorin, irinotecan, and oxaliplatin combinations in patients with previously untreated metastatic colorectal cancer. JCO. 2004;**22**:23-30. DOI: 10.1200/JCO.2004.09.046

[72] Colucci G, Gebbia V, Paoletti G, Giuliani F, Caruso M, Gebbia N, et al. Phase III randomized trial of FOLFIRI versus FOLFOX4 in the treatment of advanced colorectal cancer: A multicenter study of the Gruppo Oncologico Dell'Italia Meridionale. Journal of Clinical Oncology. 2005;**23**:4866-4875. DOI: 10.1200/JCO.2005.07.113

[73] Kerr DJ. Targeting angiogenesis in cancer: Clinical development of bevacizumab. Nature Reviews. Clinical Oncology. 2004;**1**:39-43. DOI: 10.1038/ncponc0026

[74] Efficacy of bevacizumab in first-line treatment of metastatic colorectal cancer: A systematic review and meta-analysis ScienceDirect n.d.. Available from: https://www.sciencedirect.com/science/article/abs/pii/S0959804918314370 [Accessed: April 28, 2022]

[75] da Silva WC, de Araujo VE, Lima EM, JBR DS, MRR S, PHRF A, et al. Comparative effectiveness and safety of monoclonal antibodies (Bevacizumab, Cetuximab, and Panitumumab) in combination with chemotherapy for metastatic colorectal cancer: A systematic review and meta-analysis. BioDrugs. 2018;**32**:585-606. DOI: 10.1007/s40259-018-0322-1

[76] Syed YY, McKeage K. Aflibercept: A review in metastatic colorectal cancer. Drugs. 2015;**75**:1435-1445. DOI: 10.1007/s40265-015-0444-4

[77] Verdaguer H, Tabernero J, Macarulla T. Ramucirumab in metastatic colorectal cancer: Evidence to date and place in therapy. Therapeutic Advances in Medical Oncology. 2016;**8**:230-242. DOI: 10.1177/1758834016635888

[78] Grothey A, Cutsem EV, Sobrero A, Siena S, Falcone A, Ychou M, et al. Regorafenib monotherapy for previously treated metastatic colorectal cancer (CORRECT): An international, multicentre, randomised, placebo-controlled, phase 3 trial. The Lancet. 2013;**381**:303-312. DOI: 10.1016/S0140-6736(12)61900-X

[79] De Falco V, Napolitano S, Roselló S, Huerta M, Cervantes A, Ciardiello F, et al. How we treat metastatic colorectal cancer.

ESMO Open. 2020;**4**:e000813. DOI: 10.1136/esmoopen-2020-000813

[80] Xu JX, Maher VE, Zhang L, Tang S, Sridhara R, Ibrahim A, et al. FDA Approval Summary: Nivolumab in advanced renal cell carcinoma after anti-angiogenic therapy and exploratory predictive biomarker analysis. The Oncologist. 2017;**22**:311-317. DOI: 10.1634/theoncologist.2016-0476

[81] Benson AB, Venook AP, Al-Hawary MM, Arain MA, Chen YJ, Ciombor KK, et al. Colon Cancer, Version 2.2021, NCCN Clinical Practice Guidelines in Oncology. Journal of the National Comprehensive Cancer Network. 2 Mar 2021;**19**(3):329-359. DOI:10.6004/jnccn.2021.0012

[82] Lumish MA, Cercek A. Immunotherapy for the treatment of colorectal cancer. Journal of Surgical Oncology. 2021;**123**:760-774. DOI: 10.1002/jso.26357

[83] Wang C, Fakih M. Targeting MSS colorectal cancer with immunotherapy: Are we turning the corner? Expert Opinion on Biological Therapy. 2021;**21**:1347-1357. DOI: 10.1080/14712598.2021.1933940

[84] Kloor M, von Knebel DM. The immune biology of microsatellite unstable cancer. In: Valle L, Gruber SB, Capellá G, editors. Hereditary Colorectal Cancer: Genetic Basis and Clinical Implications. Cham: Springer International Publishing; 2018. pp. 367-384

[85] Kloor M, Staffa L, Ahadova A, von Knebel DM. Clinical significance of microsatellite instability in colorectal cancer. Langenbeck's Archives of Surgery. 2014;**399**:23-31. DOI: 10.1007/s00423-013-1112-3

[86] Latham A, Srinivasan P, Kemel Y, Shia J, Bandlamudi C, Mandelker D, et al. Microsatellite instability is associated with the presence of lynch syndrome pan-cancer. Journal of Clinical Oncology. 2019;**37**:286-295. DOI: 10.1200/JCO.18.00283

[87] Goldstein J, Tran B, Ensor J, Gibbs P, Wong HL, Wong SF, et al. Multicenter retrospective analysis of metastatic colorectal cancer (CRC) with high-level microsatellite instability (MSI-H). Annals of Oncology. 2014;**25**:1032-1038. DOI: 10.1093/annonc/mdu100

[88] Gatalica Z, Vranic S, Xiu J, Swensen J, Reddy S. High microsatellite instability (MSI-H) colorectal carcinoma: A brief review of predictive biomarkers in the era of personalized medicine. Familial Cancer. 2016;**15**:405-412. DOI: 10.1007/s10689-016-9884-6

[89] Malapelle U, Parente P, Pepe F, De Luca C, Pisapia P, Sgariglia R, et al. Evaluation of micro satellite instability and mismatch repair status in different solid tumors: A multicenter analysis in a real world setting. Cell. 2021;**10**:1878. DOI: 10.3390/cells10081878

[90] Trabucco SE, Gowen K, Maund SL, Sanford E, Fabrizio DA, Hall MJ, et al. A novel next-generation sequencing approach to detecting microsatellite instability and pan-tumor characterization of 1000 microsatellite instability–high cases in 67,000 patient samples. The Journal of Molecular Diagnostics. 2019;**21**:1053-1066. DOI: 10.1016/j.jmoldx.2019.06.011

[91] Oliveira AF, Bretes L, Furtado I. Review of PD-1/PD-L1 Inhibitors in Metastatic dMMR/MSI-H Colorectal Cancer. Frontiers in Oncology. 2019;**9**:1-8

[92] Svrcek M, El-Bchiri J, Chalastanis A, Capel E, Dumont S, Buhard O, et al.

Specific clinical and biological features characterize inflammatory bowel disease–associated colorectal cancers showing microsatellite instability. JCO. 2007;**25**:4231-4238. DOI: 10.1200/JCO.2007.10.9744

[93] Patel SP, Kurzrock R. PD-L1 expression as a predictive biomarker in cancer immunotherapy. Molecular Cancer Therapeutics. 2015;**14**:847-856. DOI: 10.1158/1535-7163.MCT-14-0983

[94] Teng F, Meng X, Kong L, Yu J. Progress and challenges of predictive biomarkers of anti PD-1/PD-L1 immunotherapy: A systematic review. Cancer Letters. 2018;**414**:166-173. DOI: 10.1016/j.canlet.2017.11.014

[95] Valle L, Hernández-Illán E, Bellido F, Aiza G, Castillejo A, Castillejo M-I, et al. New insights into POLE and POLD1 germline mutations in familial colorectal cancer and polyposis. Human Molecular Genetics. 2014;**23**:3506-3512. DOI: 10.1093/hmg/ddu058

[96] Robinson PS, Coorens THH, Palles C, Mitchell E, Abascal F, Olafsson S, et al. Increased somatic mutation burdens in normal human cells due to defective DNA polymerases. Nature Genetics. 2021;**53**:1434-1442. DOI: 10.1038/s41588-021-00930-y

[97] Lal N, Beggs AD, Willcox BE, Middleton GW. An immunogenomic stratification of colorectal cancer: Implications for development of targeted immunotherapy. OncoImmunology. 2015;**4**:e976052. DOI: 10.4161/2162402X.2014.976052

[98] Kather JN, Halama N, Jaeger D. Genomics and emerging biomarkers for immunotherapy of colorectal cancer. Seminars in Cancer Biology. 2018;**52**:189-197. DOI: 10.1016/j.semcancer.2018.02.010

[99] Zhang X, Yang J, Du L, Zhou Y, Li K. The prognostic value of Immunoscore in patients with cancer: A pooled analysis of 10,328 patients. The International Journal of Biological Markers. 2020;**35**:3-13. DOI: 10.1177/1724600820927409

[100] Bruni D, Angell HK, Galon J. The immune contexture and Immunoscore in cancer prognosis and therapeutic efficacy. Nature Reviews. Cancer. 2020;**20**:662-680. DOI: 10.1038/s41568-020-0285-7

[101] Lanzi A, Sinicrope FA, Benson AB, Galon J. The consensus immunoscore in phase 3 clinical trial (N0147) and impact on patient management decisions. Oncoimmunology. n.d.;**9**:1796003. DOI: 10.1080/2162402X.2020.1796003

[102] Marliot F, Chen X, Kirilovsky A, Sbarrato T, Sissy CE, Batista L, et al. Analytical validation of the immunoscore and its associated prognostic value in patients with colon cancer. Journal for Immunotherapy of Cancer. 2020;**8**:e000272. DOI: 10.1136/jitc-2019-000272

[103] Mlecnik B, Bifulco C, Bindea G, Marliot F, Lugli A, Lee JJ, et al. Multicenter international society for immunotherapy of cancer study of the consensus immunoscore for the prediction of survival and response to chemotherapy in stage iii colon cancer. Journal of Clinical Oncology. 2020;**38**:3638-3651. DOI: 10.1200/JCO.19.03205

[104] Subrahmanyam PB, Dong Z, Gusenleitner D, Giobbie-Hurder A, Severgnini M, Zhou J, et al. Distinct predictive biomarker candidates for response to anti-CTLA-4 and anti-PD-1 immunotherapy in melanoma patients. Journal for Immunotherapy of Cancer. 2018;**6**:18. DOI: 10.1186/s40425-018-0328-8

[105] Lanzi A, Pagès F, Lagorce-Pagès C, Galon J. The consensus immunoscore: Toward a new classification of colorectal cancer. Oncoimmunology. 2020;**9**:1789032. DOI: 10.1080/2162402X.2020.1789032

[106] Wang C, Ye Y, Hu Q, Bellotti A, Gu Z. Tailoring biomaterials for cancer immunotherapy: Emerging trends and future outlook. Advanced Materials. 2017;**29**:1606036. DOI: 10.1002/adma.201606036

[107] Ciardiello F, Ciardiello D, Martini G, Napolitano S, Tabernero J, Cervantes A. Clinical management of metastatic colorectal cancer in the era of precision medicine. CA: A Cancer Journal for Clinicians. 2022;n/a:1-30. DOI: 10.3322/caac.21728

Section 6

Supportive Care

Chapter 9

Nutrition: A Natural and Promising Option in Colorectal Cancer Intervention

Olusola Bolaji Adewale

Abstract

Nutrition: a natural and promising option in colorectal cancer intervention Nutrition plays a significant role in the intervention of colorectal cancer (CRC) by decreasing the risks of colorectal carcinogenesis. Products from both plant and animal origins have been involved in the prevention and/or treatment of CRC. Intake of dietary products including fibre-rich foods, nutraceuticals, wholegrains, dairy products, and limited consumption or avoidance of red/processed meat and alcohol could reduce the risk of CRC. These nutritional compounds, in CRC intervention, could be in form of folklore/alternative medicine or isolated compounds used in the production of many chemotherapeutic agents. Monitoring of individual's nutritional status could serve as a possible preventive or therapeutic measure against CRC, majorly by interaction with intestinal microbiota, thereby potentiating host anti-cancer immune response and/or interfering with mechanisms of carcinogenesis.

Keywords: colorectal cancer, diet, intestinal microbiome, nutrition, phytochemicals

1. Introduction

The incidence of colorectal cancer (CRC), the fourth commonly diagnosed cancer and third leading cause of cancer-related deaths worldwide, is a global burden. Factors that increase the risk of CRC development include medical, hereditary, and behavioural factors. Of this, behavioural factors including dietary habits such as consumption of red/processed meat and alcohol, which can be linked to adoption of westernized way of life by developing countries, lack of physical exercise, smoking, ageing and obesity [1], as well as consumption of carbonated drinks with high sugar level and fast-foods [2]. On the contrary, the beneficial effect of nutrition is implicated in reducing the risk of CRC upon consumption of wholegrains, fibre-rich diets, dairy products, micronutrients, vegetables, fruits, and nutraceuticals [3, 4]. Also, avoidance or limited consumption of red/processed meat, alcohol and smoking could reduce the incidence or prevent CRC [3]. In other words, nutrition, either directly or indirectly, from plant or animal origin, plays a significant role in colorectal carcinogenesis.

2. Detrimental effect of nutrition

2.1 Red and processed meat

High intake of red/processed meat is linked to high risk of CRC. Red meat such as beef, pork, veal, and lamb, and preserved red meat by smoking, grilling, cooking, frying, salting, and curing are called processed meat.

2.1.1 Mechanisms

High risk of CRC with diet rich in red/processed meat (associated with low fruits, vegetables and fibre) could result from the production of heterocyclic amines and polycyclic aromatic hydrocarbons during processing at high temperatures (**Figure 1**) [5]. Haem, present in high intake of processed/red meat, could stimulate endogenous formation of potent carcinogens, N-nitroso compounds, and cytotoxic alkenals from lipid peroxidation, thereby promoting colorectal carcinogenesis [6].

2.2 High sugar/fat diet, fast foods, and sugar-sweetened drinks

Consumption of diet rich in sugar, fat, and fast foods, as well as sugar-sweetened drinks can be linked to increased risk of CRC. Fast foods and other processed foods including snacks, bakery foods and candies, are energy dense and are frequently consumed in large quantities as they are readily available. Addition of free sugars including high fructose corn syrup, sucrose to drinks and sugars present naturally in fruit juices, syrups and honey to ensure sweet taste can increase CRC risks.

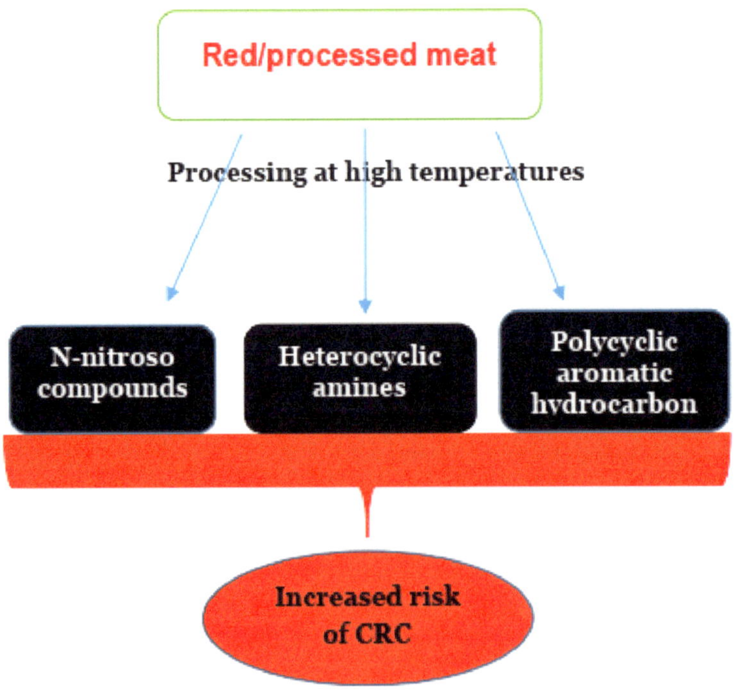

Figure 1.
Mechanisms of high intake of red and processed meat in colorectal carcinogenesis.

Therefore, drinks such as sweetened water, sodas, energy drinks, barley water, sports drinks, as well as tea-based beverages sweetened with sugars or syrups should be reduced, avoided, or replaced with sugar free drinks or drinks sweetened with artificial sweeteners [7].

2.3 Alcohol consumption

Several studies including meta-analysis, many cohort, and experimental studies, have reported the association between chronic intake of alcohol and increase in the risk of colon cancer [8, 9]. High or moderate intake of alcohol (> 12.5 grams/day) is associated with increased incidence of CRC and its mortality [10]. Although, there are discrepancies among various populations based on differences in genetic factors, body composition and other dietary factors including folate intake [8].

2.3.1 Mechanisms

The colon is one of the major organs for the distribution of orally ingested alcohol, making intracolonic level of ethanol to be equal to that of the blood level [11, 12]. At elevated level, ethanol it is converted to acetaldehyde (a known carcinogen) by colorectum cytochrome P450 2E1 (CYP 2E1), as its activity is also expressed in the colon and rectum alongside other tissues (**Figure 2**) [13]. This carcinogen, classified as group 1 carcinogen to humans by the International Agency for Research on Cancer (IARC), induces oxidative stress through an increase in the production of reactive oxygen species (ROS), as against cellular antioxidant defense system [9]. Reactive oxygen species can lead to lipid peroxidation, protein modification or bind to DNA to form carcinogenic adducts; hence, inhibition of DNA synthesis and repair mechanism, alteration in structure and function of glutathione. These could therefore, increase the proliferation of colonic mucosal [8].

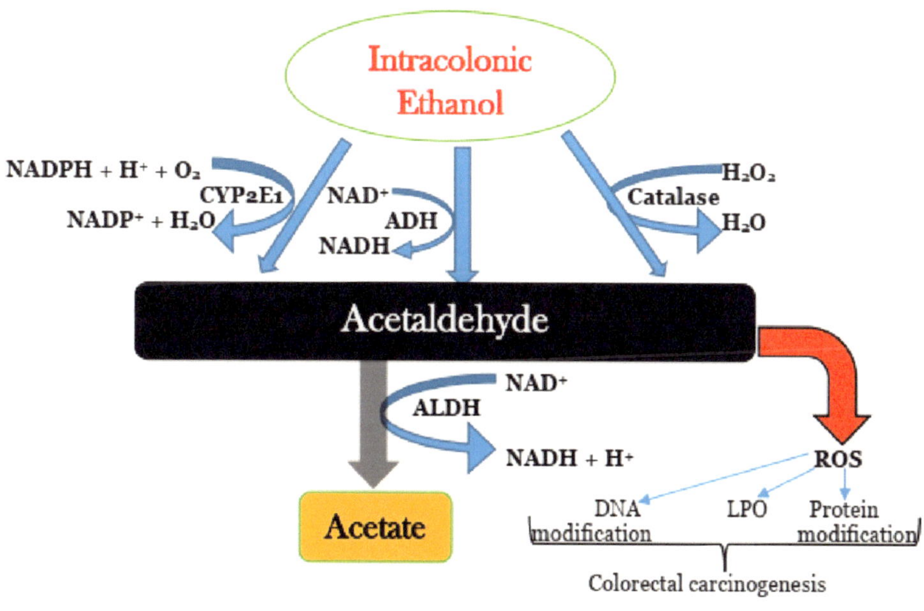

Figure 2.
Metabolism of ethanol by intracolonic bacteria and role in colorectal carcinogenesis.

Ethanol is also oxidized by bacterial alcohol dehydrogenase and catalase (expressed in the colon by colonic microbiota) to produce acetaldehyde in the colorectum [14, 15].

Acetaldehyde is therefore, accumulated in the colon (due to low activity of bacterial aldehyde dehydrogenase, which converts acetaldehyde to acetate in the colonic mucosa), and colorectal carcinogenesis is enhanced by binding to DNA and form carcinogenic DNA adducts [9, 11].

Alcohol can also act as a solvent for other dietary or environmental carcinogens into the mucosal cells, thereby inhibiting the metabolism of hormones, production of prostaglandins and lipid peroxidation [6].

Intracolonic ethanol is converted to acetaldehyde by colorectum cytochrome P450 2E1 (CYP2E1), alcohol dehydrogenase (ADH) and catalase, and the acetaldehyde is converted to acetate by aldehyde dehydrogenase (ALDH), while its accumulation results in carcinogenic DNA adducts, lipid peroxidation (LPO) or protein modification, and stimulates colorectal carcinogenesis.

2.4 Cigarette/tobacco smoking

Compounds such as acetaldehyde, aromatic amines, benzo[a]pyrene, N-nitrosamines, aromatic amines, and polycyclic aromatic hydrocarbons are carcinogens found in cigarette smoke. Nicotine and nicotine-derived nitrosamine, 4-(methylnitrosamino)-1-(3-pyridyl)-1-butanone, are known compounds present in tobacco smoke that enhance CRC metastasis by promoting cell migration and transformation of epithelial–mesenchyma [16]. These compounds could also form DNA adducts and bind to DNA, thereby causing gene mutation [17] or induce gut microbiota dysbiosis leading to colorectal carcinogenesis.

2.4.1 Mechanisms

Cigarette smoking could promote colorectal carcinogenesis due to alteration, imbalance, or disruption in gut microbiota composition (gut microbiota dysbiosis), leading to increase in stool and colonic levels of taurodeoxycholic acid (TDCA), a secondary bile acid. These changes could lead to activation of signaling pathways such as mitogen-activated protein kinase/extracellular signal-regulated protein kinase 1/2 (MAPK/ERK), interleukin 17 (IL-17) and tumour necrosis factor (TNF) in colonic epithelium, thereby promoting colonocyte proliferation [18]. Epigenetic modifications such as high microsatellite instability (MSI-H), the CpG island methylator phenotype, and the BRAF V600E mutation may reduce survival rate of CRC patient, as these have been reported to be functionally involved in colorectal carcinogenesis related to tobacco smoking. These modifications may result from (1) mutation of the glutathione S-transferase Mu 1 (GSTM1) gene, which results in impairment in the detoxification of tobacco carcinogens, thereby enhancing of carcinogenesis; (2) induction of aberrant promoter DNA methylation and silencing regulatory genes involved in tumor progression [16].

2.5 Animal fats

Studies, although limited, have linked intake of animal fats to CRC risk. A diet high in animal fats affects colonic microbiome leading to intestinal inflammation, thereby increasing the risk of CRC.

2.5.1 Mechanisms

High consumption of animal fats could increase colonic production of primary bile acids, which undergo degradation by anaerobic bacteria in the large bowel, and result in the formation of carcinogenic secondary bile acids including deoxycholic and lithocholic acids. High concentrations of these compounds could lead to increased colonocytes proliferation, through the production of ROS, thereby increasing the risk of mutation and malignant transformation [17].

Low intake or avoidance of red/processed meat, sugar/fat diet, fast foods, and sugar-sweetened drinks, alcohol, smoking, and animal fats is encouraged, as these could reduce the risk of CRC.

3. Beneficial effect of nutrition

3.1 Wholegrains

Wholegrains, including brown rice, whole-wheat bread, whole grain cornmeal, cracked wheat, and oatmeal, play a major role against CRC. Polysaccharides composition, and quantity and variety of dietary fibers present in wholegrains make them differ in their physicochemical and structural properties, as well as physiological effects [19]. Wholegrains are sources of energy, proteins, some other primary and secondary metabolites such as vitamins (especially B vitamins including folate), minerals, phytochemicals (phenolic compounds), phyto-oestrogens, and other bioactive compounds which can protect or prevent CRC [19–21]. Wholegrains are also rich source of dietary fibre, oligosaccharides and resistant starch that can influence gut environment (more explanation under dietary fibre).

3.1.1 Mechanisms

Wholegrains reduce the incidence of CRC through four mechanisms [22] by (1) the action of intestinal microbiota on dietary fibres from wholegrains in the synthesis of short-chain fatty acids, and prevents insulin resistance and serves as major source of energy (butyrate) for the colon [20], (2) phytochemicals (phenolic compounds), minerals/micronutrients, and vitamins from wholegrains have antioxidant potential capable of oxidative damage in the colon and prevents carcinogenesis [19, 20]; (3) insoluble fibre in wholegrains increases bulk of luminal contents, and dilutes potential carcinogens in the colonic epithelium to prevent colorectal carcinogenesis [23]; (4) Phytoestrogens (similar to the activities of estrogen) from wholegrains reduce risk of CRC by binding to estrogen receptors through the hormonal mechanisms [20, 21].

3.2 Dietary fibre

Dietary fibres are classified under complex carbohydrates found in plants, and are undigested in the small intestine but undergo fermentation by colonic flora [24]. This fibre is made up of non-starchy polysaccahrides which are found in fruits, vegetables, wholegrains or cereals, legumes (such as beans and lentils), plantains and tubers. Dietary fibres from pectin, guar, and oat bran are highly fermentable, while those from wheat bran and cellulose are poorly fermentable.

3.2.1 Mechanisms

Dietary fibres are fermented in the bowel by colonic microbiota to form short-chain fatty acids, such as butyrate and propionate (**Figure 3**), which have been reported to have anti-proliferative potential by inducing apoptosis and arresting of cell cycle and differentiation, and chronic inflammatory process inhibition [6, 24]. Dietary fibres can also increase faecal bulk or stool weight and frequency [24, 25], which could reduce the ability of faecal mutagens to interact with mucosa cells [24]. Examples of these are the insoluble fibres such as nuts, wheat bran, whole-wheat flour, beans, and vegetables including cauliflower, green beans and potatoes. Dietary fibres could also reduce intestinal transit time, decrease production of secondary bile acids, and reduce insulin resistance.

3.3 Dairy products and calcium supplements

High consumption of dairy products such as milk, yogurt and cheese have been linked to reduction in the incidence of CRC (Barrubés et al., 2019).

3.3.1 Mechanism

This reduction has been attributed to the presence of calcium, and other compounds such as casein, lactose, lactoferrin and butyrate present in these products, which can also increase calcium bioavailability. The role of yogurt in reducing the risk of CRC can be attributed to the presence of calcium and gut microbiome, most especially the bacteria that produces lactic acid (*Streptococcus thermophiles* and

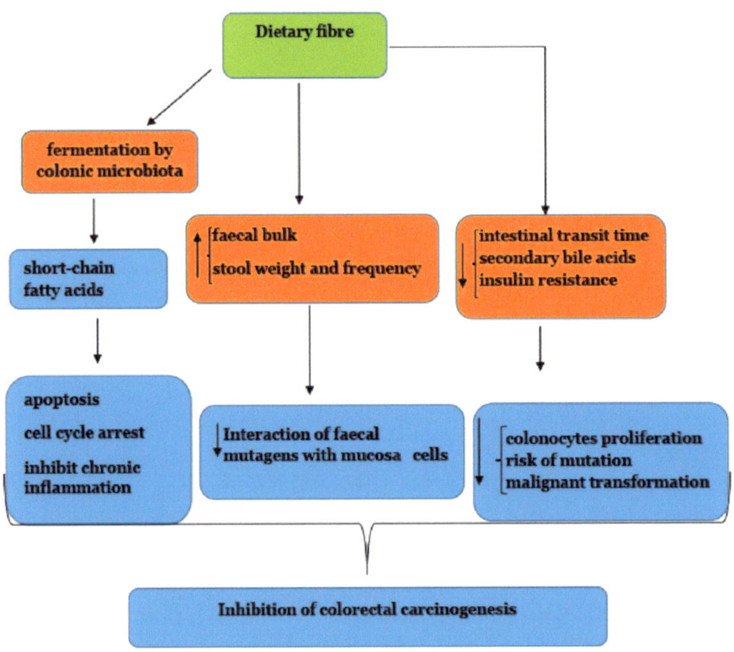

Figure 3.
Mechanisms of dietary fiber consumption and risk of colorectal cancer.

Lactobacillus bulgaricus) which bring about the reduction of soluble fecal bile acids, fecal-activated bacterial enzymes, and nitoreductase [3].

Calcium has the ability to bind free fatty acids and unconjugated bile acids, thereby reducing the toxic effects of these compounds on the colon and rectum [3]. Calcium exerts its effect by promoting cell differentiation and apoptosis, inhibiting cell proliferation, preventing colonic K-ras mutations, and inhibiting colorectal carcinogenesis induced by haem. The major limitation to this is the association of diet rich in calcium to prostate cancer [6]. In view of this, care should be taken in consumption of dairy foods, most especially those high in calcium, although there are many other bioactive constituents present in dairy foods which might contribute to its role in reducing CRC risk.

3.4 Fish and fish products

Several meta-analysis studies have reported that high fish intake (majorly fresh fish such as freshwater fish and sea fish) could reduce the risk of CRC [26–29]. Fish is known to contain long chain polyunsaturated fatty acids (PUFAs), majorly the n-3 fatty acids, including eicosapentaenoic and docosahexaenoic acids and are known to inhibit colorectal carcinogenesis [27, 30]. However, care should be taken in the consumption of processed fish such as salted, dried, smoked, and barbequed fish, as there could be an association with increased risk of CRC. This is because, dried/salted fish contains N-nitrosamines [26, 31], and fish processing at high temperatures, produce heterocyclic amines, which are carcinogenic [30].

3.4.1 Mechanism

Fish is known to be a good source of vitamin D, and vitamin D alters gene expression directly through the vitamin D receptor and induces cell differentiation and apoptosis, thereby inhibiting the initiation and progression of CRC. Fish also contains selenium, which can prevent or repair oxidative DNA damage, alter metabolism of carcinogens and regulate immune response. High intake of n-3 fatty acids reduces both the synthesis of arachidonic acid metabolites (prostaglandin E_2 and leukotriene B_4) and the expression of nuclear transcription factor κB (NF-Kb) and inducible nitric oxide synthetase (iNOS). All these processes can inhibit colorectal carcinogenesis [26, 29, 31].

3.5 Fruits and non-starch vegetables

High consumption of fruits and non-starchy vegetables have been associated with reduced risk of CRC [4]. This is due to the presence of several phytochemicals with antioxidant, anti-inflammatory, and anti-cancer properties which include vitamins, carotenoids, tocopherols, ascorbic acid, alkaloids, phenolic compounds, and intake of several other nutrients and compounds such as folate. These compounds counteract the effect of ROS by their antioxidant properties, and inhibit cellular damage and carcinogenic insults [32, 33].

3.6 Nutraceuticals and phytochemicals

Nutraceuticals, also known as functional foods, are bioactive compounds that originated from natural sources such as secondary metabolites in plant, dietary supplements, herbal products from fruits, vegetables and plants, and microorganisms or marine organisms, that are capable of preventing, treating and managing several diseases including CRC prevention and therapy [34, 35]. Phytochemicals, mainly from fruits and vegetables, possess strong antioxidant and anti-proliferative activities, and a combination of these compounds brings about their synergistic effect against several cancers [33].

3.6.1 Secondary metabolites in plants (phytochemicals)

Carotenoids such as α- and β-carotene from carrots; lycopene from grapes, papaya, and tomatoes; halocynthiaxanthin from a marine organism, *Halocynthia roretzi*, and other phytochemicals which include astaxanthin, cryoptoxanthin, xanthophyll, and zeaxanthin metabolites, have significant role as free radical scavengers and ability to induce apoptosis in CRC cells [34, 36, 37].

Polyphenols, classified into flavonoids and non-flavonoids, are group of phytochemicals which are converted by intestinal microbiota to simple phenolic acids, and are absorbed in the small intestine, thereby reducing the risk of CRC [32, 38]. Polyphenols (resveratrol, catechins, epicatechins, epigallocatechin-3 gallate (EGCG), flavanols, flavones, and isoflavones) from various sources including plants (such as green tea, grapes, turmeric, ginger), marine algae, seaweeds, and microorganisms serve as chemopreventive agents and play significant role against colorectal carcinogenesis [34, 39].

Flavonoids are dietary polyphenols that occur naturally in plant and beverages, such as fruits and vegetables, and juices, and have been associated with reduction in CRC risks [40]. Flavonoids are sub-classified into six based on their chemical structure. These include flavonols (including quercetin, myricetin, kaempferol, and isorhamnetin from sources such as tea, onions, apples, citrus, berries, and broccoli), flavones (including apigenin and luteolin from sources such as celery, perilla, lettuce, and peppers), flavanones (including hesperetin and naringenin), flavan-3-ols (including catechin, epicatechin, epigallocatechin, epicatechin-3-gallate, epigallocatechin-3-gallate from sources such as apples, cocoa, grapes, green tea, and red wine,), anthocyanins (including cyanidin, delphinidin, malvidin, pelargonidin, petunidin, peonidin from sources such as grapes, black currants, eggplant and radishes), and isoflavones (including genistein and daidzein from soy products). These compounds could prevent and reduce the risk of CRC [34, 38].

Apart from the chemopreventive role of these compounds against CRC, there are little or no side effects as compared to other CRC treatment options such as surgery, chemotherapy, and radiation.

3.6.2 Dietary supplements

Dietary supplements such as omega-3 fatty acids, vitamins (vitamin D, folate, and vitamin B complex), eugenol from honey, balm, cinnamon, clove oil, citrus, and Flos, have been reported to reduce the risk of CRC [34, 41].

3.6.3 Herbal products

Herbs and herb products have been used as a single or combination preventive or therapeutic measures for CRC. Several medicinal plants (either as extracts, juices, or diet fortified) have been studied using different experimental models. These include the use of *Crassocephalum rubens* fortified diet [42], Indian spice saffron (*Crocus sativus*), *Triticum aestivum* [43], *Camellia sinensis* [44], Chinese herbal medicines [45], and their effect against initiation and progression of CRC. These products have been reported not only to have the potential to reduce the risk of CRC but also capable of reducing the adverse reactions associated with the use of chemotherapy [45]. The preventive and therapeutic potential of these herbs, and their mechanisms of reduction in the risk of CRC could be linked to the several active compounds inherent in them [46].

3.6.4 Marine nutraceuticals

Bioactive compounds from marine organisms including acetylapoaranotin (isolated from marine *Aspergillus sp*), astaxanthin (from crab, marine animals, and *Haematococcus pluvialis*), and siphonaxanthin (from a marine green algae *Codium fragile*) have been of interest as therapeutic intervention for CRC [34], via different mechanisms.

3.7 Effect of diet on colorectal cancer patients

A hospital-based case–control study among Chinese populations, conducted in Hong Kong, revealed that current, regular, and heavy alcohol drinkers, and cigarette smokers increased risk of CRC, and avoidance of these for a long time reversed the risk [47]. A large prospective cohort study where patients were screened showed a reduction in the risk of adenoma in patients taking dietary fiber (most especially from cereal and fruit [48]. Also, in a theory-driven behavioral dietary intervention program conducted on Chinese CRC patients, improvement in diet rich in refined grain and high fibre intake, and reduction in red and processed meat was noted with no dietary deficiency and/or dietary-related anemia, which could be as a result of other sources of protein (poultry, seafood and tofu). This improvement in dietary intervention was linked to awareness on the role of diet in CRC prevention and treatment, thereby resulting in increased chances of patients' survival [49].

In a large British cohort (UK Biobank study), there was a lower risk of CRC among low meat-eaters (those that consumed processed/red meat or poultry in less than 5 times a week) when compared with the regular meat-eaters (those that consumed processed/red meat or poultry more than 5 times a week) [50]. This confirms that high risk of CRC is associated with high and regular diet of processed/red meat. In another large-scale cohort studies (UK Biobank), there was an association between high consumption of processed meat and increased risk of mortality in patients with inflammatory bowel disease, leading to high CRC risk [51, 52].

Among CRC patients in China, it was reported that low intake of poultry, seafood, processed/unprocessed red meat, could prevent high risk of CRC. However, no general agreement on high intake of white meat (fish and poultry) in reducing the risk of CRC, as contrasting results have been reported [53]. In a UK Biobank study, consumption of red/processed meat, below the UK recommended daily intake (not more than 90 g of red and processed meat a day) is suggested, as participants consuming an average of 76 g per day was associated with increased risk of CRC [54].

In the European prospective investigation into cancer and nutrition (EPIC) cohort study, no association was noted between pre-diagnostic intake of red meat or fibre and CRC survival after diagnosis, However, it was suggested that poultry intake can reduce mortality among female CRC survivors, and increased CRC-specific mortality risk with intake of processed meat. This is because dietary intake before diagnosis is assumed to predict post-diagnostic data, therefore, post-diagnostic dietary research was suggested to confirm the association [55].

There are limited clinical trials evaluating the post-surgery role of diet in CRC patients. Although, studies have shown that diet rich in red/processed meat, refined grains, sweets, and high alcohol consumption were associated with increased recurrence rates of CRC, while increased coffee consumption, dietary fiber, and vegetables, mainly light and low-fat foods, were associated with decreased CRC mortality rate [8, 56]. Also, the alternate healthy eating index-2010 (high intake of whole grains, fruits, vegetables, legumes, nuts, and long chain omega-3 fatty acids, and low intake of salt, saturated fat and red/processed meat) and moderate consumption of alcohol and lower consumption of sugar sweetened beverages and juices were associated with reduced risk of CRC mortality among women [57].

In general, more studies are suggested to investigate the role of nutrition on CRC survival (post-diagnosis), as most dietary data is currently centered on CRC prevention.

4. Conclusion

Plant-based diet, including high intake of dietary fibre, wholegrains, fruits, and vegetables, as well as animal-based diet such as fish, dairy products should be considered. Also, diets including low or avoidance of red and processed meat/fish, animal fats, cigarette smoking, alcohol, diet rich in sugar/fat, fast foods and sugar-sweetened drinks are encouraged. These are suggested to generally play significant roles in preventing CRC and as follow-up nutritional requirements for CRC patients (pre- and post-diagnosis/therapy), thereby reducing the overall risk of CRC and associated mortality.

Acknowledgements

The author acknowledges the management of Afe Babalola University, Ado-Ekiti for providing support in terms of facilities.

Conflict of interest

The author declares no conflict of interest.

DOI: http://dx.doi.org/10.5772/intechopen.106285

Author details

Olusola Bolaji Adewale
Biochemistry Program, Department of Chemical Sciences, Afe Babalola University, Ado-Ekiti, Nigeria

*Address all correspondence to: adewaleob@abuad.edu.ng

References

[1] Dekker E, Tanis PJ, Vleugels JLA, Kasi PM, Wallace MB. Colorectal cancer. The Lancet. 2019;**394**(10207):1467-1480. DOI: 10.1016/S0140-6736(19)32319-0

[2] Irabor D. Emergence of colorectal cancer in West Africa: Accepting the inevitable. South African Gastroenterology Review. 2017;**15**(1):11-16

[3] Veettil SK, Wong TY, Loo YS, Playdon MC, Lai NM, Giovannucci EL, et al. Role of diet in colorectal cancer incidence: umbrella review of meta-analyses of prospective observational studies. JAMA Network Open. 2021;**4**(2):e2037341. DOI: 10.1001/jamanetworkopen.2020.37341

[4] Chapelle N, Martel M, Toes-Zoutendijk E, Barkun AN, Bardou M. Recent advances in clinical practice: Colorectal cancer chemoprevention in the average-risk population. Gut. 2020;**69**(12):2244. DOI: 10.1136/gutjnl-2020-320990

[5] Ryan-Harshman M, Aldoori W. Diet and colorectal cancer: Review of the evidence. Canadian Family Physician Medecin de famille canadien. 2007;**53**(11):1913-1920

[6] Perera PS, Thompson RL, Wiseman MJ. Recent evidence for colorectal cancer prevention through healthy food, nutrition, and physical activity: Implications for recommendations. Current Nutrition Reports. 2012;**1**(1):44-54. DOI: 10.1007/s13668-011-0006-7

[7] Clinton SK, Giovannucci EL, Hursting SD. The World cancer research fund/american institute for cancer research third expert report on diet, nutrition, physical activity, and cancer: Impact and future directions. The Journal of Nutrition. 2020;**150**(4):663-671. DOI: 10.1093/jn/nxz268

[8] Thanikachalam K, Khan G. Colorectal cancer and nutrition. Nutrients. 2019;**11**(1):164. DOI: 10.3390/nu11010164

[9] Na H-K, Lee JY. Molecular basis of alcohol-related gastric and colon cancer. International Journal of Molecular Sciences. 2017;**18**(6):1116. DOI: 10.3390/ijms18061116

[10] Adewale OB. In vivo toxicological evaluation of peptide conjugated gold nanoparticles for potential application in colorectal cancer diagnosis. South Africa: Nelson Mandela University: Nelson Mandela Metropolitan University; 2018

[11] Salaspuro M. Microbial metabolism of ethanol and acetaldehyde and clinical consequences. Addiction Biology. 1997;**2**(1):35-46. DOI: 10.1080/13556219772840

[12] Elamin EE, Masclee AA, Dekker J, Jonkers DM. Ethanol metabolism and its effects on the intestinal epithelial barrier. Nutrition Reviews. 2013;**71**(7):483-499. DOI: 10.1111/nure.12027

[13] Teschke R. Alcoholic liver disease: Current mechanistic aspects with focus on their clinical relevance. Biomedicine. 2019;**7**(3):68. DOI: 10.3390/biomedicines7030068

[14] Jiang Y, Zhang T, Kusumanchi P, Han S, Yang Z, Liangpunsakul S. Alcohol metabolizing enzymes, microsomal ethanol oxidizing system, cytochrome P450 2E1, catalase, and aldehyde dehydrogenase in alcohol-associated liver

disease. Biomedicine. 2020;**8**(3):50. DOI: 10.3390/biomedicines8030050

[15] Rossi M, Jahanzaib Anwar M, Usman A, Keshavarzian A, Bishehsari F. Colorectal cancer and alcohol consumption—populations to molecules. Cancers. 2018;**10**(2):38. DOI: 10.3390/cancers10020038

[16] Huang YM, Wei PL, Ho CH, Yeh CC. Cigarette smoking associated with colorectal cancer survival: A nationwide, population-based cohort study. Journal of Clinical Medicine. 2022;**11**(4):913. DOI: 10.3390/jcm11040913

[17] Raskov H, Pommergaard HC, Burcharth J, Rosenberg J. Colorectal carcinogenesis--update and perspectives. World Journal of Gastroenterology. 2014;**20**(48):18151-18164. DOI: 10.3748/wjg.v20.i48.18151

[18] Bai X, Wei H, Liu W, Coker OO, Gou H, Liu C, et al. Cigarette smoke promotes colorectal cancer through modulation of gut microbiota and related metabolites. Gut. 2022:1-12. DOI: 10.1136/gutjnl-2021-325021

[19] Tayyem RF, Bawadi HA, Shehadah I, Agraib LM, Al-Awwad NJ, Heath DD, et al. Consumption of whole grains, refined cereals, and legumes and its association with colorectal cancer among jordanians. Integrative Cancer Therapies. 2016;**15**(3):318-325. DOI: 10.1177/1534735415620010

[20] Gaesser GA. Whole grains, refined grains, and cancer risk: A systematic review of meta-analyses of observational studies. Nutrients. 2020;**12**(12):3756. DOI: 10.3390/nu12123756

[21] Slavin JL. Mechanisms for the impact of whole grain foods on cancer risk. Journal of the American College of Nutrition. 2000;**19**(3 Suppl):300s-307s. DOI: 10.1080/07315724.2000.10718964

[22] Hullings AG, Sinha R, Liao LM, Freedman ND, Graubard BI, Loftfield E. Whole grain and dietary fiber intake and risk of colorectal cancer in the NIH-AARP diet and health study cohort. The American Journal of Clinical Nutrition. 2020;**112**(3):603-612. DOI: 10.1093/ajcn/nqaa161

[23] Larsson SC, Giovannucci E, Bergkvist L, Wolk A. Whole grain consumption and risk of colorectal cancer: A population-based cohort of 60,000 women. British Journal of Cancer. 2005;**92**(9):1803-1807. DOI: 10.1038/sj.bjc.6602543

[24] Zeng H, Lazarova DL, Bordonaro M. Mechanisms linking dietary fiber, gut microbiota and colon cancer prevention. World Journal of Gastrointestinal Oncology. 2014;**6**(2):41-51. DOI: 10.4251/wjgo.v6.i2.41

[25] de Wit N, Esser D, Siebelink E, Fischer A, Sieg J, Mes J. Extrinsic wheat fibre consumption enhances faecal bulk and stool frequency; a randomized controlled trial. Food & Function. 2019;**10**(2):646-651. DOI: 10.1039/C8FO01649F

[26] Xu M, Fang Y-J, Chen Y-M, Lu M-S, Pan Z-Z, Yan B, et al. Higher freshwater fish and sea fish intake is inversely associated with colorectal cancer risk among Chinese population: A case-control study. Scientific Reports. 2015;**5**(1):12976. DOI: 10.1038/srep12976

[27] Caini S, Chioccioli S, Pastore E, Fontana M, Tortora K, Caderni G, et al. Fish consumption and colorectal cancer risk: Meta-analysis of prospective epidemiological studies and review of evidence from animal studies. Cancers. 2022;**14**(3):640. DOI: 10.3390/cancers14030640

[28] Wu S, Feng B, Li K, Zhu X, Liang S, Liu X, et al. Fish consumption

and colorectal cancer risk in humans: A systematic review and meta-analysis. American Journal of Medicine. 2012;**125**(6):551-559.e555. DOI: 10.1016/j.amjmed.2012.01.022

[29] Geelen A, Schouten JM, Kamphuis C, Stam BE, Burema J, Renkema JMS, et al. Fish consumption, n-3 fatty acids, and colorectal cancer: A meta-analysis of prospective cohort studies. American Journal of Epidemiology. 2007;**166**(10):1116-1125. DOI: 10.1093/aje/kwm197

[30] Norat T, Bingham S, Ferrari P, Slimani N, Jenab M, Mazuir M, et al. Meat, fish, and colorectal cancer risk: The European Prospective Investigation into cancer and nutrition. Journal of the National Cancer Institute. 2005;**97**(12):906-916. DOI: 10.1093/jnci/dji164

[31] Pham NM, Mizoue T, Tanaka K, Tsuji I, Tamakoshi A, Matsuo K, et al. Fish consumption and colorectal cancer risk: An evaluation based on a systematic review of epidemiologic evidence among the Japanese population. Japanese Journal of Clinical Oncology. 2013;**43**(9):935-941. DOI: 10.1093/jjco/hyt094

[32] Briguglio G, Costa C, Pollicino M, Giambò F, Catania S, Fenga C. Polyphenols in cancer prevention: New insights (Review). International Journal of Functional Nutrition. 2020;**1**(2):9. DOI: 10.3892/ijfn.2020.9

[33] Liu RH. Potential synergy of phytochemicals in cancer prevention: Mechanism of action. The Journal of Nutrition. 2004;**134**(12 Suppl):3479s-3485s. DOI: 10.1093/jn/134.12.3479S

[34] Kuppusamy P, Yusoff MM, Maniam GP, Ichwan SJA, Soundharrajan I, Govindan N. Nutraceuticals as potential therapeutic agents for colon cancer: A review. Acta Pharmaceutica Sinica B. 2014;**4**(3):173-181. DOI: 10.1016/j.apsb.2014.04.002

[35] Moukette BM, Pieme AC, Biapa PCN, Njimou JR, Stoller M, Bravi M, et al. In Vitro ion chelating, antioxidative mechanism of extracts from fruits and barks of tetrapleura tetraptera and their protective effects against fenton mediated toxicity of metal ions on liver homogenates. Evidence-Based Complementary and Alternative Medicine. 2015;**2015**:14. DOI: 10.1155/2015/423689

[36] Niranjana R, Gayathri R, Nimish Mol S, Sugawara T, Hirata T, Miyashita K, et al. Carotenoids modulate the hallmarks of cancer cells. Journal of Functional Foods. 2015;**18**:968-985. DOI: 10.1016/j.jff.2014.10.017

[37] Jiang Z, Chen H, Li M, Wang W, Fan C, Long F. Association of dietary carrot/carotene intakes with colorectal cancer incidence and mortality in the prostate, lung, colorectal, and ovarian cancer screening trial. Frontiers in Nutrition. 2022;**9**:888898

[38] Chang H, Lei L, Zhou Y, Ye F, Zhao G. Dietary flavonoids and the risk of colorectal cancer: An updated meta-analysis of epidemiological studies. Nutrients. 2018;**10**(7):950. DOI: 10.3390/nu10070950

[39] Alam MN, Almoyad M, Huq F. Polyphenols in colorectal cancer: Current state of knowledge including clinical trials and molecular mechanism of action. BioMed Research International. 2018;**2018**:4154185. DOI: 10.1155/2018/4154185

[40] Li Y, Zhang T, Chen GY. Flavonoids and colorectal cancer prevention. Antioxidants. 2018;**7**:12. DOI: 10.3390/antiox7120187

[41] Hull MA. Nutritional prevention of colorectal cancer. Proceedings of the Nutrition Society. 2021;**80**(1):59-64. DOI: 10.1017/S0029665120000051

[42] Alhassan SO, Atawodi SE-O. Chemopreventive effect of dietary inclusion with Crassocephalum rubens (Juss ex Jacq) leaf on N-methyl-N-nitrosourea (MNU)-induced colorectal carcinogenesis in Wistar rats. Journal of Functional Foods. 2019;**63**:103589. DOI: 10.1016/j.jff.2019.103589

[43] Clement YN, Mahase V, Jagroop A, Kissoon K, Maharaj A, Mathura P, et al. Herbal remedies and functional foods used by cancer patients attending specialty oncology clinics in Trinidad. BMC Complementary and Alternative Medicine. 2016;**16**(1):399. DOI: 10.1186/s12906-016-1380-x

[44] Hajiaghaalipour F, Kanthimathi MS, Sanusi J, Rajarajeswaran J. White tea (Camellia sinensis) inhibits proliferation of the colon cancer cell line, HT-29, activates caspases and protects DNA of normal cells against oxidative damage. Food Chemistry. 2015;**169**:401-410. DOI: 10.1016/j.foodchem.2014.07.005

[45] Kong M-y, Li L-y, Lou Y-m, Chi H-y, Wu J-j. Chinese herbal medicines for prevention and treatment of colorectal cancer: From molecular mechanisms to potential clinical applications. Journal of Integrative Medicine. 2020;**18**(5):369-384. DOI: 10.1016/j.joim.2020.07.005

[46] Ge H, Xu C, Chen H, Liu L, Zhang L, Wu C, et al. Traditional Chinese medicines as effective reversals of epithelial-mesenchymal transition induced-metastasis of colorectal cancer: Molecular targets and mechanisms. Frontiers in Pharmacology. 2022;**13**:842295

[47] Ho JW, Lam TH, Tse CW, Chiu LK, Lam HS, Leung PF, et al. Smoking, drinking and colorectal cancer in Hong Kong Chinese: A case-control study. International Journal of Cancer. 2004;**109**(4):587-597. DOI: 10.1002/ijc.20018

[48] Kunzmann AT, Coleman HG, Huang WY, Kitahara CM, Cantwell MM, Berndt SI. Dietary fiber intake and risk of colorectal cancer and incident and recurrent adenoma in the prostate, lung, colorectal, and ovarian cancer screening trial. American Journal of Clinical Nutrition. 2015;**102**(4):881-890. DOI: 10.3945/ajcn.115.113282

[49] Lee CF, Ho JWC, Fong DYT, Macfarlane DJ, Cerin E, Lee AM, et al. Dietary and physical activity interventions for colorectal cancer survivors: A randomized controlled trial. Scientific Reports. 2018;**8**(1):5731. DOI: 10.1038/s41598-018-24042-6

[50] Watling CZ, Schmidt JA, Dunneram Y, Tong TYN, Kelly RK, Knuppel A, et al. Risk of cancer in regular and low meat-eaters, fish-eaters, and vegetarians: A prospective analysis of UK Biobank participants. BMC Medicine. 2022;**20**(1):73. DOI: 10.1186/s12916-022-02256-w

[51] Chen H, Fu T, Dan L, Chen X, Sun Y, Chen J, et al. Meat consumption and all-cause mortality in 5763 patients with inflammatory bowel disease: A retrospective cohort study. eClinicalMedicine. 2022;**47**. DOI: 10.1016/j.eclinm.2022.101406

[52] Knuppel A, Papier K, Appleby PN, Key TJ, Perez-Cornago A. Meat intake and cancer risk: Prospective analyses in UK Biobank. Proceedings of the Nutrition Society. 2020;**79**(OCE2):E115. DOI: 10.1017/S0029665120000634

[53] Chai X, Li Y, Yin Z, Wu F, Hu P, Liu X, et al. Association of meat subtypes with colorectal polyp prevalence: Finding from the lanxi pre-colorectal cancer cohort in China. Frontiers in Nutrition. 2022;**9**:833571

[54] Bradbury KE, Murphy N, Key TJ. Diet and colorectal cancer in UK Biobank: A prospective study. International Journal of Epidemiology. 2020;**49**(1):246-258. DOI: 10.1093/ije/dyz064

[55] Ward HA, Norat T, Overvad K, Dahm CC, Bueno-de-Mesquita HB, Jenab M, et al. Pre-diagnostic meat and fibre intakes in relation to colorectal cancer survival in the European Prospective Investigation into Cancer and Nutrition. British Journal of Nutrition. 2016;**116**(2):316-325. DOI: 10.1017/s0007114516001859

[56] Lewandowska A, Religioni U, Czerw A, Deptała A, Karakiewicz B, Partyka O, et al. Nutritional treatment of patients with colorectal cancer. International Journal of Environmental Research and Public Health. 2022;**19**(11): 6881. DOI: 10.3390/ijerph19116881

[57] Fung TT, Kashambwa R, Sato K, Chiuve SE, Fuchs CS, Wu K, et al. Post diagnosis diet quality and colorectal cancer survival in women. PLoS One. 2014;**9**(12):e115377. DOI: 10.1371/journal.pone.0115377

Chapter 10

Understanding Sphingolipids Metabolism in Colorectal Cancer

Pedro Nuno Brandão, Lúcia Lacerda and Marisa D. Santos

Abstract

Colorectal cancer is the fourth most frequently diagnosed cancer and one of the leading causes of cancer death around the world. Patients with locally advanced rectal cancer are treated with a combination of radiotherapy, chemotherapy, and surgery. Treatment response can be quite variable—some with complete response, while others show little or no response—and pathologic response has become a significant predictor of good oncologic outcome. The knowledge of the molecular pathways in colorectal cancer is increasing. However, unfortunately, it still fails to find some more precise method to select and tailor patients to different treatment approaches and overcome treatment resistance. Recent investigations showed that sphingolipids play an essential role in cancer biology and can influence treatment response and aggressiveness. It is of utmost importance to understand sphingolipids' metabolism in colorectal cancer and how it affects tumor biology and response to treatment.

Keywords: locally advanced rectal cancer, neoadjuvant treatment, response to treatment, biomarkers, sphingolipids metabolism

1. Introduction

Colorectal cancer is the fourth most frequently diagnosed cancer and one of the leading causes of cancer death around the World [1]. Unfortunately, despite significant advances in treatment, there has still not been a proportional improvement in survival [2, 3]. This aspect is related to diagnosing and treating neoplasms at a more advanced stage. Although considered a single entity, locally advanced colorectal cancer should be differently treated if located in the colon or mid/lower rectum [4].

In the case of locally advanced rectal cancer (LARC), in part due to its anatomical location, multimodal therapy, and neoadjuvant therapy, in particular, plays a leading role. The optimal treatment plan for patients with rectal cancer can be a complex and highly individualized process. It usually results in multimodal therapy that combines radiation therapy, chemotherapy, and surgery [5]. Although early stages can be treated with surgery alone, more advanced stages (stages II and III) typically are treated with neoadjuvant chemoradiotherapy (CRT) before surgery to decrease the risk of recurrence and optimize oncologic outcomes. The Swedish Rectal Cancer Trial, the Dutch Colorectal Cancer Group trial, and The German Rectal Cancer Group all showed that on long-term follow-up, neoadjuvant CRT was found to improve 5-year local recurrence rates, been the overall survival effect not so evident [6–8]. Response to neoadjuvant CRT can be quite variable; some have minimal response while others have a complete clinical response [9]. Pathologic response has since become an established surrogate marker of long-term survival and a useful oncologic benchmark [10, 11]. About 20% of LARC patients have a pathologic complete response. In comparison, therapeutic resistance is evident in 80% of the cases and contributes to surgical failure, disease recurrence, and poor prognosis [12]. This discrepancy is of utmost importance because one cannot forget that the associated morbidity of these strategies cannot be underestimated.

Despite increasing knowledge of the molecular signaling pathways implicated in rectal cancer, therapeutic outcomes are still only moderately successful in comparison. To change the therapeutic paradigm, LARC patients must be integrated into clinical algorithms tailoring therapy for individual patients by either identifying more effective strategies or by omitting ineffective treatments to avoid unnecessary toxicity [12, 13].

As one should note, the high rate of resistance demonstrated by the low complete response in most rectal cancer patients must lead the scientific community to explore novel molecular strategies to enhance conventional therapy.

Recent investigations showed that bioactive sphingolipids play a significant role in the colon and rectal cancer tumorigenesis, signaling mechanisms, and response to treatment as they can influence the impact and effectiveness of radio and chemotherapy. Understanding the molecular patterns and the relation between sphingolipids and CRT should provide valuable information regarding tumor survival mechanisms and, this way, pursue novel therapeutic targets.

2. Sphingolipids' metabolism and cancer

Sphingolipids are structural molecules of cell membranes with an essential role in barrier and fluidity functions [14]. They have been implicated in many physiologic and pathologic processes, such as cell growth, cell death, cell adhesion, proliferation, stress, inflammatory responses, differentiation, migration, invasion, and/or metastasis, by controlling signaling functions within the signal transduction network of cancer cell [13, 15–19]. The two central bioactive lipids, ceramide and sphingosine-1-phosphate (S1P), have opposing roles in regulating cancer cell death and survival [19]. Ceramide has been shown to mediate cell cycle arrest and cell death in response to cell stress [14, 20]. S1P has been shown to promote cell survival and proliferation [14, 18, 20, 21].

During the past decades, information regarding almost all major enzymes involved in sphingolipid metabolism was gathered, which has provided data that shows that these metabolic enzymes highly regulate the abundance of sphingolipids and their role in different biologic pathways [22]. Additional complexity derives from multiple isoforms of those enzymes that can vary in subcellular location and pH requirements, which results in different metabolic products. For instance, different ceramide synthases can produce ceramides with different fatty acid chains, which will have distinct biologic roles [12]. One should also find that different isoforms of sphingosine kinase, which generates S1P, have different localizations and functions.

Cellular stress induced by chemotherapy and/or radiation is known to cause pro-cell death mechanisms and tumor suppression, at least partly through the induction of ceramide generation [19]. On the contrary, S1P generation results in resistance to CRT. Given the importance of CRT in the treatment of LARC, understanding the relation between sphingolipids metabolism and CRT could be of utmost importance in finding new ways to treat these patients more effectively. One must also find that understanding more about the sphingolipids' metabolism may open opportunities to define potential predictive biomarkers for CRT resistance, such as S1P and glucosylceramide, as shown in previous studies with different types of tumors [23, 24].

Cellular stress induces sphingosine and/or ceramide generation by activating the de novo synthesis pathways, sphingomyelin hydrolysis, or the salvage pathway to mediate cancer cell death (**Figure 1**) [14, 25]. By contrast, many tumors exhibit increased ceramide metabolism mainly by increased activities of glycosylceramide synthase (GCS), sphingomyelin synthase (SMS), ceramide kinase (CERK), acid ceramidase (AC), and/or sphingosine kinase (SPHK), which increases the generation of sphingolipids with pro-survival functions [26, 27].

Ceramide consists of a long-chain sphingosine base and an amide-linked fatty acyl chain that varies from 14 to 26 carbons (C) in length [14, 25]. Endogenous ceramides are synthesized via the de novo pathway with the help of ceramide synthases (CERS1-6) [28], which are specialized for ceramide synthesis with different fatty acyl chain lengths. CerS or longevity assurance genes (LASS) [29, 30], a family of six members in mammals with differing tissue expression, are primarily confined to the endoplasmic reticulum (ER). Each CerS1-6 isoform has a unique tissue expression profile and predilection for a fatty acyl CoA with a specific FA chain length. Thus, depending on the CerS family member, distinct sets of ceramides with varying

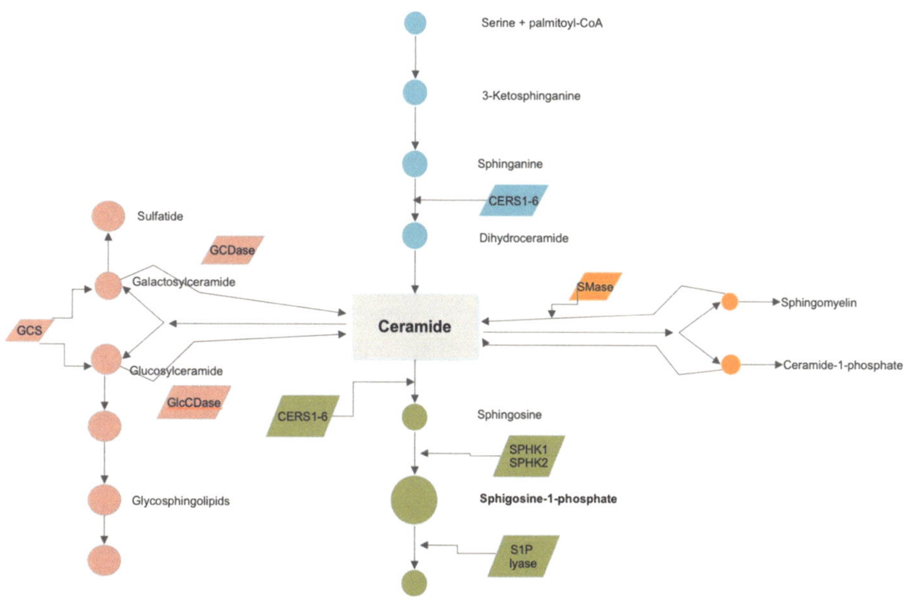

Figure 1.
Sphingolipid metabolism and some of the critical enzymes. De novo synthesis (blue) depends on CERS1-6 activity and it is the central hub of the sphingolipid pathway. Ceramide is also produced by the sphingomyelin hydrolysis (orange), which is dependent on SMase activity. The salvage pathway also relies on CERS1-6 activity (green) that can metabolize free sphingosine to ceramide. Ceramide can be converted to sulfatides by the action of galactosylceramide synthase (GCS). The complex glycosphingolipids are hydrolyzed to glucosylceramide and galactosylceramide. These lipids are then hydrolyzed by beta-glucosidases and beta-galactosidases (GCDase) to regenerate ceramide. CDase activity will metabolize ceramide to sphingosine that, in turn, will lead to S1P unbalancing the scale to a less apoptotic and pro-surviving state. S1P can be broken down by S1P lyase activity exiting the sphingolipid metabolic pathway.

chain lengths are produced [30]. With few exceptions, naturally occurring mammalian ceramides generally possess acyl chain lengths varying between C16 to C24 [31] and its biological activity has only recently become apparent.

Some studies with the administration of exogenous C16-Cer in human colon cancer cell lines showed that it resulted in programmed cell death, suggesting that an increase in endogenous production of C16-Cer could lead to the same effects [32].

Despite these results, one should note that the same ceramide analogs have entirely different effects regarding the type of histological tissue. In the head and neck squamous cell carcinoma cell line, C16:0-Cer had antiapoptotic properties [33], whereas, in HeLa cells, C16:0-ceramide worked as a proapoptotic factor [34]. Ceramides chain length is another critical factor as specific chain lengths can have different effects in different cells. Long-chain and very-long-chain ceramides have shown the opposite effect on the human colon cancer cell line [35].

Moreover, the deficiency of some ceramides may be compensated for by increased expression of others, resulting in an altered synthesis of different ceramide analogs [36].

Ceramide is also generated by sphingomyelinases (SMases, acid, neutral, or alkaline), which mediate sphingomyelin hydrolysis—by far the most abundant sphingolipid in animal cell membranes [31]—or by glucosylceramidase (GlcCDase) and galactosylceramidase (GCDase), which, respectively, catalyze glucosylceramide and/or galactosylceramide breakdown to ceramide [14, 25, 37]. In the salvage pathway, CerSs are responsible for regenerating ceramide from free sphingosine by re-acylation [38].

Ceramide is hydrolyzed by ceramidases (CDases) to yield sphingosine, which is phosphorylated by sphingosine kinases (SPHK1 and SPHK2) to generate S1P [19]. A balance between the proapoptotic properties of ceramide and the antiapoptotic properties of S1P has been termed the ceramide/S1P rheostat and is considered important in balancing cell death and survival in numerous stress situations [39]. S1P engages with five specific G protein-coupled receptors, S1PR1-5, in an autocrine or paracrine manner to elicit pro-survival signaling in various cancer cells [19, 40].

The clinical relevance of sphingolipid metabolism has been established, and it is well known, as demonstrated in the biopathological mechanisms of lysosomal storage diseases (Farber disease, Gaucher disease, Krabbe disease, and Niemann-Pick A, B disease), owing to aberrant accumulation of sphingolipids [19]. Although some of the effects of SLs appear to be cell-specific, generally, increased intracellular levels of ceramides, sphingosines, and also dihydroceramides are mostly connected with the induction of cell cycle arrest and/or cell death. In contrast, the elevated levels of S1P, ceramide-1-phosphate, glucosylceramides, and lactosylceramides seem to be associated with increased cell survival, proliferation, cell adhesion, and promotion of cell migration and/or invasion, events that are related to cancer progression [22]. Until now, the changes in S1P/Cer ratio remain the best-characterized outcome of the alterations of SL metabolism in cancer.

2.1 Biology of cancer and sphingolipid enzymes

Ceramides are essential components of cell membranes, and their presence depends on the equilibrium between production and degradation rates. Different stress stimuli, physiological or pathological, will change the way they act, usually leading to cancer cell death through various mechanisms [36] such as apoptosis, autophagy, and ER stress. In fact, as can be seen by numerous laboratory studies, the accumulation of sphingolipids represents the great majority of cell changes during apoptosis [36].

In 1993, the induction of apoptosis by ceramide was first demonstrated in leukemic cells by treatment with exogenous ceramide [41]. There are two primary pathways, an intrinsic one (mitochondrial) and an extrinsic one. While the extrinsic one results from the activation of death receptors on the cell surface, the intrinsic pathway is activated by stress stimuli like hypoxia, nutrient deprivation, or DNA damage. Cancer cells can overcome those mechanisms, escape apoptosis, and engage in pro-survival pathways [36, 42].

Despite the proapoptotic action of ceramides in cancer cells, it can also have an opposite behavior in regard to subcellular localization, the type of stress stimuli, and changes in ceramide targets [19].

The abundance of sphingolipid molecules is highly regulated by metabolic enzymes, the altered expression or activity of which has crucial roles in the induction of cancer cell death or survival [19]. 2002 was marked as the year of the discovery of the first mammalian ceramide synthase. Since then, various experiments have indicated that changing the composition of ceramide species alters cell physiology and influences pathology [43].

The discovery and cloning of CERS1-6 were key to understanding the roles of ceramides with different fatty acyl chain lengths in cancer cell signaling. CerS1 and CerS4 preferentially generate ceramide with 18–20-carbon fatty acids (C18–20-Cer), while CerS5 or CerS6 primarily generate ceramide with 14–16-carbon fatty acids (C14-16-Cer), and CerS2 selectively generates ceramides with 22–24-carbon fatty acids. CerS3 is responsible for synthesis of very-long-chain C28-32 ceramides [12].

Phenotypes observed in CerS-deficient mice suggest that ceramides with different fatty acid chain lengths have distinct biologic roles. For example, CerS1 expression was found to be repressed in head and neck cancer cells [44]; In the liver, CerS2-deficiency resulted in a compensatory generation of C16-Cer, which leads to the development of hepatocellular cancer owing to possible defects in apoptosis [45]. C16 ceramide was shown to increase apoptosis in colon cancer cells [46]. Targeting specific CerS can, in theory, shift ceramide composition in cancer cell lines resulting in different cellular responses and signaling pathways. The tissue distribution of CerS varies and likely reflects the need for specific ceramide species for proper signaling and sphingolipid homeostasis in any given tissue [29, 47].

Ceramide is also generated by the hydrolysis of sphingomyelin by SMases – acid, neutral, and alkaline – based on their pH-dependent optimal activity. Data from different studies support the hypothesis that the hydrolysis of sphingomyelin by SMases generates ceramide, which mediates cancer cell death, growth arrest, and/or tumor suppression [19]. In comparison to surrounding normal tissue, SMase activity in colorectal cancer is reduced by 75%, 50%, and 30% for alkSMase, nSMase, and aSMase, respectively [48].

There are three classes of CDases—acid, neutral, and alkaline—responsible for converting ceramide to sphingosine, which was found to be upregulated in various cancer types. Studies with prostate cancer mouse models showed tumor relapse due to radiation resistance induced by ACDase expression [49]. Neutral ceramidase (NCDase) sphingosine release is utilized for S1P biosynthesis by SPHK1 and/or SPHK2, resulting in the inhibition of cell death through reduced levels of proapoptotic ceramide. Colon cancer cells' works demonstrated that NCDase inhibition resulted in autophagy and apoptosis due to ceramide accumulation. In fact, null mice were protected from the development of colon cancer [50].

The two isoforms of sphingosine kinase, SPHK1, and SPHK2, both utilize sphingosine and generate S1P but have significant differences in subcellular localization and function [51]. SPKH1 releases S1P extracellularly, which regulates several cellular processes in an autocrine or paracrine manner, leading to pro-survival mechanisms. SPHK2 appears to have both pro and antiapoptotic functions in regard to the cell type, subcellular localization, and stimuli [51]. Increased expression of SPHK1 mRNA was indicative of poor prognosis and decreased survival in patients with various cancers [52].

SPL function represents a final path and an exit route from the sphingolipid metabolism with the hydrolysis of S1P. In fact, some studies show S1P accumulation in colon cancer tissues due to SPL downregulation [53]. On the contrary, SPL overexpression leads to increased apoptosis through reduced S1P signaling in colon cancer cells [54].

There is ample evidence suggesting that SPHK/S1P signaling pathways are associated with cancer development and metastasis (**Table 1**) [55]. Overexpression of SPHK/S1P signaling is often associated with cancer drug resistance to chemotherapy, radiation therapy, or hormonal therapies in various types of cancers [26]. It is important to note that along with SPHK1, SPHK2 is overexpressed in many human cancers, and based on its cellular localization, it can function as a pro- or antiapoptotic signaling molecule. It was suggested that knockdown of SPHK2 with siRNA or inhibition of SPHK2 activity with the selective pharmacological drugs reduces cancer cell growth, migration, and invasion [56–58] and induces apoptosis by accumulating proapoptotic ceramides. In sharp contrast, it has been recently demonstrated that mitochondrial SPHK2 is proapoptotic [55]. However, more studies need to be performed with specific SPHK2 inhibitors or mitochondrial-targeted SPHK2 that would be beneficial to identify clinically relevant functions of SPHK2.

2.2 Sphingolipids and cancer therapy

The knowledge acquired in recent years regarding sphingolipids metabolism made clear that there are quite a substantial number of different opportunities for cancer cells to escape cell death. In fact, sphingolipid metabolic pathways represent an essential branch of human and pharmacological research in pursuit of novel

Lipids	Mechanism	Functions
S1P	Intracellular Extracellular	Tumor progression
		Metastasis
		Cancer cell survival
		Cell migration
		Angiogenesis
		Inflammation
		Chemokine signaling
		Immune cell trafficking
		Epigenetic regulation

Table 1.
Significant effects mediated by S1P.

therapeutic drugs for cancer patients. About two decades ago, researchers first showed that standard-of-care treatments, for example, chemotherapeutics and radiation, modulate sphingolipid metabolism to increase endogenous ceramides, which kill cancer cells. Strikingly, resistance to these treatments has also been linked to altered sphingolipid metabolism, favoring lipid species that ultimately lead to cell survival [59]. The significant number of chemotherapeutic agents available in clinical practice is, in fact, characterized by the accumulation of sphingolipids in cells [60]. The response to stress induced by chemotherapeutic agents leads to ceramide accumulation, both by sphingomyelin hydrolysis as well as through de novo synthesis of ceramide [61], as described for daunorubicin, etoposide, and gemcitabine [60]. So, inhibiting de novo pathway enzymes leads to decreased ceramide levels, reducing the cytotoxicity of the chemotherapeutics and finally their overall efficacy. In the phase II clinical trial, elevated serum levels of C18 ceramide were markedly associated with improved response to gemcitabine plus doxorubicin combination therapy in patients with recurrent head and neck cancers [62].

Interestingly, altered ceramide levels are not the only biological connection between sphingolipids and chemotherapy; glucosylceramides are increased in breast cancer and in patients who were resistant to chemotherapy. The enzyme that generates glucosylceramide is upregulated in several different tumor types such as lung cancer, breast cancer, and colorectal cancer [63].

Ceramide levels can also be diminished by the action of CDase enzymes which converts ceramide to sphingosine, which, in turn, can be transformed to S1P. *In vitro* and *in vivo* studies have shown that by overexpressing ACDase, tumors are more aggressive and resistant to chemotherapies [64].

In essence, when too much ceramide accumulates and the metaphorical balance overflows, the cell dies (**Figure 2**).

In regard to radiotherapy, one of the first discoveries of the role of ceramide in cell death in radiation subjects was the rapid hydrolysis of sphingomyelin to ceramide by SMase [65]. Notably, ceramide was shown to be the major mediator of cellular stress after radiation exposure [66]. Besides sphingomyelin hydrolysis, raised ceramide levels can also be achieved by induction of de novo synthesis in response to radiation, as seen in Scarlatti F. *et al. in vitro* study with radiation-resistant DU145 prostate cancer cells. Those cells were treated with resveratrol resulting in resensitization to radiation by stimulating the de novo pathway, a finding that was validated when sphingolipid synthesis inhibitors blocked sensitization and reverted DU145 cells to radiation-resistant status [67].

Lastly, ceramide cell levels in response to radiation are also increased by ceramide synthase activity [68]. The current knowledge is that ceramide levels are firstly increased by sphingomyelin hydrolysis and then by CerS activity, 8 to 24 h after radiation therapy [69]. These data suggest that ceramide generation in cancer cells in response to chemotherapy and radiotherapy has an important role in tumor suppression.

Bacterial resistance to antibiotic drugs was first described after the discovery that penicillin prompted bacteria to develop defense mechanisms culminating in the expression of an array of efflux transporters in the outer cell wall [70]. The broad range of substrates used by these transport proteins resulted in coining the term multidrug resistance (MDR) as pathogens can limit the accumulation of diverse drugs targeted against them [31, 71]. Some cancer types harbor intrinsic MDR, most probably due to exogenous expression of drug efflux transport proteins in the tissue of origin. Other cancer types acquire MDR through prolonged

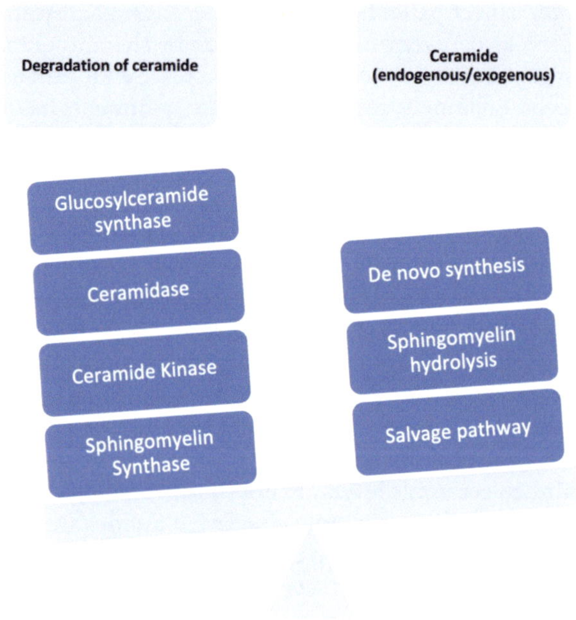

Figure 2.
The accumulation of ceramide (endogenous and exogenous) and degradation of ceramide.

or repeated treatment with chemotherapeutic drugs [72]. An altered glycosphingolipid profile in cancerous versus non-cancerous cells was observed in cell lines transformed by chemicals or viruses and impacted cell growth, intercellular recognition, and cell adhesivity. The conversion of ceramide to glucosylceramide by GCS has been shown to mediate drug resistance in various cancers [23]. Importantly, drug sensitivity was restored when GCS was inhibited or downregulated [73], but not all studies exhibit the dependence of drug resistance on CGS/CluCer [74]. SPHK1 overexpression was reported at intrinsic or acquired resistance to cetuximab in CRC cell lines, xenograft mouse models, and tumors obtained from patients [24] and S1PR1 inhibition using FTY720 sensitized resistant CRC cells and tumors to cetuximab [24]. Hence, while CGS and SPHK1/2 are potential therapeutic targets to overcome drug resistance, increased accumulation of their sphingolipid products—glucosylceramide and S1P, respectively—might be potential predictive biomarkers for chemotherapy resistance in various cancers [19]. Descriptive lipidomic studies may help to identify potential lipid markers of distinct rectal cancer stages.

3. Sphingolipids and colorectal cancer

3.1 Sphingolipids' levels in plasma and tumor tissue

The last decade was fruitful in the investigation of the metabolic switch during tumorigenesis [75]. Lipids are central in different cellular levels of physiology that go from plasmatic and membrane organization, plasticity, and signaling mechanisms [76–78].

Data from the literature indicate that the equilibrium between ceramides of various chain lengths is crucial for cell fate [35]. As noted before, the S1P/Cer ratio changes remain the best-characterized outcome of the alterations of SL metabolism in cancer.

The amount of new information and knowledge regarding sphingolipids in colorectal cancer can hardly be systematized. The best option is to follow the sphingolipids' metabolic pathways and see which alterations are present in cancer cells.

Ceramides and their proportion are different in plasma of patients with CRC and tumor tissue compared with plasma and tissue control levels. On the other hand, plasma ceramide concentration is not directly related to ceramide concentration in tumor tissue. One must also be aware that different chain lengths can have different actions regarding cell localization and the microenvironment. Chen et al. demonstrated increased levels of C16:0 and C24:0 ceramides and reduced levels of both C18 and C20 ceramides in colorectal tumor tissues [79–81]. Levels of C22:0 ceramide were unchanged [80]. Those results were in line with the protein expression and enzymatic activity of SCD1 (Stearoyl-CoA desaturase-1), a key conversion enzyme that regulates lipogenesis. SCD1 inhibition impairs the proliferation of cancer cells probably by cellular endogenous ceramide signals mediation [80]. Another study showed an increased amount of S1P and C14:0 compared to normal tissue and a significantly lower amount of C18:0 and C20:0, as previously noted [36].

The plasma profile of sphingolipids appears to be different than in tissues with the highest concentration in the plasma for C24:0-ceramide and C24:1-ceramide [36]. The concentration for C22:0, C16:0-ceramides, and S1P is smaller but significant [36]. Another study, however, showed significantly higher concentration levels of C16, C18, C18:1, and C24:1-ceramide than those of controls and lower levels of C24-sphingomyelin; there was a relation between these results and stage IV CRC. These results are limited by the small sample size and retrospective design of the study [82]. Markowski et al. divided the patients into two groups regarding their stage and showed that a higher tumor content of C20:0 and C24:0-ceramide was present in the TNM III + IV group. In plasma, there was a statistically significant relation between CRC patients in TNM stage III + IV and higher levels of C16:0 and C18:1-ceramides. Their data raise the possibility that it could be possible to distinguish patients between early and advanced stages based on this model [36]. Taken together, one must note that plasma ceramide concentration is not directly related to ceramide concentration in tumor tissue.

In another study with patients with pulmonary and hepatic metastasis submitted to radiotherapy, it was observed that although pre-treatment levels of ceramides did not correlate with response to treatment, patients with complete response had higher post-treatment total plasma ceramide levels than non-responders [83].

Lymph node invasion was shown to have a positive correlation with C24 ceramide levels in CRC tumor tissues [79]. It was also demonstrated that Sphingosine 1-phosphate (S1P) signaling pathways were associated with lymphangiogenesis [84].

3.2 Sphingolipids enzymes in colorectal cancer

3.2.1 Pro-ceramide metabolic pathways

As mentioned before, sphingolipids' metabolism is regulated through a complex equilibrium between different enzymes' actions, which will, in the end, change the balance between ceramide and S1P. For example, different enzymes will provide different ceramides, with different actions depending on the tissue and subcellular localization.

The discovery and cloning of CERS1–6 were crucial for understanding the roles of ceramides with different fatty acyl chain lengths in cancer cell signaling. Hartmann et al. showed that overexpression of CerS4 and CerS6 in HCT-116 human colon cancer cells inhibits cell proliferation by upregulation of long-chain ceramides C16:0, C18:0, and C20:0. In contrast, upregulation of CerS2 and concomitant increase of C24:0 and C24:1 promotes cell proliferation [35].

Jang et al. revealed that all four CerS genes were significantly upregulated in CRC tissues compared with corresponding normal tissues [85]. CERS6 overexpression reduced the proliferation of CRC cells and induced apoptosis, whereas CERS2 overexpression increased the proliferation of CRC cells [35]. Regardless of the mechanism, overexpression of CERS2 and CERS6 decreased the viability of CRC cell lines tested [85]. CerS6-generated C16 ceramide was shown to increase apoptosis in colon cancer cells [46].

CERS5-ko mice showed significantly larger colon tumors than CERS5-wt mice [86]. Another study showed that strong CERS5 staining correlated with poor prognosis in patients with CRC [87]. CERS4 and CERS5 were also found to be upregulated in colon cancer prior to apoptosis induction and down-regulated after apoptosis induction in colon cell lines [88].

The importance of ceramide levels in cancer cells was also demonstrated in studies with ceramide analogs such as LCL-30, the cationic water-soluble analog of C16-ceramide. LCL-30 accumulates in cells' mitochondria and induces mitochondrial swelling, decreases membrane potential, caspase activation, and ultimately cell death [89, 90]. The same group also tested its actions in colon carcinoma cell line CT-26 as an *in vivo* model of colorectal cancer, demonstrating that LCL-30 was cytotoxic to CT-26 cells [90].

Adiseshaiah et al. also showed that injection of nanoliposomal C6-ceramide, an autophagy inducer, in combination with vinblastine, decreased tumor growth in comparison to the individual treatments [75]. The authors used the colon cancer xenograft model (LS174T) and showed that the combination treatment resulted in statistically significant suppression of tumor growth compared to a single treatment. The rationale behind the study was that cancer cells might evade anticancer therapy by inducing autophagy, so blocking it should improve therapeutic response.

It is undoubtedly that microenvironment will largely influence cancer cells' fate during their life cycle. Cancer cell progression is associated with tumorigenic M2 macrophages. Ceramide-treated macrophages were shown to induce the switching of macrophage polarization toward the pro-inflammatory M1-phenotype. Ceramide also abolished macrophage-induced epithelial-mesenchymal transition and migration of colorectal cancer cells [91]. Other studies have demonstrated that M1 and M2 macrophages can switch phenotypes and lipids have the potential to modulate their function and phenotypes [92, 93]. Ceramides act as an intracellular second messenger and membrane component [94]. Araujo Junior et al. have demonstrated that ceramide can reduce M2 phenotype and block migration of cancer cells, suggesting that targeting ceramide in the tumor microenvironment could, in theory, reduce tumor progression and potential for metastasis of colon cancer cells [91].

Ceramide is also generated by the hydrolysis of sphingomyelin by SMases—acid, neutral, and alkaline—based on their pH-dependent optimal activity.

The activities of neutral and alkaline SMase were highest in the ascending colon and decreased in the sigmoid colon and rectum, whereas no significant difference was found for acidic SMase activity at all locations [48]. Markowski et al. also examined the relationship of sphingolipids levels in CRC tissue on tumor localization and documented that, albeit complex and ambiguous, the number of total ceramides was lowest in sigmoid and cecum tumors and the largest in rectal tumors [36]. SMase activity was found to be decreased in colorectal carcinomas, mainly alkaline SMase activity, which results in lowered cellular levels of ceramide. In comparison to surrounding normal tissue, SMase activity in colorectal cancer is reduced by 75%, 50%, and 30% for alkSMase, nSMase, and aSMase, respectively [48].

3.2.2 Pro-S1P metabolic pathways

So, on one side of the balance, we can identify the mechanisms responsible for ceramide raised levels; however, on the other side, we should pay attention to the antagonist mechanisms leading to the degradation of ceramide in detriment to S1P and their transitory metabolites.

Among the five ceramidases identified to date [95], neutral CDase is predominantly expressed in the colon and is involved in the metabolism of dietary sphingolipids [96]. It was shown that inhibition of NCDase induces an increase of ceramide in colon cancer cells, decreasing cell growth and increasing apoptosis [50, 81]. Coant et al. also showed that deletion of NCDase protected mice from the onset and progression of colorectal cancer C16:0 ceramide levels were increased. The inhibition of NCDase leads to inhibition of the WNT/β-catenin pathway [81]. HT 29 colon cancer cells treated with NCDase inhibition were accompanied by decreased survival, increased apoptosis, and autophagy [50]. Animal studies also showed that inhibition of NCDase delayed tumor growth, with increased ceramide and reduced tumor cell proliferation [50]. Taken together, NCDase appears to be an important target for new therapeutic strategies.

Studies in mice have demonstrated that oral administration of plant-type sphingolipids increased colonic Sphingosine-1-phosphate lyase (SPL) levels and reduced S1P levels, cytokine levels, and tumorigenesis, indicating that SPL can prevent transformation and carcinogenesis [53]. These studies suggest that dietary sphingolipids can have a role in colon cancer prevention in opposition to high-fat diets that possibly increase the risk of colorectal cancer. SPL is highly expressed in normal intestinal and colonic epithelium, however, it is downregulated in CRC cells and in early adenomatous lesions of Min mice [54]. SPL expression promotes apoptosis through a cascading mechanism that involves p53, p38, PIDD, and caspase-2; however, it is not clear how this interaction occurs [54]. SPL activity provides an exit route from sphingolipid metabolism via the rapid hydrolysis of S1P. SPL appears to be downregulated at the protein level in colon cancer tissues, and SPL silencing promoted colon carcinogenesis, which occurred via S1P accumulation and/or S1PR signaling [53]. On the contrary, SPL overexpression leads to increased apoptosis through reduced S1P signaling in colon cancer cells [54].

The two isoforms of sphingosine kinase, SPHK1, and SPHK2, utilize sphingosine and generate S1P but have significant differences in subcellular localization and function [51]. Sphingosine kinases (SPHK1 and 2) are overexpressed in many cancers, including colorectal cancer, compared with normal mucosa [97]. The expression levels of SPHK1 and 2 were also high in liver metastases compared with matched normal colon tissues. SPHK1 and SPHK2 are observed in different places within the cell; SPHK1 in the cytosol while SPHK2 was detected in both cytosol and nucleus [97]. SPHKs seem to have a role in promoting the metastatic potential of colorectal cancer cells [97]. FTY-720, an S1P receptor antagonist, reduces cell migration and invasion and significantly decreases cellular proliferation in all cell lines tested [97].

3.3 Sphingolipids, treatment resistance, and new strategies

5-Fluorouracil (5-FU) is one of the first-line chemotherapy agents' in colorectal cancer and despite its efficacy, drug resistance is still an important limitation. Jung et al. conducted a lipidomic analysis showing that resistance to 5-FU is associated with the up-regulation of sphingomyelin and the down-regulation of CERS [98].

SPHK1 contribution to cetuximab resistance in colorectal cancer was investigated. The authors found overexpressed and overactivated SPHK1 in colorectal cancer cells with intrinsic or acquired resistance to cetuximab [24]. It was also documented that treatment of resistant cells with FTY-720 resulted in resensitization to cetuximab both *in vitro* and *in vivo* [24]. This association could be a new therapeutic strategy to overcome chemotherapy resistance and also a biomarker of interest for cetuximab resistance.

In another study involving SPHK2, the authors found that using ABC294649, a novel SPHK2 inhibitor, resulted in growth inhibition and apoptosis of CRC cells, with S1P depletion and ceramide incrementation. Also, exogenously-added S1P inhibited ABC294640 cell effects. The authors also described that ABC294649 sensitized 5-FU and cisplatin-mediated anti-HT-29 cell activity. This agent could be an important anti-CRC weapon, and it is also available in an oral formulation [58]. Xun et al. demonstrated in HT-29 cell lines that SphK2 inhibition (ABC294640) resulted in S1P depletion and ceramide incensement with consequent cell lethality. Oral administration dramatically inhibited H-29 xenograft growth in nude mice [58].

SphK inactivation induces the accumulation of S1P precursors, including sphingosine and ceramide, causing cell apoptosis and growth arrest [99].

Activity in primary cancer cells was also tested. SphK2 expression was different between patients, however, ABC294640 activity was negatively associated with SphK2 expression level [58].

Glucosylceramide synthase (GCS), a ceramide-metabolizing enzyme, has been demonstrated to be overexpressed in CRC tissues compared with non-CRC tissues. Wang et al. documented that high-expression GCS patients were associated with significantly higher lymph node metastasis than the low CGS expression group [63].

GCS has been associated with several studies that documented its role in chemotherapy resistance [63, 100]. Oxaliplatin-resistant cells demonstrated increased expression of GCS protein compared to the parental cell line, with increased levels of glucosylceramide (GlcCer) [100]. Madigan et al. also showed that inhibition of GCS expression resulted in the reduction of ClcCer levels with restored sensitivity to oxaliplatin. Oxaliplatin-resistant CRC cells also expressed lower ceramide levels compared to parental cells. In fact, the conversion of ceramide to glucosylceramide by GCS represents an essential mechanism for limiting ceramide accumulation [101]. It was also shown that the rate of GCS was higher in patients receiving neoadjuvant chemotherapy than in non-CRC tissues, raising the possibility that chemotherapy drugs might induce the high expression of GCS and increase the risk of MDR [63]. The authors hypothesized that oxaliplatin treatment might result in reduced ceramide levels compared to oxaliplatin-sensitive cells. C16-ceramide was the only species to differ significantly between the two cell lines. Higher sphingomyelin levels were found in the positive nodes of colorectal cancer patients compared to the negative lymph nodes [102].

In recent years, a few new pharmacologic strategies have been used in laboratory and clinical trials. Fenretinide (preclinical; reduces de novo synthesis with dihydroceramide accumulation), Safingol (association with irinotecan, preclinical; SPHK1 inhibitor), Ceramide nanoliposomes (association with tamoxifen, preclinical; apoptosis promoter by ceramide accumulation), α-GalCer (preclinical; α- galactosylceramide-pulsed antigen-presenting cells), and Fingolimod (association with sphingosine and cetuximab, preclinical; functional antagonist of the sphingosine-1-phosphate receptor (S1PR) and structural analog of sphingosine) [60, 103] are the most important in colorectal cancer with exciting and promising results.

4. In summary

Sphingolipids are structural molecules of cell membranes with an essential role in barrier and fluidity functions. They have been implicated in many physiologic and pathologic processes, such as cell growth, cell death, adhesion, proliferation, stress, inflammatory responses, differentiation, migration, invasion, and/or metastasis.

The sphingolipids play an essential role in cancer biology and influence treatment response and aggressiveness. It also happens in colorectal cancer and may be interesting in developing an individualized treatment plan for LARC.

Nevertheless, the molecule's action interpretation is complicated, given the complexity of sphingolipid's metabolism with several activations and counter-regulation pathways. In addition, there are isoforms whose action is different depending on the location in the cell and the type of tissues in which they occur. Finally, the balance among ceramides has also essential for the activity response.

However, we can state that in general terms, there are two central bioactive lipids, ceramides and sphingosine-1-phosphate (S1P), which have opposing roles in regulating cancer cell death and survival. Ceramides have been shown to mediate cell cycle arrest and cell death in response to cell stress. Also, the equilibrium between ceramides of various chain lengths is crucial for cell fate. On the other hand, S1P has been shown to promote cell survival and proliferation.

Thus, the increase in specific ceramides in the tumor may correspond to a lower aggressiveness or effective response to the therapy instituted. In comparison, the rise in S1P in the tumor will correspond to a greater aggressiveness of tumor resistance to the treatment.

In this perspective, the measurement of ceramides and S1P may be of interest to assess the aggressiveness of a particular tumor. Nevertheless, on the other hand, we can try to interfere with the amount of these elements present in the tumor to modify tumor resistance to conventional therapy.

From published studies, it appears that sphingolipids' metabolism in tumor tissue is unsettled in colorectal cancer.

Ceramides and their proportion are different in plasma of patients with CRC and tumor tissue compared with plasma and tissue control levels. On the other hand, plasma ceramide concentration is not directly related to ceramide concentration in tumor tissue.

The knowledge gathered in the past decade can lead us to new ways of treating CCR patients, trying to overcome treatment resistance, and, in the end, achieving higher response rates and improved global life expectancy.

In conclusion, the knowledge of tumor sphingolipids metabolism may be essential in colorectal cancer treatment. Unfortunately, the studies about this issue are small and few. Therefore, investigation in this area is needed.

Conflict of interest

The authors declare no conflict of interest.

Author details

Pedro Nuno Brandão[1,2]*, Lúcia Lacerda[2,3,4] and Marisa D. Santos[1,2]

1 Colorectal Surgery Unit, University of Porto Hospital Center, Porto, Portugal

2 UMIB - Unit for Multidisciplinary Research in Biomedicine (ICBAS, University of Porto), Porto, Portugal

3 Medical Genetics Center, University of Porto Hospital Center, Porto, Portugal

4 ITR - Laboratory for Integrative and Translational Research in Population Health, University of Porto, Porto, Portugal

*Address all correspondence to: pedronunobg@gmail.com

References

[1] Bray F, Ferlay J, Soerjomataram I, et al. Global cancer statistics 2018: GLOBOCAN estimates of incidence and mortality worldwide for 36 cancers in 185 countries. CA: a Cancer Journal for Clinicians. 2018;**68**:394-424

[2] NCCN. Rectal cancer: NCCN Version 2.2019 Clinical Practice Guideline in Oncology. NCCN Guidelines.

[3] Bailey CE, Hu CY, You YN, et al. Increasing disparities in the age-related incidences of colon and rectal cancers in the United States, 1975-2010. JAMA Surgery. 2015;**150**:17-22

[4] Johns LE, Houlston RS. A systematic review and meta-analysis of familial colorectal cancer risk. The American Journal of Gastroenterology. 2001;**96**:2992-3003

[5] Kleiman D, Guillem J. The Management of Rectal Cancer. In: Current Surgical Therapy. 12th ed. 2017. pp. 224-234

[6] Folkesson J, Birgisson H, Pahlman L, et al. Swedish rectal Cancer trial: Long lasting benefits from radiotherapy on survival and local recurrence rate. JCO. 2005;**23**:5644-5650

[7] Van Gijn W, Marijnen CAM, Nagtegaal ID, et al. Preoperative radiotherapy combined with total mesorectal excision for resectable rectal cancer: 12-year follow-up of the multicentre, randomised controlled TME trial. The Lancet Oncology. 2011;**12**:575-582

[8] Sauer R, Liersch T, Merkel S, et al. Preoperative versus postoperative chemoradiotherapy for locally advanced rectal cancer: Results of the German CAO/ARO/AIO-94 randomized phase III trial after a median follow-up of 11 years. Journal of Clinical Oncology. 2012;**30**:1926-1933

[9] Glynne-Jones R, Wyrwicz L, Tiret E, et al. Rectal cancer: ESMO clinical practice guidelines for diagnosis, treatment and follow-up. Annals of Oncology. 2017;**28**:iv22-iv40

[10] Rödel C, Martus P, Papadoupolos T, et al. Prognostic significance of tumor regression after preoperative chemoradiotherapy for rectal cancer. Journal of Clinical Oncology. 2005;**23**:8688-8696

[11] Park IJ, You YN, Agarwal A, et al. Neoadjuvant treatment response as an early response indicator for patients with rectal cancer. Journal of Clinical Oncology. 2012;**30**:1770-1776

[12] Camp ER, Patterson LD, Kester M, et al. Therapeutic implications of bioactive sphingolipids: A focus on colorectal cancer. Cancer Biology and Therapy. 2017;**18**:640-650

[13] García-Barros M, Coant N, Truman JP, et al. Sphingolipids in colon cancer. Biochimica et Biophysica Acta - Molecular and Cell Biology of Lipids. 2014;**1841**:773-782

[14] Hannun YA, Obeid LM. Principles of bioactive lipid signalling: Lessons from sphingolipids. Nature Reviews Molecular Cell Biology. 2008;**9**:139-150

[15] Hannun YA. Functions of ceramide in coordinating cellular responses to stress. Science. 1996;**274**:1855-1859

[16] Nikolova-Karakashian MN, Rozenova KA. Ceramide in stress

response. Advances in Experimental Medicine and Biology. 2010;**688**:86-108

[17] Stancevic B, Kolesnick R. Ceramide-rich platforms in transmembrane signaling. Frontiers in Membrane Biochemistry. 2010;**584**:1728-1740

[18] El Alwani M, Wu BX, Obeid LM, et al. Bioactive sphingolipids in the modulation of the inflammatory response. Pharmacology and Therapeutics. 2006;**112**:171-183

[19] Ogretmen B. Sphingolipid metabolism in cancer signalling and therapy. Nature Reviews Cancer. 2017;**18**:33-50

[20] Hannun YA, Obeid LM. Many ceramides. Journal of Biological Chemistry. 2011;**286**:27855-27862

[21] Maceyka M, Milstien S, Spiegel S. Sphingosine-1-phosphate: The Swiss army knife of sphingolipid signaling. Journal of Lipid Research. 2009;**50**:S272

[22] Hannun YA, Obeid LM. Sphingolipids and their metabolism in physiology and disease. Nature Reviews Molecular Cell Biology. 2018;**19**:175-191

[23] Liu Y-Y, Yu JY, Yin D, et al. A role for ceramide in driving cancer cell resistance to doxorubicin. The FASEB Journal. 2008;**22**:2541-2551

[24] Rosa R, Marciano R, Malapelle U, et al. Sphingosine kinase 1 overexpression contributes to cetuximab resistance in human colorectal cancer models. Clinical Cancer Research. 2013;**19**:138-147

[25] Hannun Y, Bell R. Lysosphingolipids inhibit protein kinase C: Implications for the sphingolipidoses. Science. 1987;**235**:670-674

[26] Pyne NJ, Pyne S. Sphingosine 1-phosphate and cancer. Nature Reviews Cancer. 2010;**10**:489-503

[27] Morad SAF, Levin JC, Shanmugavelandy SS, et al. Ceramide-antiestrogen nanoliposomal combinations-novel impact of hormonal therapy in hormone-insensitive breast cancer. Molecular Cancer Therapeutics. 2012;**11**:2352-2361

[28] Pewzner-Jung Y, Ben-Dor S, Futerman AH. When do lasses (longevity assurance genes) become CerS (ceramide synthases)? Insights into the regulation of ceramide synthesis. Journal of Biological Chemistry. 2006;**281**:25001-25005

[29] Levy M, Futerman AH. Mammalian ceramide synthases. IUBMB Life. 2010;**62**

[30] Mullen TD, Hannun YA, Obeid LM. Ceramide synthases at the Centre of sphingolipid metabolism and biology. Biochemical Journal. 2012;**441**:789-802

[31] Lee WK, Kolesnick RN. Sphingolipid abnormalities in cancer multidrug resistance: Chicken or egg? Cellular Signalling. 2017;**38**:134-145

[32] Tylichová Z, Slavík J, Ciganek M, et al. Butyrate and docosahexaenoic acid interact in alterations of specific lipid classes in differentiating colon cancer cells. Journal of Cellular Biochemistry. 2018;**119**:4664-4679

[33] Senkal CE, Ponnusamy S, Manevich Y, et al. Alteration of ceramide synthase 6/C 16-ceramide induces activating transcription factor 6-mediated endoplasmic reticulum (ER) stress and apoptosis via perturbation of cellular Ca 2+ and ER/golgi membrane network. Journal of Biological Chemistry. 2011;**286**:42446-42458

[34] Sassa T, Suto S, Okayasu Y, et al. A shift in sphingolipid composition from C24 to C16 increases susceptibility to

apoptosis in HeLa cells. Biochimica et Biophysica Acta - Molecular and Cell Biology of Lipids. 2012;**1821**:1031-1037

[35] Hartmann D, Lucks J, Fuchs S, et al. Long chain ceramides and very long chain ceramides have opposite effects on human breast and colon cancer cell growth. International Journal of Biochemistry and Cell Biology. 2012;**44**:620-628

[36] Markowski AR, Błachnio-Zabielska AU, Guzińska Ustymowicz K, et al. Ceramides profile identifies patients with more advanced stages of colorectal cancer. Biomolecules. 2020;**10**. DOI: 10.3390/biom10040632

[37] Ogretmen B, Hannun YA. Biologically active sphingolipids in cancer pathogenesis and treatment. Nature Reviews Cancer. 2004;**4**:604-616

[38] Garcia-Ruiz C, Morales A, Fernández-Checa JC. Glycosphingolipids and cell death: One aim, many ways. Apoptosis. 2015;**20**:607-620

[39] Proia RL, Hla T. Emerging biology of sphingosine-1-phosphate: Its role in pathogenesis and therapy. Journal of Clinical Investigation. 2015;**125**:1379-1387

[40] MacEyka M, Spiegel S. Sphingolipid metabolites in inflammatory disease. Nature. 2014;**510**:58-67

[41] Obeid LM, Linardic CM, Karolak LA, et al. Programmed cell death induced by ceramide. Science. 1993;**259**:1769-1771

[42] Sharma A, Boise LH, Shanmugam M. Cancer metabolism and the evasion of apoptotic cell death. Cancers. 2019;**11**. DOI: 10.3390/cancers11081144

[43] Park JW, Park WJ, Futerman AH. Ceramide synthases as potential targets for therapeutic intervention in human diseases. Biochimica et Biophysica Acta - Molecular and Cell Biology of Lipids. 2014;**1841**:671-681

[44] Koybasi S, Senkal CE, Sundararaj K, et al. Defects in cell growth regulation by C18:0-ceramide and longevity assurance gene 1 in human head and neck squamous cell carcinomas. Journal of Biological Chemistry. 2004;**279**:44311-44319

[45] Pewzner-Jung Y, Brenner O, Braun S, et al. A critical role for ceramide synthase 2 in liver homeostasis II. Insights into molecular changes leading to hepatopathy. Journal of Biological Chemistry. 2010;**285**:10911-10923

[46] White-Gilbertson S, Mullen T, Senkal C, et al. Ceramide synthase 6 modulates TRAIL sensitivity and nuclear translocation of active caspase-3 in colon cancer cells. Oncogene. 2009;**28**:1132-1141

[47] Wegner MS, Schiffmann S, Parnham MJ, et al. The enigma of ceramide synthase regulation in mammalian cells. Progress in Lipid Research. 2016;**63**:93-119

[48] Hertervig E, Nilsson Å, Nyberg L, et al. Alkaline sphingomyelinase activity is decreased in human colorectal carcinoma. Cancer. 1997;**79**:448-453

[49] Cheng JC, Bai A, Beckham TH, et al. Radiation-induced acid ceramidase confers prostate cancer resistance and tumor relapse. The Journal of Clinical Investigation. 2013;**123**. DOI: 10.1172/JCI64791

[50] García-Barros M, Coant N, Kawamori T, et al. Role of neutral ceramidase in colon cancer. FASEB Journal. 2016;**30**:4159-4171

[51] Neubauer HA, Pitson SM. Roles, regulation and inhibitors of sphingosine kinase 2. FEBS Journal. 2013;**280**:5317-5336

[52] Zhang Y, Wang Y, Wan Z, et al. Sphingosine kinase 1 and cancer: A systematic review and meta-analysis. PLoS One. 2014;**9**. DOI: 10.1371/journal.pone.0090362

[53] Degagné E, Pandurangan A, Bandhuvula P, et al. Sphingosine-1-phosphate lyase downregulation promotes colon carcinogenesis through STAT3-activated microRNAs. Journal of Clinical Investigation. 2014;**124**:5368-5384

[54] Oskouian B, Soonyakumaran P, Borowsky AD, et al. Sphingosine-1-phosphate lyase potentiates apoptosis via p53- and p38-dependent pathways and is down-regulated in colon cancer. Proceedings of the National Academy of Sciences of the United States of America. 2006;**103**:17384-17389

[55] Hait NC, Maiti A. The role of Sphingosine-1-phosphate and Ceramide-1-phosphate in inflammation and Cancer. Mediators of Inflammation. 2017;**2017**. DOI: 10.1155/2017/4806541

[56] Neubauer HA, Pham DH, Zebol JR, et al. An oncogenic role for sphingosine kinase 2. Oncotarget. 2016;**7**:64886-64899

[57] Lee E, Jung J, Jung D, et al. Inhibitory effects of novel SphK2 inhibitors on migration of Cancer cells. Anti-Cancer Agents in Medicinal Chemistry. 2017;**17**. DOI: 10.2174/1871520617666170213124856

[58] Xun C, Chen MB, Qi L, et al. Targeting sphingosine kinase 2 (SphK2) by ABC294640 inhibits colorectal cancer cell growth in vitro and in vivo. Journal of Experimental & Clinical Cancer Research: CR. 2015;**34**:94

[59] Shaw J, Costa-Pinheiro P, Patterson L, et al. Novel sphingolipid-based Cancer therapeutics in the personalized medicine era. Advances in Cancer Research. 2018;**140**:327-366

[60] Companioni O, Mir C, Garcia-Mayea Y, et al. Targeting sphingolipids for Cancer therapy. Frontiers in Oncology. 2021;**11**. DOI: 10.3389/fonc.2021.745092

[61] Beckham TH, Cheng JC, Marrison ST, et al. Interdiction of sphingolipid metabolism to improve standard Cancer therapies. In: Advances in Cancer Research. Academic Press Inc.; 2013. pp. 1-36

[62] Saddoughi SA, Garrett-Mayer E, Chaudhary U, et al. Results of a phase II trial of gemcitabine plus doxorubicin in patients with recurrent head and neck cancers: Serum C 18-ceramide as a novel biomarker for monitoring response. Clinical Cancer Research. 2011;**17**:6097-6105

[63] Wang C, Liu JN, Xu L, et al. Expression and significance of glucosylceramide synthase in colorectal carcinoma tissues. European Review for Medical and Pharmacological Sciences. 2014;**18**:3632-3637

[64] Beckham TH, Lu P, Cheng JC, et al. Acid ceramidase-mediated production of sphingosine 1-phosphate promotes prostate cancer invasion through upregulation of cathepsin B. International Journal of Cancer. 2012;**131**:2034-2043

[65] Haimovitz-Friedman A, Kan CC, Ehleiter D, et al. Ionizing radiation acts on cellular membranes to generate ceramide and initiate apoptosis.

Journal of Experimental Medicine. 1994;**180**:525-535

[66] Modrak DE, Gold DV, Goldenberg DM. Sphingolipid targets in cancer therapy. Molecular Cancer Therapeutics. 2006;**5**:200-208

[67] Scarlatti F, Sala G, Ricci C, et al. Resveratrol sensitization of DU145 prostate cancer cells to ionizing radiation is associated to ceramide increase. Cancer Letters. 2007;**253**:124-130

[68] Vit JP, Rosselli F. Role of the ceramide-signaling pathways in ionizing radiation-induced apoptosis. Oncogene. 2003;**22**:8645-8652

[69] Carroll B, Donaldson JC, Obeid L. Sphingolipids in the DNA damage response. Advances in Biological Regulation. 2015;**58**:38-52

[70] Munita JM, Arias CA. Mechanisms of antibiotic resistance. Microbiology Spectrum. 2016;**4**. DOI: 10.1128/microbiolspec.VMBF-0016-2015

[71] Hyde SC, Emsley P, Hartshorn MJ, et al. Structural model of ATP-binding proteing associated with cystic fibrosis, multidrug resistance and bacterial transport. Nature. 1990;**346**:362-365

[72] Leonard GD, Fojo T, Bates SE. The role of ABC transporters in clinical practice. The Oncologist. 2003;**8**(5):411-424

[73] Liu Y, Han T, AE GI, et al. Ceramide glycosylation potentiates cellular multidrug resistance. The FASEB Journal. 2001;**15**:719-730

[74] Prinetti A, Basso L, Appierto V, et al. Altered sphingolipid metabolism in N-(4-Hydroxyphenyl)-retinamide-resistant A2780 human ovarian carcinoma cells. Journal of Biological Chemistry. 2002;**278**:5574-5583

[75] Adiseshaiah PP, Clogston JD, McLeland CB, et al. Synergistic combination therapy with nanoliposomal C6-ceramide and vinblastine is associated with autophagy dysfunction in hepatocarcinoma and colorectal cancer models. Cancer Letters. 2013;**337**:254-265

[76] Marimpietri D, Brignole C, Nico B, et al. Combined therapeutic effects of vinblastine and rapamycin on human neuroblastoma growth, apoptosis, and angiogenesis. Clinical Cancer Research: An Official Journal of the American Association for Cancer Research. 2007;**13**:3977-3988

[77] Mariño G, Fernández AF, López-Otín C. Autophagy and aging: Lessons from progeria models. Advances in Experimental Medicine and Biology. 2010;**694**:61-68

[78] Pattingre S, Bauvy C, Carpentier S, et al. Role of JNK1-dependent Bcl-2 phosphorylation in ceramide-induced macroautophagy. The Journal of Biological Chemistry. 2009;**284**:2719-2728

[79] Chen L, Chen H, Li Y, et al. Endocannabinoid and ceramide levels are altered in patients with colorectal cancer. Oncology Reports. 2015;**34**:447-454

[80] Chen L, Ren J, Yang L, et al. Stearoyl-CoA desaturase-1 mediated cell apoptosis in colorectal cancer by promoting ceramide synthesis. Scientific Reports. 2016:6. DOI: 10.1038/srep19665

[81] Coant N, Garciá-Barros M, Zhang Q, et al. AKT as a key target for growth promoting functions of neutral ceramidase in colon cancer cells. Oncogene. 2018;**37**:3852-3863

[82] Separovic D, Shields AF, Philip PA, et al. Altered levels of serum ceramide, sphingosine and sphingomyelin are

associated with colorectal cancer: A retrospective pilot study. Anticancer Research. 2017;**37**:1213-1218

[83] Dubois N, Rio E, Ripoche N, et al. Plasma ceramide, a real-time predictive marker of pulmonary and hepatic metastases response to stereotactic body radiation therapy combined with irinotecan. Radiotherapy and Oncology. 2016;**119**:229-235

[84] Aguirre-Portolés C, Fernández LP, De Molina AR. Precision nutrition for targeting lipid metabolism in colorectal cancer. Nutrients. 2017;**9**. DOI: 10.3390/nu9101076

[85] Jang SW, Park WJ, Min H, et al. Altered mRNA expression levels of the major components of sphingolipid metabolism, ceramide synthases and their clinical implication in colorectal cancer. Oncology Reports. 2018;**40**:3489-3500

[86] El-Hindi K, Brachtendorf S, Hartel JC, et al. Ceramide synthase 5 deficiency aggravates dextran sodium Sulfate-induced colitis and Colon carcinogenesis and impairs T-cell activation. Cancers. 2020;**12**. DOI: 10.3390/cancers12071753

[87] Fitzgerald S, Sheehan KM, Espina V, et al. High CerS5 expression levels associate with reduced patient survival and transition from apoptotic to autophagy signalling pathways in colorectal cancer. The Journal of Pathology. Clinical Research. 2015;**1**:54-65

[88] Mojakgomo R, Mbita Z, Dlamini Z. Linking the ceramide synthases (CerSs) 4 and 5 with apoptosis, endometrial and colon cancers. Experimental and Molecular Pathology. 2015;**98**:585-592

[89] Dindo D, Dahm F, Szulc Z, et al. Cationic long-chain ceramide LCL-30 induces cell death by mitochondrial targeting in SW403 cells. Molecular Cancer Therapeutics. 2006;**5**:1520-1529

[90] Dahm F, Bielawska A, Nocito A, et al. Mitochondrially targeted ceramide LCL-30 inhibits colorectal cancer in mice. British Journal of Cancer. 2008;**98**:98-105

[91] de Araujo Junior RF, Eich C, Jorquera C, et al. Ceramide and palmitic acid inhibit macrophage-mediated epithelial–mesenchymal transition in colorectal cancer. Molecular and Cellular Biochemistry. 2020;**468**:153-168

[92] Remmerie A, Scott CL. Macrophages and lipid metabolism. Cellular Immunology. 2018;**330**:27-42

[93] Talamonti E, Pauter AM, Asadi A, et al. Impairment of systemic DHA synthesis affects macrophage plasticity and polarization: Implications for DHA supplementation during inflammation. Cellular and Molecular Life Sciences. 2017;**74**:2815-2826

[94] Wang SW, Hojabrpour P, Kolesnick RN, et al. Regulation of ceramide generation during macrophage apoptosis by ASMase and de novo synthesis. Biochimica et Biophysica Acta. 2015;**1851**:1482-1489

[95] Mao C, Obeid LM. Ceramidases: Regulators of cellular responses mediated by ceramide, sphingosine, and sphingosine-1-phosphate. Biochimica et Biophysica Acta. 2008;**1781**:424-434

[96] Coant N, Hannun YA. Neutral ceramidase: Advances in mechanisms, cell regulation, and roles in cancer. Advances in Biological Regulation. 2019;**71**:141-146

[97] Jafari N, Drury J, Morris AJ, et al. De novo fatty acid synthesis-driven sphingolipid metabolism promotes metastatic potential of colorectal cancer. Molecular Cancer Research. 2019;**17**:140-152

[98] Jung JH, Taniguchi K, Lee HM, et al. Comparative lipidomics of 5-fluorouracil–sensitive and –resistant colorectal cancer cells reveals altered sphingomyelin and ceramide controlled by acid sphingomyelinase (SMPD1). Scientific Reports. 2020;**10**. DOI: 10.1038/s41598-020-62823-0

[99] Dimanche-Boitrel M-T, Rebillard A, Gulbins E. Ceramide in chemotherapy of tumors. Recent Patents on Anti-Cancer Drug Discovery. 2011;**6**:284-293

[100] Madigan JP, Robey RW, Poprawski JE, et al. A role for ceramide glycosylation in resistance to oxaliplatin in colorectal cancer. Experimental Cell Research. 2020;**388**. DOI: 10.1016/j.yexcr.2020.111860

[101] Messner MC, Cabot MC. Glucosylceramide in humans. Advances in Experimental Medicine and Biology. 2010;**688**:156-164

[102] Merchant TE, Diamantis PM, Lauwers G, et al. Characterization of malignant colon tumors with 31P nuclear magnetic resonance phospholipid and phosphatic metabolite profiles. Cancer. 1995;**76**:1715-1723

[103] Janneh AH, Ogretmen B. Targeting sphingolipid metabolism as a therapeutic strategy in Cancer treatment. Cancers. 2022;**14**:2183